Measurement in Elderly Chronic Care Populations

Measurement in Elderly Chronic Care Populations

Jeanne A. Teresi, EdD, PhD

M. Powell Lawton, PhD

Douglas Holmes, PhD

Marcia Ory, PhD

Editors

 Springer Publishing Company

Springer Publishing Company, Inc.
536 Broadway
New York, NY 10012-3955

Cover design by: Margaret Dunin

97 98 99 00 01 / 5 4 3 2 1

Library of Congress Cataloging-in-Publication Data

Measurement in elderly chronic care populations / Jeanne Teresi ...
    [et al.], editors.
        p.   cm.
    Reprinted from Journal of mental health and aging, v. 2, no. 3,
(winter, 1996) with title: Measurement issues in older chronic care
populations.
    Includes bibliographical references and index.
    ISBN 0-8261-9990-9
    1. Nursing home patients—Mental health.   2. Geriatric psychiatry.
I. Teresi, Jeanne.
    [DNLM: 1. Geriatric Assessment.   2. Chronic Disease—in old age.
WT 30 M484 1997]
RC451.4.N87M43   1997
618.97'689075—DC 21
DNLM/DLC
for Library of Congress   97-28766
                                                 CIP

Measurement in Elderly Chronic Care Populations

Editors

Jeanne A. Teresi, PhD, EdD, Hebrew Home for the Aged at Riverdale,
Research Division, Columbia University Stroud Center,
New York State Psychiatric Institute, Office of Mental Health

M. Powell Lawton, PhD, Polisher Institute, Philadelphia Geriatric Center,
Temple University

Douglas Holmes, PhD, Hebrew Home for the Aged at Riverdale,
Research Division

Marcia Ory, PhD, National Institute on Aging

Contributors

Robert C. Abrams, MD The New York Hospital—Cornell Medical Center, Payne Whitney Clinic and Westchester Division

Steven M. Albert, PhD, MS Gertrude H. Sergievsky Center, College of Physicians and Surgeons, Columbia University

Kathryn Bayles, PhD National Center for Neurogenic Communication Disorders, Department of Speech and Hearing Sciences, University of Arizona

Cornelia Beck, PhD, RN, FAAN College of Nursing, University of Arkansas for Medical Sciences

Jamila Bookwala, PhD Kent State University

Margaret Calkins, PhD IDEAS, Inc., Cleveland

Denis A. Evans, MD Rush Institute on Aging, Rush Presbyterian—St. Luke's Medical Center

Gerald L. Glandon Rush-Presbyterian-St. Luke's Medical Center, New York

Douglas Holmes, PhD Hebrew Home for the Aged at Riverdale, New York

Ann Hurley, DNSc, RN Geriatrics Research Education Clinical Center, E. N. Rogers Memorial Veterans Hospital, Bedford, Massachusetts

Ira R. Katz, MD, PhD Department of Psychiatry, University of Pennsylvania, Philadelphia, Pennsylvania

Jennie Jacobs Kronenfeld, PhD School of Health Administration and Policy, Arizona State University, Tempe, Arizona

M. Powell Lawton, PhD Polisher Institute, Philadelphia Geriatric Center, Temple University, Nashville, Tennessee

David A. Lindeman, PhD Rush-Presbyterian-St. Luke's Medical Center, New York

John N. Morris, PhD Department of Social Research, Hebrew Rehabilitation Center, Boston

Shirley A. Morris   Department of Social Research, Hebrew Rehabilitation Center, Boston

Alan R. Morse, PhD, JD   President-Elect, the Jewish Guild for the Blind

Jason T. Newsom, PhD   Portland State University

Marcia Ory, PhD   National Institute on Aging

Patricia Parmelee, PhD   Polisher Research Institute, Philadelphia Geriatric Center, Philadelphia, Pennsylvania

Anton Porsteinsson, MD   Department of Psychiatry, University of Rochester Medical Center, Monroe Community Hospital, Rochester, New York

Bruce P. Rosenthal, OD, FAAO   Chief, Low Vision Programs, The Lighthouse

Valorie Shue, BA   College of Nursing, University of Arkansas for Medical Sciences

Richard Schulz, PhD   University of Pittsburgh

Philip Sloane, MD, MPH   University of North Carolina

Pierre N. Tariot, MD   Department of Psychiatry, University of Rochester Medical Center, Monroe Community Hospital, Rochester, New York

Jeanne A. Teresi, EdD, PhD   Hebrew Home for the Aged at Riverdale, Columbia University Stroud Center, and New York State Psychiatric Institute, Office of Mental Health

Linda Teri, PhD   University of Washington Medical Center, Seattle, Washington

Ladislav Volicer, MD, PhD   Geriatrics Research Education Clinical Center, E. N. Rogers Memorial Veterans Hospital, Bedford, Masssachusetts

Myron F. Weiner, MD   University of Texas Southwestern Medical Center, Dallas, Texas

Gerald D. Weisman, PhD   University of Wisconsin, Milwaukee

Peter J. Whitehouse, MD, PhD   Editor, *Alzheimer's Disease and Associated Disorders: An International Journal;* Alzheimer Center, University Hospitals of Cleveland

Foreword

Defining and Measuring Outcomes in Research on Alzheimer's Disease and Related Chronic Conditions: An Interdisciplinary Communication and Collaborative Challenge

This book provides an excellent review of measures used to assess individuals in chronic care settings. This work is timely as we seek to enrich our understanding of the how such individuals live their lives and whether our environments and programs satisfactorily address their needs and enhance their quality of life. In the later stages of dementia, such individuals often are neglected by the broader research community. This book represents not just a summary of current approaches but a step in the evolution of our understanding of assessment including that of important noncognitive symptoms; such symptoms are perhaps more disabling than the purely cognitive symptoms, and contribute frequently to impairment in quality of life for both patient and caregiver.

This book is appearing at a time when several other national and international projects are examining approaches to outcomes research in dementia. This supplement will contribute to current research on the impact of clinical interventions whether they be a new drug, novel program, or innovative modification in the environment. Families and payers are asking for better assessments of the effects of new intervention initiatives. As an interdisciplinary community of scholars, it is critical that we respond to these questions from families and policy makers. This response must include an awareness of other related activities, such as the following, that address similar topics.

A conference was held in Washington on September 11–12, 1996, to review the state of the art in outcomes measurement in dementia research. This is a topic that has long been neglected by the broader research community. Sponsored by the Alzheimer Association, the Agency for Health Care Policy and Research, the Advisory Panel on Alzheimer's Disease to the Department of Health and Human Services, the National Institute of Aging, the National Institute of Nursing Research, the National Institute of Mental Health, and the Department of Veterans Affairs, this conference had as its purpose the identification and resolution of difficult conceptual and methodological questions that arise in selecting and measuring the effectiveness of interventions to treat Alzheimer's disease and related disorders. This conference was part of the final project of the national advisory panel, seeking to examine comprehensively the therapeutic goals that we should establish at different stages of dementia. Unfortunately, the panel is phasing out just at the time when coordination of national efforts may be most critical.

A second project related to the focus of this special issue is the Instrument Protocol Committee of the National Institute of Aging Cooperative Study. This group has been designing and conducting studies of medications used to improve the symptoms of patients with Alzheimer's disease. It has developed new measures of cognition, behavior, activities of daily living, and related topics including some appropriate for severely demented patients. Drug studies are being conducted more often today than even just a few years ago; there is increased need to assess people as a basis for differential placement both within and outside of institutions. The need to assess people at all levels of cognitive impairment emphasizes the need for researchers to be aware of related attempts to improve the assessment of intervention outcomes.

In this time of financial constraints on health care, we must develop more efficient cross-field collaboration or at least be aware of parallel activities. Too long have unrecognized tensions existed between those who advocate the development of biological solutions and those who look to psychosocial answers. This tension can stimulate creativity, and provide the opportunity to identify and celebrate with society the sharing of such common goals as improving the quality of lives of clients and families. Alzheimer's disease research and program development is in some jeopardy because of limitations on research and clinical funding. We must learn of new ways to think about collaborative relationships among biologists, clinicians, and care system developers. Old conflicts between scientists and families over balancing the priorities of improving care and finding a cure, and between "hard" and "soft" science are not only stale but destructive as we attempt to provide answers for society about the growing problem of dementia. Planning efforts should be open and honest in establishing expectations for future progress.

The growing problem of dementia is not only a problem for the United States. Japan, Europe, and other populous countries, such as China, also are confronted with rapidly aging populations. The search for more effective drugs is already a global process as multinational companies develop international strategies. The International Working Group for the Harmonization of Dementia Drug Guidelines is examining the use of outcome measures in worldwide drug trials and attempting to bring harmony to the approaches recommended by national regulatory agencies, such as the Food and Drug Administration in the United States, the European Medicines Evaluation Agency in Europe, and the Ministry of Health and Welfare in Japan. So, too, each one of these world regions is developing new plans for long-term care. Thus, cross-national sharing of outcomes assessment approaches for services and programs is needed as well. Internationally, we have much to share across intellectual and cultural boundaries, and across geographic boundaries as well.

As a member of the national advisory panel, chairperson of the International Harmonization Group and of the program committee of the Washington Outcomes Conference, and Editor of *Alzheimer's Disease and Associated Disorders: An International Journal*, I congratulate the guest editors of this special issue, and I am pleased to announce that our international journal will be publishing the articles of the other outcomes-related activities described earlier in the coming year.

PETER J. WHITEHOUSE, MD, PHD

Preface

Measurement of Older Chronic Care Populations

This book contains reviews of measures that can be used in chronic care settings among individuals whose assessment is complicated because of factors such as frailty, perception and communication problems, and advanced cognitive impairment. Although the 1994 *Annual Review of Gerontology and Geriatrics* (Lawton & Teresi, 1994) was a review of assessment measures for use with older people in general, there are few reviews of measures for use with chronic care populations. However, a 1994 supplement to the *Alzheimer's Disease and Associated Disorders: An International Journal* (Holmes, Ory, & Teresi, 1994) outlined a conceptual orientation to assessment among the chronic care population. Based on the experiences of investigators from the National Institute on Aging collaborative studies of dementia care and members of the national Workgroup on Research and Evaluation of Special Care Units (WRESCU), several groups of difficult-to-assess individuals were identified and different approaches to assessment discussed. Underlining the importance of measurement in chronic care settings, a forthcoming special issue (see the Foreword by Whitehouse) focuses on methodological issues in the measurement of outcome domains among a subset of the chronic care population: persons with dementia.

This book contains reviews of many outcome domains as well as of other areas of function relevant to chronic care populations. These include cognition, communication, vision, behavior, personality, depression, affect, physical and functional capacity, informal and formal supports and caregiving, the environment, quality of life and service inputs, and costs of care. We are pleased with this effort because, in addition to representation by internationally recognized authors, we were fortunate to have an equally expert group of associate editors whose tireless efforts helped to improve the quality of this volume.

As the life span is extended, more individuals will experience chronic illness and disability that affects their quality of life and that of those around them. Better assessment methods are needed for identifying functional disorders that may be amenable to intervention and for treatment efficacy studies. As an example of treatment efficacy, investigation of new drugs aimed at enhancing cognitive function require long-term tracking with assessment measures that can address adequately the potential range of decline. Many measures are inadequate for this task; alternative methods that extend the assessable range of cognitive function are reviewed in this book. Other chronic conditions are currently treatable, if detected. For example, vision is difficult to assess among this population using standard approaches; alternative methods for identifying low vision are reviewed here, so that appropriate corrections can be made. Similarly, depression can be treated if properly recognized; standard approaches fall short when applied to individuals who are frail, fatigued, or moderately to severely cognitively impaired.

There is a burgeoning interest in measures that will more accurately describe and predict the status of individuals from chronic care populations. The authors think that this set of reviews will aid researchers and clinicians in the selection of such measures.

ACKNOWLEDGMENT. The articles appearing in this volume are an outgrowth of the planning and development activities coordinated by WRESCU, a national group of professionals conducting research dealing with the care of elderly persons with dementing illness. WRESCU operates with support from the National Alzheimer Center of the Hebrew Home for the Aged at Riverdale, the Helen Bader Foundation, the Retirement Research Foundation, and the National Institute on Aging.

JEANNE A. TERESI, EdD, PhD
M. POWELL LAWTON, PhD
DOUGLAS HOLMES, PhD
MARCIA ORY, PhD

REFERENCES

Holmes, D., Ory, M., & Teresi, J. (Eds.). (1994). Special dementia care: Research, policy and practice issues. *Alzheimer's Disease and Associated Disorders: An International Journal, 8* (Suppl. 1).

Lawton, M.P., & Teresi, J. A. (Eds.). (1994). *Annual review of gerontology and geriatrics: Vol. 14. Focus on assessment techniques.* New York: Springer Publishing Co.

Chapter 1

Cognitive Assessment Measures for Chronic Care Populations

Jeanne A. Teresi and Denis A. Evans

CONCEPTUAL ORIENTATION TO THE MEASUREMENT OF COGNITION AMONG CHRONIC CARE POPULATIONS

This chapter is a review of selected cognitive assessment measures for use with individuals from chronic care populations. Such individuals may be very frail, very old, have sensory disorders, advanced dementia, or suffer from multiple health conditions or disabilities. Because the chronic care population encompasses a broad range of cognitive disabilities, assessment instruments should be sensitive across a spectrum of impairment levels. Accurate assessment is important for adequate care planning, charting the possible decline trajectories for families and other caregivers, and for differentiating among subtypes of dementia and pseudodementias.

Some of the issues discussed subsequently were also those considered by a consortium of investigators from the National Institute on Aging (NIA) Collaborative Studies: Special Care Units for Alzheimer's Disease (Ory, 1994) and summarized in a supplement to the *Journal of Alzheimer Disease and Associated Disorders* (Holmes, Ory, & Teresi, 1994). The conceptual issues related to cognitive assessment summarized subsequently, are discussed in more detail in an article by Teresi, Lawton, Ory and Holmes (1994).

Among persons with advanced cognitive impairment, there are different "measurement populations:" (a) persons with impaired consciousness who are not alert; (b) persons who are arousable and alert, but unable to perform simple commands and with variable ability to communicate; (c) persons who are alert, arousable, and able to communicate, but provide nonratable (e.g., rambling, incoherent) responses to questions, and (d) persons who provide ratable but incorrect responses to most test items. Those with severe cognitive impairment are usually rated at the highest stages of impairment on typical staging measures (e.g., 6 or 7 on the Global Deterioration Scale; Reisberg, Ferris, de Leon & Crook, 1982, or 5 on the Clinical Dementia Rating; Hughes,

Acknowledgment. This effort was partially funded by the National Institute on Aging (NIA), grants AG08948, Impacts of Special Care Units in Nursing Homes; AH10315, Longitudinal Study of four types of Alzheimer's Disease Special Care Units; AG10330, Coordinating Center to the NIA Collaborative Studies of Special Care Units for Alzheimer's Disease.

Berg, Danziger, Coben, & Martin, 1982). Because the chronic care population also includes many individuals with mild to moderate cognitive impairment, the ideal measure would be applicable across these levels. The focus of this review, however, is on measures that have been developed for use, or have been widely used, among individuals with more advanced cognitive impairment.

Although a large proportion of the chronic care population exhibits some degree of cognitive impairment, it is among those with severe communication disorder that specific measurement problems arise. The problem of nontestable persons is referred to in the measurement literature as the floor effect (scoring very poorly, e.g., 0–10 on the Mini-Mental State Examination [MMSE]; Folstein, Folstein, & McHugh, 1975). Preliminary data from the New York site of the NIA collaborative studies (a probability sample of nursing home residents, Teresi, Holmes, & Ramirez, 1996) indicate that 7% of the sample were not alert or arousable; 18% were arousable but could not follow simple commands; and although an additional 5% could respond to questions, the responses were unratable on more than half of the items. Finally, an additional 13% scored in the 0 to 10 range on the MMSE, and almost half (47%) were in stages 6 or 7 on the Global Deterioration Scale (GDS) (Reisberg, Ferris, De Leon, & Crook, 1982). Across the NIA Collaborative sites, 27% to 30% of residents were either incapable of arousal (11%-15%) or unable to follow simple commands (14%-16%). These data suggest that almost one third of the nursing home residents were untestable, and that almost half would experience severe floor effects using standard assessment instruments, such as the MMSE. Although the proportion of untestable and low-scoring individuals are lower in adult day health care and home care populations, there are still appreciable numbers of individuals in these settings who are difficult to assess (Teresi, Holmes, & Ramirez, 1996).

APPROACHES TO MEASUREMENT

Methods for measuring cognitive impairment include self-report (direct assessment), observation, informant report, and medical record review including the collection of information based on administrative data sets. Direct cognitive assessment can be expressed as psychometric screening, more intensive neuropsychological testing, global clinical ratings, or staging methodologies. Direct cognitive screening measures have been the primary approach to cognitive assessment; however, recent attention has focused on the use of other approaches, such as informant reports or observation when dealing with advanced dementia. Moreover, there is a trend in the literature on assessment of advanced dementia toward examining noncognitive constructs, which reflect sequelae of cognitive impairment. Instruments developed for assessing severe cognitive impairment measure, in addition to cognitive function, incapacity in activities of daily living (ADL), physical and social function, and communication (Ritchie & Ledesert, 1991) or neurological signs (Franssen, Kluger, Torossian, Reisberg, 1993). The latter, some of which have been found to be more prevalent in the latest stage of illness (Franssen, Kluger, Torossian, & Reisberg, 1993) include (a) release signs (primitive reflexes), such as paratonia (involuntary resistance to passive movement), sucking reflex, hand grasp, and snout and blink reflexes; (b) extrapyramidal signs (rigidity, abnormal movements), such as arm swing, walking speed, step length, and erect posture; and (c) pyramidal signs (jaw-jerk, foot clonus, and extensor plantar reflexes).

FOCUS OF THIS REVIEW

The focus of this review is on directly administered psychometric measures. However, the authors more briefly discuss each of the other methodologies, with specific reference to recent reviews or to promising or new measures. They confine the review to measures that can be used with later-stage dementia, as there are numerous reviews of measures for the less cognitively impaired. The neuropsychological and communication batteries used with severe cognitive impairment are discussed elsewhere by Bayles in this book. The authors also do not review the cognitive battery from the Consortium to Establish a Registry for Alzheimer's Disease (CERAD) for two reasons. First, it includes several well-known cognitive measures reviewed elsewhere (Morris, Mohs, Rogers, Fillenbaum, & Heyman, 1988). Second, its utility for measuring cognitive impairment in persons with communication disorders, sensory impairments, or advanced dementia has not been determined (Morris et al., 1989), although preliminary evidence suggests that measures of naming, fluency, and constructional ability were more discriminatory than were memory and recall tasks when differentiating among all levels (mild, moderate, and severe) of dementia (Welsh et al., 1991, 1992). Another popular derivative measure not reviewed here, but used in many multisite studies in Europe, is the CAMCOG (Roth et al., 1986), which contains 67 items measuring memory, praxis, language, and abstract thinking, and includes the MMSE. Although not originally developed for use with later stage cognitive impairment, it recently has been suggested as a measure that can be used with aphasic patients because it has been claimed to have more items that are less dependent on language than do other such measures. However, in one study of ischemic stroke patients (Kwa et al., 1996), none of the severely aphasic could be tested with the measure, and only about one half (46%) of those with discernible aphasia were capable of being assessed.

When available, the authors have identified the summary statistics used in the psychometric development of the measures. The authors note several problems relevant to their interpretation. Some investigators did not consider study design in calculating coefficients (e.g., use of mixed [fixed rater] effects models) to estimate interrater reliability when an intraclass correlation coefficient using a random effects model would have been more appropriate, or use of Pearson correlations to estimate association between raters, without providing evidence of the parallelism of the two ratings.

DIRECT PSYCHOMETRIC MEASURES

Standard Brief Cognitive Measures

There are several well-known, relatively brief cognitive measures, including the MMSE (Folstein, Folstein, & McHugh, 1975), the Blessed Information-Memory-Concentration Test (Blessed, Tomlinson, & Ross, 1968), the Comprehensive Assessment and Referral Evaluation Mental Status Questionnaire (Golden, Teresi, & Gurland, 1984), the Kahn-Goldfarb Mental Status Questionnaire (Kahn et al., 1960), and the

Short Portable Mental Status Questionnaire (Pfeiffer, 1975). These measures are commonly referred to in the literature as *screening measures*; however, the authors will not use this term, which connotes a first-stage screening process to identify possible cases for follow-up with more comprehensive second-stage neuropsychological assessment, thus enhancing sensitivity in the detection of dementia. In the current context, this distinction is inappropriate because the authors are examining a population where the disease is fairly common and where further assessment is often problematic because of severe communication disorder, frailty, or comorbidity.

Although the authors provide a description of each of the brief measures, the reader is referred to a review by Albert (1994), for detailed data regarding their psychometric properties. For additional reviews of the MMSE, see Tombaugh and McIntyre (1992). All reviewers note the problem of floor effects of the MMSE (and other so-called screening measures) for use with advanced impairment, or for charting longitudinal change through severe stages of dementia. For example, Sclan and colleagues (1990) present data showing mean MMSE scores of 6.5 ($SD = 6.05$) for individuals at GDS (Reisberg, Ferris, de Leon, & Crook, 1982) stage 6 and mean scores of 0 for those at stage 7. The authors argue that 30% to 50% of the course of AD is unmeasurable using traditional cognitive tests. Studies have also found lower specificity of the MMSE for very old persons (Osterweil, Mulford, Syndulko, & Martin, 1994) and for the frail (Anthony, LeResche, Niaz, Von Korff, & Folstein, 1982). Lower scores have been observed for individuals with sensory impairments (Uhlmann, Teri, Rees, Mozlowski, & Larson, 1989) and with loss of motor function resulting from physical impairments (Kafonek et al., 1989).

1. *Blessed Information-Memory-Concentration Test.* The Blessed-Information-Memory-Concentration Test contains 27 items measuring orientation, memory, and calculation/attention. Typical items are "cannot spell own name," "does not recall dates for World War I," "does not know correct hour of the day," "does not count backward correctly from 20 to 1."

2. *Mental Status Questionnaires (Kahn-Goldfarb Mental Status Questionnaire, CARE Mental Status Questionnaire, and Short Portable Mental Status Questionnaire).* These three measures each contain 10 similar items measuring orientation to person, place, and time. Typical items are "does not know year of birth," "does not know today's date," "does not recall interviewer's name," "does not recall name of current president."

3. *MMSE and its modifications.* The MMSE contains 20 items measuring the degree of cognitive impairment in the areas of orientation, attention and calculation, registration, recall and language, as well as the ability to follow verbal and written commands. Recall or short-term memory is measured by asking the respondent to recall a list of three objects memorized earlier. Typical orientation items are "cannot name nursing home or place s/he is in," "cannot name state s/he is in," "does not know the current year." Attention is measured by asking the respondent to spell the word "World" backward or to calculate "serial 7s." Language is measured by object-naming tasks and those requiring the interviewee to follow directions (e.g., folding a piece of paper).

Factor analytic studies of the MMSE among nursing home residents have suggested that expansion of the MMSE may be useful (Abraham et al., 1994), as embodied in the Modified Mini-Mental State (3MS) (Teng & Chui, 1987), which assesses additional constructs: delayed and remote memory, language fluency and abstraction. Other modifications include additional items, intended to increase the range of item difficulties, and replacement of educationally biased items (serial 7s with counting backward from 5 to 1). The 3MS was recently compared with the MMSE and the Mattis Dementia Rating Scale (DRS) (Mattis, 1976) using a sample of 120 nursing home residents (Nadler et al., 1995). Interrater reliabilities for the MMSE and 3MS were both .99, using Pearson correlations between two raters. Test-retest reliability was .92 for the 3MS and .85 for the MMSE; the respective Cronbach's α's were .90 and .84. Both the 3MS and the DRS had a wider distribution of score ranges than did the MMSE. At standard cutting scores, the 3MS and DRS had higher sensitivity and negative predictive values, but slightly lower positive predictive value and considerably lower specificity. At optimal cuts, the DRS was superior to both the MMSE and 3MS in terms of all summary statistics; the 3MS was somewhat more sensitive than the MMSE and had slightly better negative predictive value, but was slightly worse than the MMSE in terms of specificity and positive predictive value. However, there were no significant differences among the measures in terms of receiver operating characteristics (ROC) curve analyses. All measures produced a relatively high number of false positives in the nursing home sample, associated with lower education, higher age, and history of depression. Other research has also identified cultural differences as a contributor to false-positive classification (Gurland, Wilder, Cross, Teresi, & Barrett, 1992). These variables may need to be factored into classification algorithms based on cognitive measures when used among chronic care populations.

Measures That Can Be Used for Assessment of Frail, Very Old, or Severely Demented Populations

The remainder of this review focuses predominantly on measures that can be used to assess individuals with advanced cognitive impairment, although a few are also sensitive at milder impairment levels.

Severe Impairment Batteries

The authors provide only a partial review of the severe impairment batteries because they are reviewed in the article by Bayles in this volume and in a recent review by Albert (1994).

1. *The Severe Impairment Battery* (SIB) (Saxton, McGonigle-Gibson, Swihart, Miller, & Boller, 1990; Saxton & Swihart, 1989). This battery measures 9 constructs with the following six subscales: Attention, Orientation, Memory, Language, Visuoperception, and Construction; additional items measure social skills, praxis, and name recognition. A later version of the test is available from National Rehabilitation Services. Interrater reliabilities calculated on behalf of 11 subjects, estimated using Pearson correlations, ranged from .87 to 1.00; test-retest correlations ranged from .22 for Construction and .36 for Orientation to .86 for the other subscales. The test-retest correlation for the total scale was .85. The correlations between components of the SIB and the MMSE ranged from .16 to .77, with the total score correlating .74 with the MMSE; scale intercorrelations were in the moderate range with a few exceptions, indicating lack of redundancy. Analysis of 15 subjects with 0 to 4 MMSE scores showed a range of 15 to 114 of a possible range of 152 on the SIB total, reflecting the ability of the SIB to produce more variability in scale scores. Conversely, the authors report that the scale does

not have utility for individuals scoring higher than 9 on the MMSE or higher than 90 on Mattis DRS (Saxton & Swihart, 1989).

   2. *Test for Severe Impairment* (TSI) (Albert & Cohen, 1992). This test contains 24 items measuring memory, language, conceptualization, and motor performance; the scale range is from 0 to 24. Albert (1994) reports several reliability statistics (test-retest $r=.96$; internal consistency $\alpha=.90$). No interrater reliability is presented. The measure correlated .83 with the MMSE. The TSI was used in a study of 272 long-term care residents (Morris et al., 1994) and compared with the Cognitive Performance Scale (CPS), a global staging measure based on the Minimum Data Set (MDS) (Morris et al., 1990), and described subsequently. The TSI correlated .73 with the MMSE among persons scoring 0 to 10 on the MMSE. The TSI showed increased variability in scale scores over the MMSE for the moderately (MMSE mean=6.9, $SD=6.9$; TSI mean=12.0, $SD=7.8$) and severely impaired (MMSE mean=5.1, $SD=5.3$; TSI mean=12.5, $SD=9.1$) (stages 4 and 5 out of 6 stages). However, there was little advantage of the TSI over the MMSE for stage 6 (very severe impairment) (MMSE mean=.4, $SD=.9$; TSI mean=1.5, $SD=3.0$). In examining the TSI scores of those with MMSE scores of 0 to 10, there is no advantage to the TSI over the MMSE at any of the three most advanced CPS stages (means and SDs are almost identical).

   It is difficult to interpret the relatively high correlations (.74 and .83) between the severe impairment batteries and the MMSE. Depending on the sample used, such high correlations might suggest statistical redundancy, although Saxton and colleagues reported a lower correlation (.43) between the SIB and the MMSE for the 0 to 4 group. Preliminary evidence for extending measurement in the moderate to severe range through use of the severe impairment batteries appears promising; however, the utility of the batteries for assessing more advanced later stage impairment is unclear. More extensive psychometric analyses, with larger sample sizes are needed. Additionally, a better theoretical link to standard neuropsychological constructs is needed because the theoretical foundations of these measures have been questioned (Zandi, 1994). Finally, these measures are not useful for assessing individuals at higher functioning levels, making them less attractive for some research, such as the NIA Collaborative Studies, where both higher and lower functioning individuals were assessed. (See also the article by Bayles in this issue.)

Reverse Piagetian Models and Measures

Because it has been observed that visual recognition memory is one of the most well-preserved functions in dementia (Church & Wattis, 1988), awareness of the environment may be one of the last cognitive skills to be lost. The Piagetian model permits measurement of presymbolic and primitive symbolic function, focusing on sensorimotor function and awareness of environmental cues (Piaget, 1977). According to this conceptualization, there is a hierarchical organization of cognitive function; the infant moves from the most primitive (sensory motor stage) to the preoperative or concrete operations, to a more formal operations phase. Although there may be some value to application of such scales in the search for a "reversed progression," the theoretical validity of the reverse Piagetian model as applied to elderly persons with cognitive impairment has been questioned on the grounds that the model fails to account for previously learned, automatic behaviors (Thornbury, 1993; Zandi, 1994). Additionally, the empirical validity of an ordinal reverse progression in functional decline has been challenged (Cohen-Mansfield, Werner, & Reisberg, 1995; Eisdorfer et al., 1992).

1. *Ordinal Scale for Psychological Development* (OSPD) (Uzgris & Hunt, 1975) *and Modified Ordinal Scale for Psychological Development* (M-OSPD) (Auer & Reisberg, in press; Auer, Sclan, Yaffee & Reisberg, 1994; Sclan, Foster, Reisberg, Franssen & Welkowitz, 1990). Measures developed for testing infant function have been applied to individuals with dementia. For example, Sclan and colleagues (1990) applied the OSPD (Uzgris & Hunt, 1975), which measures function from birth to age 2, to 26 GDS stage 6 and 7 patients. The authors found that although nonzero scores were achieved in stage 7, scores on most subscales were near zero. However, there was some variation for the total scale score, with a mean score of 9.67 (SD=11.83). In a later partial replication study of the M-OSPD (Auer, Sclan, Jaffee, & Reisberg, 1994), which included the original study subjects plus additional subjects (n=70), similar results were obtained. However, it was shown that relatively more variability and nonzero scores were observed among early, rather than later, stage 7 subjects. Most information loss occurred in stages 7d, 7e, and 7f of the Functional Assessment Staging Test (FAST) (Reisberg, 1988), but even for these advanced stage 7 patients, the mean was well above zero (8.4, SD=9.7). Interrater reliability, using the Pearson correlation coefficient was .97; internal consistency, estimated using Cronbach's alpha was .95 for the total scale and .75 to .98 for subscales; the Spearman correlation coefficient between the M-OSPD and FAST was -.77, providing evidence of convergent validity with a functional measure of cognitive impairment.

Most recently, two interrater reliability studies were conducted among individuals with severe dementia (GDS stages 6 and 7 in the nursing home and 5 to 7 in the community) in two settings: nursing home and community. These studies yielded high intraclass correlation coefficients (ICC), calculated using a two-way random effects model (Auer & Reisberg, in press). The coefficients for the nursing home and community samples, respectively, were Object Permanence (.97, .96), Means-Ends (.93, .41), Causality (.98; .28); Spatial Relations (.94, .95), Schemes (.97, .77), and Total Score (.99, .96). The authors attribute the low ICCs for two of the subscales to severe ceiling effects in the community sample; they propose further studies that would include community residents with a broader range of disability. With respect to the Means End and Causality subscales, 74% and 86%, respectively, of the community sample received a ceiling score, although most subjects were at stage 6. This suggests that it might also be fruitful to include items with a broader range of item difficulties. Because the authors emphasize using a semistructured format (e.g., using the test examiner or a spouse as the test object when assessing ability to "trace an object moving through an arc of 180 degrees"), it may be necessary to reestablish interrater reliability if studies are conducted with different investigators.

2. *Hierarchical Dementia Scale* (HDS) (Cole & Dastoor, 1983). The HDS (Cole & Dastoor, 1983, 1987) constitutes another application of the hierarchical reverse Piagetian model. The HDS was developed using 20 of a set of cognitive constructs identified by experts. Items measuring each construct were generated and ordered in a hierarchical fashion from 1 to 10, with 10 representing highest function. The rank order of item difficulty was examined in an iterative fashion, developing a "Guttman"-type ordinal positioning. However, it is unclear what statistical procedures were used to estimate item difficulties or to achieve ordinality. Each subscale is administered using a header-contingency approach; the item set is entered at an estimated level of impairment, and testing is continued up or down the subscale until two consecutive items are correct. The remaining (easier) items are then assumed to be correct. The scale maximum is 200; the authors suggest that a score of 160 connotes mild dementia, whereas a score of 0 to 39 is indicative of severe dementia.

According to Ronnberg and Ericsson (1994), who performed secondary psychometric analysis of the scale, it measures nine domains: orientation, observation, memory, praxis, gnosis, language, concentration, cognition, and motor (prefrontal) function. The authors claim that the test resembles the DRS (Mattis, 1976) in terms of hierarchical arrangement but is composed of easier items. The original test authors (Cole & Dastoor, 1983) report that the constructs measured (presumably within these nine domains) are *orienting* (greetings, handshake); *prefrontal* (tactile prehension to oral tactile reflex); *ideomotor* (commands to reverse hands to open mouth); *looking* (finding images to looks at picture); *ideational* (imaginary match and candle to open door); *denomination* (nominal aphasia to deformed words); *comprehension (verbal and written)* (close eyes and touch left ear to open mouth); *registration* (spoon, candle, scissors, button, whistle to spoon); *gnosis* (superimposed words to response to touch-pinch); *reading* (paragraph to the letter M), *orientation* (date to first name); *construction* (four block diagonal to circle), *concentration* (serial 7s to counting 1 to 10); *calculation* (43–17 to 3+1); *drawing* (cube to scribble); *motor* (none to lateral restriction of eye movement); *remote memory* (amount of pension to place of birth); *writing (form and content)* (flowing style to scribble, no impairment to missing three to four words); *similarities* (airplane-bicycle to orange-banana), *recent memory* (all five to any one).

The original authors examined 50 patients with either Alzheimer's disease or multi-infarct dementia. Using the HDS, two examiners independently assessed each person; both the Blessed Dementia Scale and the Crichton Geriatric Rating Scale were also used. Patients were reassessed 15 days later. EEG values for the dominant occipital α frequency were recorded. Observed scores on the HDS were 11 to 191, with a mean of 113 (SD=50). Interrater reliability was .89; test-retest was .84 (methods of calculation are not provided). Cronbach's α was .97. Interrater reliabilities across subscales range from .54 for orienting to .87 for ideational (eight subscales have interrater reliabilities of less than .70). The correlation of the HDS with the Blessed was .72 and .74 with the Chrichton Scale. The electroencephalogram frequency correlated .57 with the scale.

A later study of the psychometric properties of the scale (Ronnberg & Ericsson, 1994) compared the HDS to the MMSE and CDR. Fifty subjects from two residential settings were diagnosed using *Diagnostic and Statistical Manual of Mental Disorders* (3rd ed.) (DSM III) R/NINCDS-ADRDA criteria. The mean time for administration was 26 minutes; five persons initially refused, experiencing a negative reaction to the test; they were later able to complete the test. Interrater reliability was calculated using Cohen's κ; relationships of HDS scores to other scale scores were ascertained using Spearman's rank order correlation coefficient. Twenty-one subjects were evaluated for test-retest and interrater reliability. Test-retest reliability was .96 over a 2- to 3-week interval. The κ for the subscales ranged from .76 to .96. The mean scores were 104 (SD=43) and the range from 23 to 157. Of those with MMSE scores of 0, 6 received scores on the HDS. All subjects were CDR stage 3. The correlation between CDR and HDS was -.71; the correlation of HDS to MMSE was .86. The authors conclude that subscales 3 to 15 are indicative of severe dementia for those scoring 0 on the MMSE. Patients with mild dementia can have deteriorated recent memory, whereas those with severe impairment were found to have preserved orienting behaviors. The authors suggest that cultural factors may influence the writing and calculation subscales, sensory-motor impairment influences performance-based items, and vision impairment is a problem for writing and visual discrimination items.

Cognitive Batteries Intended for Use Across a Range of Disability Including Advanced-Stage Cognitive Impairment

1. *The Alzheimer's Disease Assessment Scale* (ADAS) (Rosen, Mohs, & Davis, 1984) One of the most widely used measures in clinical trials involving individuals with Alzheimer's disease is the ADAS (Rosen, Mohs, & Davis, 1984). The ADAS contains a cognitive subscale (ADAS-COG), which measures memory (three task areas worth 27 error points), language (five task areas worth 25 error points), praxis (two task areas worth 10 error points), and orientation worth 8 error points; the range is from 0 to 70. Administration time is about $\frac{1}{2}$ hour. Another version, the ADAS-Late Version (ADAS-L), was developed by the same authors to assess individuals with advanced dementia (Kincaid et al., 1995).

ADAS-COG: The interrater reliability of the ADAS-COG is reported as .99; the test-retest as .92 (Olin & Schneider, 1995). The method of computation is not provided. Olin and Schneider (1995) performed a factor analysis using a varimax orthogonal rotation; three factors were identified: language (commands, language, comprehension, word finding); memory (word recall, word recognition, orientation, remembering test instructions, object naming); praxis (constructional, ideational praxis). Eigenvalues were 5.01, 1.13, .95, respectively, suggesting that the 11-item set could also be considered unidimensional. Using repeated measures (multivariate analysis of variance), all factors showed significant differences in changes for experimental (Tacrine) versus control group subjects. However, there was no differential gain for any one factor scale over another, also arguing for use of a single summary score.

The ability of the ADAS to discriminate among four different severity levels of cognitive impairment was examined by Zec and colleagues (1992). Using cutoffs on the MMSE of 0 to 9 for severe impairment and 24 or higher for no or very mild impairment, they found large and significant differences on the ADAS-COG among most groups, concluding that the measure is useful for measurement across a range of cognitive impairment levels. The ADAS-COG correlated -.76 with the MMSE, suggesting good convergent construct validity. The authors compared effect sizes to those reported by Christensen, Hadzi-Pavlovic, and Jacomb (1991) for other cognitive measures; they report a favorable result for the ADAS-COG (effect sizes of 3.5 for the whole group, 5.5 for the very mild, 3 for the mild, 5.3 for the moderate, and 9.5 for the severe) as contrasted with 2.9 for the MMSE and 3.3 for the Buschke Selective Reminding Test), although again based on a relatively small sample size.

Several studies have been conducted assessing the predictive validity of the ADAS. For example, Stern and colleagues (1994) found that, on average, the ADAS maximum was reached 8 months after the Blessed maximum was reached, suggesting that the ADAS holds some advantage in the assessment of persons with advanced cognitive impairment. The authors conclude that the ADAS cognitive subscale was more sensitive to mild and severe deficits than was the Blessed, but that the ability to detect treatment effects with the ADAS is better for mild to moderately impaired individuals than for the very mild or very severely impaired. They also conclude that although studies of treatment effects need not have a design that is matched for age of onset, gender, or family history, treatment groups must be matched on severity of disease because there are different rates of change across severity levels. Recently, it also has been suggested that groups should be matched on education, as persons who did not complete high school performed significantly worse on many of the subscales (Doraiswamy et al., 1995).

ADAS-L: The belief that measures that assess more than just cognitive constructs are critical to the assessment of severe cognitive impairment has given rise to the development of scales that also contain behavioral and functional (e.g., ADL) items or subscales. One such measure is the ADAS-L (Kincaid et al., 1995), which obtains data from the assessor based both on observations of the person and on interviews with caregivers. There are 20 items in four sections: (a) six direct assessment tests of memory, language, praxis, and orientation; (b) six assessor ratings of psychiatric and cognitive impairment, and four ratings of cognitive impairment and interpersonal skills based on caregiver reports and four items rating ADL (source unspecified). The scale ranges from 0 (no impairment) to 81. In one study of geriatric schizophrenics (Harvey et al., 1992), the intraclass correlation coefficient (methods of estimation unspecified) ranged from .52 to .94, with the exception of two low baserate items. The median ICC was .83. The authors performed a three-factor principal components factor analysis with varimax rotation. They claim that three meaningful factors were extracted: cognition, self-care/motor, and pathological thinking/depression. However, results suggest unidimensionality: the eigenvalues are 10.4, 1.8, and 1.1, respectively; the first factor explains 52% of the variance, and the other two 9% and 6%, respectively. Moreover, because oblique rotation was not performed and loadings of all items on all factors are not presented, it is difficult to evaluate the analyses, however, a test of scree would probably be more consistent with a unidimensional interpretation, given the size of the eigenvalues and the fact that the last factor contained only two items.

A discriminant function analyses, conducted separately for the MMSE and the ADAS-L, using the five CDR categories as outcomes, yielded almost identical overall correct classifications for the MMSE and ADAS-L (62.3%, 60.5%). The ADAS-L performed worse than did the MMSE in terms of correct classifications for CDR stage 0 to .5 (3.8% vs. 61.5%); stage 3 (severe) (58.2% vs. 75.3%). It performed better at stage 1 (mild) (85.7% vs. 62.3%) and stage 4 (profound) (91.7%, 0%). The authors indicate that use of only the cognitive items improves classification at the mild stage.

These data do not make a convincing case for the use of the ADAS-L over the MMSE because, although there was a substantial gain in predictive accuracy over the MMSE for the profound stage, the measure was less accurate at the severe stage. However, if used in conjunction with more standard psychometric tests, incremental classification accuracy might be achieved at the profound stage.

2. *Executive Interview* (EXIT) (Royall, Mahurin, & Gray, 1992). Royall and colleagues (1993) define executive functions as "those cognitive processes which orchestrate relatively simple ideas, movements, or actions into complex, goal-directed behaviors" (p. 1813). The authors suggest that without these organizing functions, ADLs will not be integrated but will break into task segmentation. Executive cognitive dysfunction can be associated with frontal lobe lesions or other similar damage, and may be prominent in schizophrenics with negative features, persons with subcortical stroke, and some individuals with depression, Parkinson's disease, and Alzheimer's disease (Royall et al., 1993).

EXIT items measure the following constructs: frontal release, motor or cognitive preservation, verbal intrusion, disinhibition, loss of spontaneity, imitation behavior, environmental dependency, utilization behavior. There are 25 tasks, such as *repeating sequences of numbers and letters* (1-A); *word fluency* (name as many words starting with A as you can); *design fluency, anomalous sentence repetition; thematic perception; memory/distraction; interference; automatic behavior* (rotating elbow; pushing on palm); *grasp reflex; social habit; motor impersistence* (stick out your tongue and say, "aah"); *snout reflex; finger-nose-finger task; go-no-go; echopraxia* (command to touch ear while examiner is touching nose;

examiner slaps hand); *Luria hand sequences* (palm-fist; slap, fist, cut); *grip task; complex commands; serial order reversal* (months of year backward); *counting* (count fish); *utilization behavior* (holds up pen); *imitation behavior* (flexes wrist). Items with "low item-class correlations" were excluded. The interview takes 10 minutes, and scores range from 0 to 50, with 50 indicative of greater impairment. The author reports an interrater reliability coefficient (Pearson's *r*) of .90 for 30 subjects rated by two physicians.

The EXIT, the MMSE, and a behavioral measure were administered to 40 subjects (10 from each of four settings ranging from retirement apartments to skilled nursing facilities). Exclusion criteria included inability to follow simple commands or sensory/physical impairments. The EXIT was highly correlated with the MMSE (-.85), with a test of sustained attention (.82), and with traditional measures of executive function (Trailmaking A .82; Trailmaking B, .83). The measure also distinguished significantly among the four levels of care in terms of mean values, whereas the MMSE scores were similar across more independent levels (containing more mildly impaired residents.) The measure has been found to be associated with disturbed behavior: Royall, Mahurin, and Cornell (1995) reported a correlation of .79 between the EXIT and the Nursing Home Behavior Problem Scale. The authors claim that the measure is able to discriminate across both mild as well as severe levels of cognitive impairment, and that the measure distinguishes subcortical from cortical cognitive impairment and is useful in differentiating cognitive impairment because of depression from impairment resulting from other disorders. They claim that, in contrast to the EXIT, the MMSE underestimates dementia level of cognitive impairment in subcortical cases, and that the NINCDS mislabels subcortical disorders as primary degenerative dementia. However, the distinction between subcortical and cortical dementia has been questioned (Whitehouse, 1986), in part, because of findings showing damage to both cortical and subcortical areas of the brain in some Alzheimer's disease patients (Boller, Mizutani, Roessman, & Gambetti, 1980) and AD changes at autopsy among some patients with Parkinson's disease (Katzman, 1992), and, in part, because of the difficulty distinguishing clinically among subgroups purportedly characterized as cortical or subcortical (Mayeux et al., 1981; Paolo et al., 1995a).

In a second examination of the EXIT (Royall et al., 1993), the authors studied 21 elderly independent living subjects, 37 residential care elderly, 46 intermediate care elderly, and 40 schizophrenic inpatients. They report that the instrument is more sensitive to mild cognitive impairment than is the MMSE, as evidenced by the finding that 53% of those who scored higher than 23 on the MMSE had impairment in executive function. The EXIT was not superior to the MMSE in terms of correlations with level of care. Of interest is that the correlation for the MMSE and the Executive Interview was -.80 for the elderly sample, but only -.48 for the schizophrenic subsample. The high correlation between the MMSE and the Executive Function measure among the elderly, of whom a higher proportion are cognitively impaired, calls into question the definition of the construct. After correction for attenuation resulting from unreliability, the correlation among the measures would be very high, suggesting that the measures are statistically redundant. One would hope for better discriminant validity between measures of executive function and measures of different constructs. The authors claim that the correlation implies that the MMSE is measuring executive function. However, one could argue the opposite. Perhaps the executive function measure is really just a measure of other neuropsychological constructs measured by the MMSE.

3. *Neurobehavioral Cognitive Status Examination* (NCSE) (Kiernan, Mueller, Langston, & Van Dyke, 1987). The NCSE assesses several constructs: orientation, attention, spontaneous speech, comprehension, repetition, naming, constructional ability, memory, calcula-

tions, similarities, judgments, by asking a screening question in each area and performing further testing if failure on the item is observed. Initial examination of the measure showed sensitivity superior to that of the MMSE for classifying cognitive impairment resulting from focal cerebral lesions among a sample of neurosurgical patients. However, a later study of elderly on an acute care geriatric unit (Fields et al., 1992) showed greater sensitivity of the NCSE over the MMSE at the price of much worse specificity and positive predictive value. One third of the sample could not complete either measure because of severe communication impairment, and several moderately impaired individuals either could not cooperate to the point of finishing the measure or took a long time for completion (e.g., among those who could complete the NSCE, it took over twice as long to administer as the did the MMSE, and required good hearing and vision). Conversely, based on use of the scale among 503 geropsychiatric inpatients, Wiederman and Morgan (1995) concluded that it shows promise as a screening measure; however, information is not provided about completion rates and complications associated with administration.

4. *Mattis Dementia Rating Scale* (DRS) (Mattis, 1976; Psychological Assessment Resources [PAR], 1988); *Research Mattis Dementia Rating Scale.* The DRS (Mattis, 1976; PAR, 1988) is a widely used neuropsychological test of cognitive impairment across a range of cognitive disability and types of impairment. During 1995, several articles appeared describing the validity of the DRS for varying purposes, such as differentiating between Alzheimer's and Parkinson's diseases, between so-called cortical and subcortical (e.g., Parkinson's and Huntington's diseases) dementias, and for use with geropsychiatric patients or for detecting mild dementia. Investigators have found that performance of individuals with Huntington's disease was more impaired on the Initiation subtest, whereas that of Alzheimer's patients was more impaired on the Memory subtest (Rosser & Hodges, 1994; Salmon et al., 1989) Paolo and colleagues (1995a) also found that the Alzheimer's patients performed worse than did patients with Parkinson's disease on the Memory subscale, whereas the Parkinson's disease patients performed worse on Construction (probably because of motor impairments characteristic of the disease); however, they report that the correct classification rate, based on discriminant function analyses, was only 72% to 74% relative to a 50% base rate, indicating weak clinical validity for discriminating the disease states.

The original authors report test-retest reliability of .97 (Coblentz et al., 1973). Other authors report internal consistencies for the subscales ranging from .75 to .95 (Vitaliano et al., 1984) and high split-half reliability (.90) for the total measure (Gardner et al., 1981). A recent investigation, using unadjusted DRS scores estimated the sensitivity of the DRS, using the CDR as the gold standard, at .92 for an Alzheimer's group and .90 for a Parkinson's group. The specificities were .91 and .71, respectively (correct classification rates were .91 and .75; Paolo et al., 1995b). Monsch and colleagues (1995) used age- and education-adjusted scores in a ROC analysis among a sample of outpatients and normal elderly. The sensitivity was .98 and specificity .97; a cross-validation with community resident elderly yielded sensitivity of .91 and specificity of .93.

The original version of the DRS is available through Psychological Assessment Resources (PAR). An adaptation, the NIA Research Mattis Dementia Rating Scale (R-MDRS) was modified to capture the severity of impairments existing among the institutionalized elderly. No item wordings were changed; however, the R-MDRS further delineates "nonresponses," specifically, responses that are not ratable because of a respondent's (a) inability to attend to or comprehend a question, (b) refusal to answer a question or perform a task, or (c) physical or perceptual impairment. An arousal screen was added to the beginning of the measure. Items are arranged in order of difficulty from easy to difficult or difficult to easy, in a header-contingency format. If several easy items are missed, it is assumed that more difficult items would not be answered correctly.

The Attention Scale consists of 19 items designed to measure attention. Typical items involve repeating a series of digits forward and backward, following two successive commands, and imitating simple commands.

The Initiation and Perseveration Scale consists of 11 items designed to test an individual's ability to begin, switch, and end a task. Typical items are "name all the things you can find or buy in a supermarket," "name all the things I [the interviewer] am wearing," and "say 'bee-key-gee' four times."

The Construction Scale consists of 6 items measuring an individual's ability to reproduce a series of designs (i.e., four vertical lines, a diamond in a square, and a signature).

The Conceptualization Scale consists of 32 items testing ability to detect similarities or differences among verbal and visual stimuli. Typical items involve identification of similarities or differences among sets of figures, determining abstract or concrete similarities among objects. For example, the subject is presented with three designs and asked to indicate which is most similar and later, which is different.

The Memory Scale consists of 20 items designed to measure orientation, recall, and recognition. Typical items are "What is the day of the week?"; "Who is governor now?"; and "What is the name of the city we are in right now?"

Preliminary data (Teresi, 1995) from the SCU Collaborative Studies (Ory, 1994) indicates that internal consistencies for scales were good, ranging from .76 to .87 for Attention across sites, .63 to .70 for Initiation and Perseveration, .84 to .91 for Construction, .76 to .88 for Memory, and .91 to .95 for the Total Scale. The least amount of missing data (an average of about 37%) was observed on the Attention subscale, contrasted with other subscales where the range was 18% to 61%. Most missing data occurred among subjects at GDS stage 6 (31% to 50% of missing data across sites) or stage 7 (27% to 50%). The main reasons for nontestability was the absence of verbal response to questions (18% to 26% across sites), active psychotic state (0% to 16%), and other verbal but unintelligible response (19% to 37%). Collectively, 35% to 74% were scorable on the DRS. However, the Attention subscale performed better, with 43% to 80% scorable. It was possible to assess 73% of GDS (Reisberg, Ferris, de Leon, & Crook, 1982) stage 6 and 11% of stage 7 on Attention subscale and 67% of GDS stage 6, and 7% of stage 7 on the R-MDRS Total Scale. For the Attention subscale, an additional 20% (net gain) in proportion assessed over the MMSE was observed. For the total score, an additional one third of those who gave no response to the MMSE or whose responses were not ratable obtained a R-MDRS score, but no gains were observed among the nonarousable, and few gains were observed among those who could not complete simple commands. These findings are similar to others (Nadler et al., 1995) who observed a better range of scores on the DRS than the 3MS or the MMSE.

In one longitudinal investigation of the MMSE, the Blessed Information-Memory and Concentration (IMC) (Blessed, Tomlinson, & Roth, 1968) and the Dementia Rating Scale (DRS) (Mattis, 1976), the DRS evidenced appreciably greater sensitivity to change among the severely demented (Salmon et al., 1990). The authors attribute the increased capability for detection of longitudinal change among the more severely impaired to the presence of some items with lower item difficulties and to the incorporation of items measuring attention, which is preserved until late stages of dementia. However, as Claman and Radebaugh (1991) report, conference participants in an NIA international workshop on clinical trials in Alzheimer's disease concluded that more work on instrumentation is needed to measure cognitive decline over time better.

GLOBAL STAGING METHODOLOGIES

Although we do not review staging measures here, there has been renewed interest in the use of global staging methodologies among chronic care populations. (For a review of staging measures for chronic care populations, see Reisberg, Sclan, Franssen, Kluger, & Ferris, 1994.) Staging measures include the GDS (Reisberg, Ferris, de Leon, & Crook, 1982) and the Clinical Dementia Rating (CDR) (Hughes, Berg, Danziger, Coben, & Martin, 1982). Based on a combination of direct assessment, observation, and informant report, these measures are potentially useful for making functional statements about individuals, particularly those with advanced dementia and communication disorders. For example, an analyses (Juva et al., 1994) of the CDR in comparison with the MMSE and an ADL scale found that the CDR corresponded better with a measure of ADL impairment (κ=.46) than did the DSM III (κ=.33). Although there is some tautology in the relationship (ADL is a prominent feature of the CDR ratings, and kappas were used instead of a more appropriate sensitivity analyses against a "gold standard"), these findings suggest that staging measures may have utility in predicting both cognitive status as well as the more clinically relevant functional status. Additionally, unpublished findings (NIA Coordinating Center, 1995) from the recent NIA collaborative studies of dementia special care (Ory, 1994) have shown that relatively fewer missing data are observed for staging measures than for cognitive test measures.

OBSERVATIONAL MEASURES

Most of the observation measures do not focus on cognitive impairment but include several cognitive items within item sets that are primarily intended to measure behaviors. Most of these measures will thus not be reviewed here because the primary focus is behavior, and they are reviewed in the article by Tariot and colleagues in this issue. For another recent review of such measures, see Teri and Logsdon (1995).

1. *The Neurobehavioral Rating Scale* (NRS) (Levin et al., 1987). The NRS is one observational measure that contains a relatively large proportion of cognitive items. The scale contains many items from the Brief Psychiatric Rating Scale (Overall & Gorham, 1988), augmented by cognitive items. The NRS contains 28 items observational items rated after a 45-minute structured interview. Items are rated on a 6-point behaviorally anchored metric ranging from 0 (not present) to 6 (extremely severe). Typical cognitive items are "inattention/reduced alertness"; "disorientation"; "conceptual disorganization"; "memory deficits"; "comprehension deficit"; "speech articulation defect"; "expressive deficit"; and "fluent aphasia." A principal components factor analysis with varimax rotation yielded a 7-item cognitive factor; reported interrater reliability (calculated using averaged Spearman rank-order correlations across three pairs of raters), assessed with respect to 15 patients with

dementia, was .88 for the Cognition factor (Sultzer, Berissford, & Gunay, 1995). Before assessing the utility of this cognitive subscale, more extensive factor analyses using other solutions and cross-validation samples are needed. Further, interrater reliability analyses needs to be conducted with a larger number of subjects.

2. *Eschelle Comportement et Adaptation* (ECA) (Ritchie & Ledesert, 1991). The ECA is an observational measure for completion by caregivers who have frequent contact with the person, following a process involving observation, and, if necessary, direct questioning. Cronbach's αs for five subscales are Language (.6), Social Integration (.5), Occupation and Orientation (.4), Physical Independence (.7), and Mobility (.7). These coefficients are relatively low, given what appears to be adequate item distributions. Most subscales were found to have a wide range of scores among the 20% severely impaired individuals who score zero on the MMSE; the ECA was significantly correlated with the MMSE; however, no coefficient is provided. Most items are rated on a severity scale with anchored responses. For example, writing ability has the following anchors: "writes short notes or letter, writes several sentences, writes a single sentence, writes own name, unable to write." A problem with this and other items is that no codes are provided for incapacity because of noncognitive reasons, such as physical disability.

INFORMANT-BASED MEASURES

Informant-based scales frequently focus on functional sequelae of Alzheimer's disease, and because they obtain information from a staff or informal caregiver, they do not require language skills for completion. Jorm (1996) reviews the advantages of informant-based measures: assessment of domains relevant to everyday function; capability for assessment using mail or telephone surveys; avoidance of possibly unpleasant direct cognitive testing and possible culture bias; and use with nontestable subjects. Disadvantages include difficulties encountered in securing a reliable informant, and inability to assess adequately neuropsychological constructs that may be necessary for specific diagnoses.

Based on his review, Jorm (1996) concluded that most factor analyses reflect unidimensionality; high internal consistencies (.71 to .97) have been observed; test-retest correlations range from 61 to .97, with the exception of one measure); interinformant correlations, reported for only three of the measures ranged from .60 to 1.0. Correlations of informant scales with measures, such as the MMSE or Blessed, have ranged from .37 to .78. However, most correlations were in the range of .40 to .60, indicating only moderate agreement and considerable possibility of inaccurate assessment. Most informant measures evaluated for correlation with education and premorbid ability appeared to be independent; however, two were manifestly not independent, and not all scales were examined in this way; thus, more research is needed to examine the influence of culture and education on informant measures of cognitive impairment.

There are several informant-based scales, reviewed recently by Jorm (1996); however, none was designed specifically for use among individuals with advanced dementia. Therefore, the authors review only one scale (see later), intended for use with severely impaired individuals. However, one additional widely investigated informant measure, the Informant Questionnaire on Cognitive Decline in the Elderly (IQCODE) (Jorm & Jacomb, 1989), should be noted.

1. *IQCODE* (Jorm & Jacomb, 1989) This measure, which assesses changes in cognitive performance over the previous decade, has been shown to have high reliability, to be convergent with the MMSE, and to be unaffected by premorbid intelligence, education, and physical capacity of the subject; however, the measure has been reported to be influenced by other noncognitive factors (Jorm et al., 1996). A recent analyses (Mulligan, Mackinnon, Jorm, Giannakopoulos, & Michel, 1996) of ROCs of three different methodologies for assessing cognitive impairment: informant assessment, direct assessment, and antisaccadic eye movements showed that the informant (IQCODE) and direct assessment methodologies were statistically equivalent in terms of relationship to diagnosis.

2. *Bedford Alzheimer Nursing Scale-Severity subscale* (BANS-S). (Volicer, Hurley, Lathi & Kowall, 1994) The BANS-S, completed by nursing staff, is intended for use with individuals with severe impairment. Seven items, sleeping, speech, dressing, eating, mobility, muscles, and eye contact, are rated on a 4-point continuum. A typical rating, for muscles, is "very flexible and has full joint motion; somewhat flexible, with some joint motion; somewhat rigid; contracted." The subscale, developed using an *n* of 69, was reported to have internal consistencies across three sites and two raters ranging from .64 to .80; Pearson correlations between two pairs of raters ranged from .82 to .87. Construct validity coefficients with the Test for Severe Impairment was -.65 at baseline and -.50 at 3-month follow-up. Baseline and follow-up correlations with a Language Assessment measure were -.62 and -.44, respectively, and -.31 and -.14 with the MMSE. The measure correlated .56 and .41 with the KATZ measure of ADL. Thus, the measure has good convergent validity with measures of severe impairment but less impressive divergent validity with measures of ADL. The measure correlated .44 with density of neurofibrillary tangles in area CA2, .49 in CA3, .33 in CA1, and 0 in CA4. No information on the correlation of the other measures with autopsy results is presented.

MEDICAL RECORDS AND ADMINISTRATIVE DATA SETS

The authors briefly describe in this section two MDS-based measures of cognition. One is a global staging measure (which is included here instead of in the section on staging measures because it is based on an administrative data set rather than on direct clinical assessments), and the second is a psychometric measure developed using MDS items.

The Cognitive Performance Scale (CPS) (Morris et al., 1994)*; and Minimum Data Set-Cognition* (MDS-COG) (Hartmaier, Sloane, Guess, & Koch, 1994) is a seven-category measure, described by the authors as a hierarchical cognitive performance rating scale. The measure uses responses to five MDS items: two dichotomous items (comatose, short-term memory impairment); and three multipoint items (cognitive skills for decision making, understood by others, ADL Self-Performance in Eating). These five items have interrater reliabilities (using trained research nurses) ranging from .77 to .94. The η^2 for the CPS in relation to the MMSE was .75. Other research with the CPS, using a random sample of 200 residents from 8 nursing homes in North Carolina, showed sensitivity of .94, specificity of .94, and area under the (ROC) curve of .96. (Hartmaier et al., 1995). The authors conclude that "when performed by a trained research nurse using recommended protocols," the CPS is a valid cognitive status measure.

The Cognitive Performance Measure was examined (Hartmaier, Sloane, Guess, & Koch, 1994) in relation to the GDS cognitive staging measure (Reisberg, Ferris, de

Leon, & Crook, 1982). The weighted κ was .41. Agreement between the CPS and GDS across stages ranged from 0% for stages 3 and 4 to 50% for stages 1 and 7. By collapsing stages of the GDS, the authors were able to increase the weighted κ to .76, but report that the percent agreement for stages 5 and 7 remained low. To improve agreement, the authors used logistic regression to determine additional items predictive of each GDS stage. The CPS was expanded to 8 items, scored on a continuous (0 to 10) scale. Eight cognitive (short- and long-term memory, location of room, knows he or she is in a nursing home, orientation, and decision making), communication and ADL (dressing self-performance) items were included. The weighted κ with the GDS was .82 (.80 for a cross-validation subsample) for the new measure (MDS-COG), which had greater agreement (65% with GDS stage 5 and 86% for GDS stage 7) than did the CPS. The sensitivity and specificity with the MMSE was .95 and .88, respectively; the positive and negative predictive values were .96 and .85, respectively. It would appear that the MDS-COG, when used by trained research or clinical nursing staff, shows promise as a severity measure of cognitive status.

However, one caveat is that the item reliabilities reported previously are for the sample as a whole. The authors of the MDS have found lower interrater reliability among the cognitively impaired, as contrasted with the cognitively intact for items assessing communication, sensory ability and functional status/continence (Phillips, Chu, Morris, & Hawes, 1993). Calculating an overall index of nonreliability (the sum of all items for which perfect agreement was not achieved), average disagreement among all 40 items examined in these domains was 7 of 40 items for the intact and 10 of 40 for the impaired. They found that the negative effects of cognitive dysfunction on reliability was greatest for the items assessing communication (one of the areas included in the CPS and MDS-COG) and sensory impairments, despite use of two trained research nurse assessors. Of concern was the finding that the most reliable of items across the entire nursing home sample of 147 nursing homes were the least reliable when applied to the cognitively impaired.

DISCUSSION

The authors have reviewed four approaches to cognitive assessment among individuals from chronic care populations; these include direct psychometric testing, observation, informant reporting, and use of medical record data. We also have described four groups of individuals with advanced cognitive impairment typically found in chronic care populations. Psychometric testing cannot be used with the first two of these groups (individuals who are not arousable or who cannot follow simple commands). At the end stage of illness, it may be the case that only functional status and neurological signs rather than cognitive domains are measurable; however, more research is needed to determine whether this is so and to better define the point at which assessment is no longer possible. Global staging measures that combine observation, informant reports, and chart data have been recommended as the only way to obtain information about cognitive status among those with advanced cognitive impairment or severe communication disorder. However, in the author's view, methods and sources of data gathering should remain independent. If different types of data are to be collected, they should be collected using distinct, separate measures, or with columns provided for independent coding of each data element by source; a final global rating might be a consensus opinion based on review of information (collected in a standardized format) across the sources.

The chronic care population includes individuals with a broad spectrum of cognitive disability and comorbid conditions; the ideal cognitive measure would perform adequately among mild to moderately impaired as well as among the severely impaired individuals. There is a need to (a) determine more about the interrelationships among different approaches to measurement, (b) examine the relative capability of the measures at varying cognitive impairment severity levels, (c) examine the relative predictive ability of each approach, and (d) develop a better blend of theoretical definitions of constructs with their empirical operationalization.

REFERENCES

Auer, S. R., & Reisberg, B. (in press). Reliability of the Modified Ordinal Scales of Psychological Development (M-OSPD): A cognitive assessment battery for severe dementia. *International Psychogeriatrics.*

Auer, S. R., Sclan, S. G., Yaffe, R. A., & Reisberg, B. (1994). The neglected half of Alzheimer disease: Cognitive and functional concomitants of severe dementia. *Journal of the American Geriatrics Society, 42,* 1266-1272.

Abraham, I. L., Manning, C. A., Snustad, D. G., Brashear, H. R., Newman, M. C., & Wofford, A. B. (1994). Cognitive screening of nursing home residents: Factor structures of the Mini-Mental State Examination. *Journal of the American Geriatrics Society, 42,* 750-756.

Albert, M. S. (1994). Brief assessments of cognitive function in the elderly. In M. P. Lawton & J. A. Teresi (Eds.), *Annual review of gerontology and geriatrics: Vol. 14. Focus on assessment techniques* (pp. 93-106). New York: Springer Publishing Co.

Albert, M., & Cohen, C. (1992). The test for severe impairment: An instrument for the assessment of patients with severe cognitive dysfunction. *Journal of the American Geriatrics Society, 40,* 449-453.

Anthony, J. C., LeResche, L., Niaz, U., Von Korff, M. R., & Folstein, M. F. (1982). Limits of the Mini-Mental State as a screening test for dementia and delirium among hospital patients. *Psychological Medicine, 12,* 397-408.

Blessed, G., Tomlinson, B. E., & Roth, M. (1968). The association between quantitative measures of dementia and of senile change in the cerebral gray matter of elderly subjects. *British Journal of Psychiatry, 114,* 797-811.

Boller, F., Mizutani, T., Roessman, U., & Gambetti, P. (1980). Parkinson disease, dementia and Alzheimer disease: Clinicopathological correlations. *Annals of Neurology, 41,* 485-490.

Christensen, H., Hadzi-Pavlovic, D., & Jacomb, P. (1991). The psychometric differentiation of dementia from normal aging: a meta analysis. *Psychological Assessment, 3,* 147-155.

Church, M., & Wattis, J. P. (1988). Psychological approaches to the assessment and treatment of old people. In J. P. Wattis & I. Hindmarch (Eds.), *Psychological assessment of the elderly* (pp. 151-179). New York: Churchill Livingstone.

Claman, D. L., & Radebaugh, T. S. (1991). Neuropsychological assessment in clinical trials of Alzheimer's disease. *Alzheimer Disease and Associated Disorders, 5*(Suppl. 1), S49-S56.

Coblentz, J. M., Mattis S., Zingesser, L. H., Kassoff, S. S., Wisniewski, H. M., & Katzman, R. (1973). Presenile dementia: Clinical aspects and evaluation of cerebrospinal fluid dynamics. *Archives of Neurology, 29,* 299-308.

Cohen-Mansfield, J., Werner, P., & Reisberg, B. (1995). Temporal order of cognitive and functional loss in a nursing home population. *Journal of the American Geriatrics Society, 43,* 974-978.

Cole, M., & Dastoor, D. (1983). The Hierarchic Dementia Scale. *Journal of Clinical Experimental Gerontology, 5,* 219-234.

Cole, M., & Dastoor, D. (1987). A new hierarchic approach to the measurement of dementia. *Psychosomatics, 28,* 298-304.

Doraiswamy, P. M., Krishen, A., Stallone, F., Martin, M. D., Potts, N. L., Metz, M. D., & DeVeaugh-Geiss, J. (1995). Cognitive performance on the Alzheimer's Disease Assessment Scale. *Neurology, 45,* 1980-1984.

Eisdorfer, C., Cohen, D., Paveza, G. J., Ashford, J. W., Luchins, D. J., Gorelick, P. B., Hirschman, R. S., Freels, S. A., Levy, P. S., Semla, T. P., & Shaw, H. A. (1992). An empirical evaluation of the Global Deterioration Scale for staging Alzheimer's Disease. *American Journal of Psychiatry, 149,* 190-194.

Fields, S. D., Fulop, G, Sachs, C. J., Strain, J., & Fillit, H. (1992). Usefulness of the neurobehavioral cognitive status examination in the hospitalized elderly. *International Psychogeriatrics, 4,* 93-102.

Folstein, M. F., Folstein, S. E., & McHugh, P. R. (1975). Mini-Mental State: A practical guide for grading the cognitive state of patients for the clinician. *Journal of Psychiatric Research, 12,* 189-198.

Franssen, E. H., Kluger, A., Torossian, C. L., & Reisberg, B. (1993). The neurologic syndrome of severe Alzheimer's disease: Relationship to functional decline. *Archives of Neurology, 50,* 1029-1039.

Gardner, R. F., Oliver-Munoz, S., Fisher, L., & Empting, L. (1981). Mattis Dementia Rating Scale: Internal reliability using a diffusely impaired population. *Journal of Clinical Neuropsychology, 3,* 271-275.

Golden, R., Teresi, J., & Gurland, B. (1984). Development of indicator-scales for the Comprehensive Assessment and Referral Evaluation interview schedule. *Journal of Gerontology, 39,* 138-146.

Gurland, B. J., Wilder, D. E., Cross, P. E., Teresi, J. A., & Barrett, V. W. (1992). Screening scales for dementia: Toward reconciliation of conflicting cross-cultural findings. *International Journal of Geriatric Psychiatry, 7,* 105-113.

Hartmaier, S. L., Sloane, P. D., Guess, H. A., & Koch, G. G. (1994). The MDS Cognition Scale: A valid instrument for identifying and staging nursing home residents with dementia using the minimum data set. *Journal of the American Geriatrics Society, 42,* 1173-1179.

Hartmaier, S. L., Sloane, P. D., Guess, H. A., Koch, G. G., Mitchell, C. M., & Phillips, C. D. (1995). Validation of the Minimum Data Set Cognitive Performance Scale: Agreement with the Mini-Mental State Examination. *Journal of Gerontology: Medical Sciences, 50,* M128-M133.

Harvey, P. D., Davidson, M., Powchik, P., Parrella, M., White, L., & Mohs, R. C. (1992). Assessment of dementia in elderly schizophrenics with structured rating scales. *Schizophrenia Research, 7,* 85-90.

Holmes, D., Ory, M., & Teresi, J. (Eds.). (1994). Special dementia care: Research, policy and practice issues. *Alzheimer's Disease and Associated Disorders: An International Journal, 8*(Suppl. 1).

Hughes, C. P., Berg, L., Danziger, W. L., Coben, L. A., & Martin, R. L. (1982). A clinical scale for the staging of dementia. *British Journal of Psychiatry, 140,* 566-572.

Jorm, A. F. (1996). Assessment of cognitive impairment and dementia using informant reports. *Clinical Psychology Review, 16,* 51-73.

Jorm, A. F., Broe, G. A., Creasey, H. Sulway, M. R., Dent, O., Fairley, M. J., Kos, S. C., & Tennant, C. (1996). Further data on the validity of the Informant Questionnaire on Cognitive Decline in the Elderly (IQCODE). *International Journal of Geriatric Psychiatry, 2,* 131-139.

Jorm, A. F., & Jacomb, P. A. (1989). The Informant Questionnaire on Cognitive Decline in the Elderly (IQCODE): Sociodemographic correlates, reliability, validity and some norms. *Psychological Medicine, 19,* 1015-1022.

Juva, K., Sulkava, R., Erkinjuntti, T., Ylikoski, R., Valvanne, J., & Tilvis, R. (1994). Staging the severity of dementia: Comparison of clinical (CDR, DSM-III-R), functional (ADL, IADL) and cognitive (MMSE) scales. *Acta Neurologica Scandinavica, 90,* 293-298.

Kafonek, S., Ettinger, W. H., Roca, R., Kittner, S., Taylor, N., & German, P. S. (1989). Instruments for screening for depression and dementia in a long-term care facility. *Journal of the American Geriatrics Society, 37,* 29-34.

Kahn, R., Goldfarb, A., Pollack, M., & Peck, A. (1960). The relationship of mental and physical status in institutionalized aged persons. *American Journal of Psychiatry, 117,* 326-328.

Katzman, R. (1992). Diagnosis and management of dementia. In R. Katzman & J. Rowe (Eds.), *Principles of geriatric neurology* (pp. 167-206). Philadelphia: F. A. Davis.

Kiernan, R. J., Mueller, J., Langston, J. W., & Van Dyke, C. (1987). The Neurobehavioral Cognitive Status Examination: A brief but differentiated approach to cognitive assessment. *Annals of Internal Medicine, 107,* 481-485.

Kincaid, M. M., Harvey, P. D., Parella, M., White, L., Putman, K. M., Powchik, P., Davidson, M., & Mohs, R. C. (1995). Validity and utility of the ADAS-L for measurement of cognitive and functional impairment in geriatric schizophrenic inpatients. *The Journal of Neuropsychiatry and Clinical Neurosciences, 7,* 76-81.

Kwa, V. I. H., Limburg, M., Voogel, A. J., Teunisse, S., Derix, M. M. A., & Hijdra, A. (1996). Feasibility of cognitive screening of patients with ischaemic stroke using the CAMCOG. *Journal of Neurology, 243,* 405-409.

Levin, H. S., High, W. M., Goethe, K. E., Sisson, R. A., Overall, J. E., Rhoades, H. M., Eisenberg, H. M., Kalisky, Z., & Gary, H. E. (1987). The Neurobehavioral Rating Scale: Assessment of the behavioral sequelae of head injury by the clinician. *Journal of Neurology, Neurosurgery and Psychiatry, 50,* 183-193.

Mattis, S. (1976) Mental status examination for organic mental syndrome in the elderly patient. In L. Bellak & T. B. Karasu (Eds.), *Geriatric psychiatry: A handbook for psychiatrists and primary care physicians* (pp. 77-121). New York: Grune & Stratton.

Mayeux, R., Stern, Y., Rosen, J., & Benson, D. F. (1981). Is "subcortical dementia" a recognizable clinical entity? *Annals of Neurology, 14,* 278-283.

Monsch, A. U., Bondi, M. W., Salmon, D. P., Butters, N., Thal, L. J., Hansen, L. A., Wiederholt, W. C., Cahn, D. A., & Klauber, M. R. (1995). Clinical validity of the Mattis Dementia Rating Scale in detecting dementia of the Alzheimer's type. *Archives of Neurology, 52,* 899-904.

Morris, J. C., Heyman, A., Mohs, R., Hughes, M. S., van Belle, G., Fillenbaum, G., Mellits, E. D., & Clark, C. (1989). The Consortium to Establish a Registry for

Alzheimer's Disease (CERAD): 1. Clinical and neuropsychological assessment of Alzheimer's disease. *Neurology, 39,* 1159-1165.

Morris, J. C., Mohs, R., Rogers, H., Fillenbaum, G., & Heyman, A. (1988). CERAD clinical and neuropsychological assessment of Alzheimer's disease. *Psychopharmacological Bulletin, 24,* 641-651.

Morris, J. N., Fries, B. E., Mehr, D. R., Hawes, C., Phillips, C., Mor, V., & Lipsitz, L. A. (1994). MDS Cognitive Performance Scale. *Journal of Gerontology: Medical Sciences, 49,* M174-M182.

Morris, J. N., Hawes, C., Fries, B. E., Phillips, C. D., Mor, V., Katz, S., Murphy, K., Drugovich, M. L., & Friedlob, A. S. (1990). Designing the National Resident Assessment Instrument for Nursing Homes. *The Gerontologist, 39,* 293-307.

Mulligan, R., Mackinnon, A., Jorm, A. F., Giannakopoulos, P., & Michel, J. (1996). A comparison of alternative methods of screening for dementia in clinical settings. *Archives of Neurology, 53,* 532-536.

Nadler, J. D., Relkin, N. R., Cohen, M. S., Hodder, R. A., Reingold, J., & Plum, F. (1995). Mental status testing in the elderly nursing home population. *Journal of Geriatric Psychiatry and Neurology, 8,* 177-183.

Olin, J. T., & Schneider, L. S. (1995) Assessing response to tacrine using the factor analytic structure of the Alzheimer's Disease Assessment Scale (ADAS)—cognitive subscale. *International Journal of Geriatric Psychiatry, 10,* 753-756.

Ory, M. (1994). Dementia special care units: The development of a national research initiative. *Alzheimer's Disease and Associated Disorders: An International Journal, 8*(S1), S389-S394.

Osterweil, D., Mulford, P., Syndulko, K., & Martin, M. (1994). Cognitive function in old and very old residents of a residential facility: Relationship to age, education, and dementia. *Journal of the American Geriatrics Society, 42,* 766-773.

Overall, J. E., & Gorham, D. R. (1988). Introduction—The Brief Psychiatric Rating Scale (BPRS): Recent developments in ascertainment and scaling. *Psychopharmacology Bulletin, 24,* 97-99.

Paolo, A. M., Troster, A. I., Glatt, S. L., Hubble, J. P., & Koller, W. C. (1995a). Differentiation of the dementias of Alzheimer's and Parkinson's disease with the Dementia Rating Scale. *Journal of Geriatric Psychiatry Neurology, 8,* 184-188

Paolo, A. M., Troster, A. I., Glatt, S. L., Hubble, J. P., & Koller, W. C. (1995b). Influence of demographic variables on the Dementia Rating Scale. *Journal of Geriatric Psychiatry Neurology, 8,* 38-41.

Pfeiffer, E. (1975). A short portable mental status questionnaire for the assessment of organic brain deficit in elderly patients. *Journal of the American Geriatrics Society, 23,* 433-441.

Phillips, C. D., Chu, C. W., Morris, J. N., & Hawes, C. (1993). Effects of cognitive impairment on the reliability of geriatric assessments in nursing homes. *Journal of the American Geriatrics Society, 41,* 136-142.

Piaget, J. (1977). *The origins of intelligence in children.* New York: International University Press.

Psychological Assessment Resources, Inc. (1988). *Dementia Rating Scale.*

Reisberg, B. (1988). Functional Assessment Staging (FAST). *Psychopharmacology Bulletin, 24,* 653-655.

Reisberg B., Ferris, S. H., de Leon, M. J., & Crook, T. (1982). The Global Deterioration Scale for assessment of primary degenerative dementia. *American Journal of Psychiatry, 139,* 1136-1139.

Reisberg, B., Sclan, S. G. Franssen, E., Kluger, A., & Ferris, S. (1994). Dementia staging in chronic care populations. *Alzheimer Disease and Associated Disorders: An International Journal, 8*(S1), S188-S205.

Ritchie, K., & Ledesert, B. (1991). *International Journal of Geriatric Psychiatry, 6,* 217-226.

Ronnberg, L., & Ericsson, K. (1994). Reliability and validity of the Hierarchic Dementia Scale. *International Psychogeriatrics, 6,* 87-93.

Rosen, W. G., Mohs, R. C., & Davis, K. L. (1984). A new rating scale for Alzheimer's disease. *American Journal of Psychiatry, 141,* 1356-1364.

Rosser, A. E., & Hodges, J. R. (1994). The Dementia Rating Scale in Alzheimer's disease, Huntington's disease and progressive supranuclear palsy. *Journal of Neurology, 241,* 531-536.

Roth, M., Tyme, E., Mountjoy, C. Q., Huppert, F. A., Hendrie, A., Verma, S., Goddard, R. (1986). CAMDEX: A standardized instrument for the diagnosis of mental disorders in the elderly with special reference to the early detection of dementia. *British Journal of Psychiatry, 149,* 698-709.

Royall, D. R., Mahurin, R. K., & Cornell, J. (1995). Effect of depression on dementia presentation: Qualitative assessment with the Qualitative Evaluation of Dementia (QED). *Journal of Geriatric Psychiatry and Neurology, 8,* 4-11.

Royall, D. R., Mahurin, R. K. & Gray, K. F. (1992). Bedside assessment of executive cognitive impairment: The Executive Interview. *Journal of the American Geriatrics Society, 40,* 1221-1226.

Royall, D. R., Mahurin, R. K., True, J. E., Anderson, B., Brock, I. P., Freeburger, L., & Miller, A. (1993). Executive impairment among the functionally dependent: Comparisons between schizophrenic and elderly subjects. *American Journal of Psychiatry, 150,* 1813-1819.

Salmon, D. P., Kwo-on-Yuen, P. F., Heindel, W. C., Butters, N., & Thal, L., (1989). Differentiation of Alzheimer's disease and Huntington's disease with the Dementia Rating Scale. *Archives of Neurology, 46,* 1204-1208.

Salmon, D. P., Thal, L. J., Butters, N., & Heindel, W. C. (1990). Longitudinal evaluation of dementia of the Alzheimer type: A comparison of 3 standardized mental status examinations. *Neurology, 40,* 1225-1230.

Saxton, J., McGonigle-Gibson, K. L., Swihart, A. A., Miller, V. J., & Boller, F. (1990). Assessment of the severely impaired patient: Description and validation of a new neuropsychological test battery. *Psychological Assessment: A Journal of Consulting and Clinical Psychology, 2,* 298-303.

Saxton, J., & Swihart, A. (1989). Neuropsychological assessment of the severely impaired elderly patient. *Clinics in Geriatric Medicine, 5,* 531-543.

Sclan, S. G., Foster, J. R., Reisberg, B., Franssen, E., & Welkowitz, J. (1990). Application of Piagetian measures of cognition in severe Alzheimer's disease. *Psychiatric J. University of Ottawa, 15,* 4, 223-228.

Stern, R. G., Mohs, R. C., Davidson, M., Schmeidler, J., Silverman, J., Kramer-Ginsberg, E., Searcey, T., Bierer, L., & Davis, K. (1994). A longitudinal study of Alzheimer's disease: Measurement, rate, and predictors of cognitive deterioration. *American Journal of Psychiatry, 151,* 390-396.

Sultzer, D. L., Berisford, M. A., & Gunay, I. (1995). The Neurobehavioral Rating Scale: Reliability in patients with dementia. *Journal of Psychiatric Research, 29,* 185-191.

Tombaugh, T. N., & McIntyre, N. J. (1992). The Mini-Mental Status Examination: A comprehensive review. *Journal of the American Geriatrics Society, 40,* 922-935.

Teng, E. & Chui, H. C. (1987). The Modified Mini-Mental State Exam. *Journal of Clinical Psychiatry, 48,* 314-318.

Teresi, J. (1995). *Preliminary psychometric on the cognitive measures prepared by the Coordinating Center to the National Institute on Aging Collaborative Studies of Special Dementia Care.*

Teresi, J., Holmes, D., & Ramirez, M. (1996). *Personal Home Care in New York City: Characteristics of recipients; degree and costs of service use; and comparison with matched groups of nursing home residents* (Report to the United Hospital Fund).

Teresi, J., Lawton, P., Ory, M., & Holmes, D. (1994). Overview of measurement issues in chronic care populations. *Alzheimer's Disease and Associated Disorders: An International Journal, 8*(Suppl. 1): S144-S183.

Teri, L., & Logsdon, R. G. (1995). Methodologic issues regarding outcome measures for clinical drug trials of psychiatric complications in dementia. *Journal of Geriatric Psychiatry and Neurology, 8*(Suppl. 1), S8-S17.

Thornbury, J. M. (1993). The use of Piaget's theory in Alzheimer's disease. *The American Journal of Alzheimer's Care and Related Disorders & Research,* 16-21.

Uhlmann, R. F., Teri, L., Rees, T. S., Mozlowski, K., & Larson, E. B. (1989). Impact of mild to moderate hearing loss on mental status testing: Comparison of standard and written Mini-Mental State Examinations. *Journal of the American Geriatric Society, 37,* 223-228.

Uzgiris, I., & Hunt, J. M. V. (1975). Assessment in infancy: Ordinal scales of psychological development. Urbana: University of Illinois.

Vitaliano, P. P., Breen, A. R., Russo, J., et al. (1984). The clinical utility of the Dementia Rating Scale for assessing Alzheimer patients. *Journal of Chronic Diseases, 37,* 743-753.

Volicer, L., Hurley, A. C., Lathi, D. C., & Kowall, N. W. (1994). Measurement of severity in advanced Alzheimer's disease. *Journal of Gerontology: Medical Sciences, 49,* M223-M226.

Welsh, K., Butters, N., Hughes, J., Mohs, R., & Heyman, A. (1991). Detection of abnormal memory decline in mild cases of Alzheimer's disease using CERAD neuropsychological measures. *Archives of Neurology, 48,* 278-281.

Welsh, K., Butters, N., Hughes, J., Mohs, R. & Heyman, A. (1992). Detection and staging of dementia in Alzheimer's disease: Use of the neuropsychological measures developed for the Consortium to Establish a Registry for Alzheimer's Disease (CERAD). *Archives of Neurology, 49,* 448-452.

Whitehouse, P. J. (1986). The concept of subcortical and cortical dementia: Another look. *Annals of Neurology, 19,* 1-6.

Wiederman, M., & Morgan, C. D. (1995). Neruobehavioral Cognitive Status Exam (NCSE) with geriatric inpatients. *Clinical Gerontologist, 15,* 35-47.

Zandi, T. (1994). Comments on measurement of severe dementia. *Alzheimer Disease and Associated Disorders, 8,* S1, S206-S208.

Zec, R. F., Landreth, E. S., Vicari, S. K., Feldman, E., Belman, J., Andrise, A., Robbs, R., Kumar, V., & Becker, R. (1992). Alzheimer Disease Assessment Scale: Useful for both early detection and staging of dementia of the Alzheimer type. *Alzheimer Disease and Associated Disorders, 6,* 89-102.

Chapter 2

Measurement of Communicative Function in Cognitively Impaired Older Adults

Kathryn Bayles

Communicative function can be defined as the sharing of information by means of a symbol system, of which language is but one. To know a language is to know the symbols and the rules for combining them for particular purposes. Language users have internalized the phonologic, syntactic, semantic, and pragmatic rules used to share information. Cognition can be defined as the processes for creating, manipulating, and storing knowledge including perception, attention, reasoning, and memory. Clearly, language is one type of stored knowledge. The use of language knowledge depends on the integrity of perceptual and memorial systems; therefore, the measurement of communicative function requires consideration of the integrity of perceptual and memorial systems as well as linguistic knowledge and processes.

Individuals can have circumscribed cognitive impairments that have minimal or no effect on their ability to produce language and communicate. However, when cognitive impairment is substantial, the ability to communicate is affected. Of concern in this chapter are individuals who are cognitively impaired as a result of age-related dementing diseases. These individuals always have communicative disorders because by definition dementia constitutes broad-based cognitive impairment.

The diagnosis of dementia requires the presence of intellectual deficits sufficient to interfere with social and occupational functions. According to the *Diagnostic and Statistical Manual of Mental Disorders* (4th ed., American Psychiatric Association, 1994) the primary feature of dementia is the development of multiple cognitive deficits that include memory disorder and at least one of the following: aphasia, apraxia, agnosia, or disturbance in executive function.

Dementia is a syndrome with many causes, the most common of which is the irreversible neurodegenerative process known as Alzheimer's disease (AD). Other common irreversible causes are vascular disease that eventuates in multiple infarctions, Lewy Body disease, and Parkinson's disease (PD). These common dementia-producing

Acknowledgment. This work was supported, in part, by National Multipurpose Research and Training Center Grant DC-01409 from the National Institute on Deafness and Other Communication Disorders. Cheryl Tomoeda and Jody Wood assisted in the preparation of this article.

conditions are progressive, and affected individuals will suffer inexorable decline in communicative function. All of these diseases produce a serious effect on memory, thereby altering the ability to communicate. This fact is fundamental to understanding why certain measures of language/communicative function are better than others for documenting the effects of dementing diseases.

As the population of cognitively impaired elders has grown, professionals have become increasingly aware of the need to measure disease effects as a prelude to planning effective care. In fact, the Omnibus Budget Reconciliation Act (OBRA, 1987) requires that all long-term care residents be evaluated in relation to communicative and cognitive functions, as well as others, within the first 6 days of their residency if the facility is to qualify for Medicare coverage of residents. Additionally, the law requires that a resident care plan be developed and on file in the patient's chart by the 14th day of residency. Typically, communicative and cognitive functions of residents are screened, and if problems are detected, in-depth evaluation follows. Data about communicative function are given to the nurse responsible for amassing the required information about the resident's status. OBRA also states that screening and comprehensive assessment should be done with measurement tools that are reliable and valid. A few measures have been designed specifically to evaluate the communicative function of dementia patients; however, many other measures of communicative function have been administered to dementia patients. This chapter begins with a critical review of the instruments designed specifically for evaluating communicative function of cognitively impaired adults. Thereafter, other communication measures that have been given to dementia patients are discussed.

MEASURES DESIGNED TO EVALUATE COMMUNICATIVE FUNCTION IN COGNITIVELY IMPAIRED ADULTS

Two measures of communicative function that were designed for use with cognitively impaired adults that are now in wide use are the Arizona Battery for Communication Disorders of Dementia (ABCD) (Bayles & Tomoeda, 1993) and the Functional Linguistic Communication Inventory (FLCI) (Bayles & Tomoeda, 1994). Another measure designed for cognitively impaired adults, which contains a subset of items related to communicative function, is the Severe Impairment Battery (SIB) (Saxton, McGonigle-Gibson, Swihart, Miller, & Boller, 1990).

Arizona Battery for Communication Disorders of Dementia

The ABCD was designed to provide professionals a method for screening or comprehensively evaluating linguistic communication and related processes. The battery comprises 14 subtests that evaluate 5 constructs: linguistic expression, linguistic comprehension, verbal episodic memory, mental status, and visuospatial construction.

The standardization sample consisted of 272 individuals: 86 AD subjects, 62 nondemented PD subjects, 8 demented PD subjects, 86 age-matched normal elders, and 30 young normal subjects. All subjects met the following criteria for participation: spoke English as a first language, could read, had no history of drug or alcohol abuse, had no previous neurological or psychiatric disorder, had visual acuity sufficient to read 18-point font print, and had speech discrimination skills sufficient to pass a speech discrimination screening test with 80% or better accuracy.

All AD subjects met the National Institute of Neurological and Communicative Disorders and Stroke-Alzheimer's Disease and Related Disorders Association (NINCDS-ADRDA) diagnostic criteria for probable AD (McKhann et al., 1984). Excluded were individuals with evidence or history of diabetes, hypertension, myocardial infarction, epilepsy, stroke, focal brain lesion, grade III or IV retinopathy, head injury associated with loss of consciousness, depression, psychosis, neoplastic disease in the last 5 years, and scores of 12 or greater on the Hamilton Depression Rating Scale (Hamilton, 1967), a cutoff score above which depression is considered present (Lazarus, Newton, Cohler, Lesser, & Schweon, 1987). All AD subjects scored less than 4 on the modified Hachinski Ischemic Scale (Rosen, Terry, Fuld, Katzman, & Peck, 1980), a scale used to screen individuals for vascular disease.

All PD subjects were participants in a longitudinal study of disease effects on memory and language and were diagnosed by the same neurologist. Those PD subjects with a rating on the Global Deterioration Scale (GDS) (Reisberg, Ferris, de Leon, & Crook, 1982) of 3 or greater were classified as demented.

The older normal control subjects lived in the community, and some were participants in a senior citizens' nutrition program. The young normal control subjects were recruited from high schools and the student body at the University of Arizona. All subjects were rated with the GDS; their ratings and demographic characteristics have been reported in Table 2.1. Subjects also were given the Mini-Mental State Examination (MMSE) (Folstein, Folstein, & McHugh, 1975) and the Block Design subtest of the Wechsler Adult Intelligence Scale–Revised (WAIS-R) (Wechsler, 1981).

Intergroup comparisons were made of the raw, summary, construct, and total overall scores for each subject group. Generally subtest performance distinguished mild dementia patients from normal elderly subjects and moderate from mild dementia patients at statistically significant levels. When raw scores were converted to summary scores, significant differences again were found between the groups. Similar results were obtained for construct scores and the total overall score.

Performance of United Kingdom subjects on ABCD. The ABCD was administered to AD patients, normal elders and young normal individuals who reside in the United Kingdom (UK) (Armstrong, Bayles, Borthwick, & Tomoeda, 1996). When comparisons were made between the performance of US and UK dementia patients, no significant differences were observed with a single exception, moderate UK AD subjects performed significantly poorer on the recognition memory subcomponent of the Word Learning Subtest, likely because they were more severe.

When the performances of US and UK normals were compared, the only significant differences were on the Concept Definition and Object Description Subtests with US subjects performing better. These differences were speculated to result from the cultural tendency of American subjects to be more verbally assertive.

Validity. To evaluate the criterion validity of the ABCD, the performance of the normal elderly subjects was used to establish a cutoff value for each subtest below which an individual could be considered to have performed subnormally. The selected value approximated the 5th centile of normal performance, meaning that 95% of

TABLE 2.1 Demographic Characteristics of Subjects in the ABCD Study

Variable		Young NC	Old NC	Mild AD	Mod. AD	NPD	DPD
Sex							
Male	*N=*	13	26	20	25	40	5
Female	*N=*	17	60	21	20	22	3
Handedness							
Right	*N=*	26	84	39	42	57	8
Left	*N=*	4	2	1	1	2	0
Both	*N=*	0	0	1	2	3	0
GDS Rating							
1	*N=*	30	86	0	0	28	0
2	*N=*	0	0	0	0	34	0
3	*N=*	0	0	7	0	0	5
4	*N=*	0	0	34	0	0	1
5	*N=*	0	0	0	30	0	1
6	*N=*	0	0	0	15	0	1
Age							
	M	20.29	70.44	76.74	75.01	70.14	73.18
	SD	(3.12)	(17.07)	(8.55)	(18.67)	(7.37)	(7.60)
Education							
	M	13.50	13.72	14.15	12.65	14.42	15.12
	SD	(2.40)	(2.64)	(3.56)	(4.09)	(2.74)	(3.31)
Estimated IQ							
	M	105.30	111.04	113.18	109.60	112.69	115.43
	SD	(7.18)	(7.19)	(8.72)	(10.16)	(7.21)	(9.47)

Reprinted from Bayles, K. A. & Tomoeda, C. K. (1993). *Arizona Battery for Communication Disorders of Dementia.* Tucson: Canyonlands Publishing, by permission. Copyright 1993 by Canyonlands Publishing, Inc.

normals achieved a higher score. Using the χ^2 statistic, the null hypothesis was tested that equal proportions of normal elders, and mild AD and moderate AD subjects fell below the specified cutoff value. As can be seen in Table 2.2, the tests were found highly efficacious for screening for mild AD. The most effective were the verbal episodic memory tasks: Story Retelling–Delayed and the Free Recall score from Word Learning. Using Story Retelling–Delayed, 92% of normals, 83% of mild AD subjects, and 100% of moderate AD subjects were identified.

In another analysis of validity, the ABCD performance of 50 AD patients from the standardization study was correlated with performance on three established measures of dementia severity: the MMSE, the Block Design subtest of the WAIS-R, and the Global Deterioration Scale score. The correlation between ABCD performance and these test scores was measured by the probability for concordance statistic; results reflected high correlations between the ABCD subtests and these measures. A similar procedure undertaken using ABCD summary scores yielded the same results.

Reliability. The ABCD was administered to 20 of the AD subjects on two occasions, 1 week apart. The strength of association between the two test presentations was measured using the Pearson product-moment correlation and Kendall's τ (b). Results of these analyses showed high test-retest reliability. Virtually no learning effect was observed.

TABLE 2.2 Success of ABCD Subtests in Screening for AD

CONSTRUCT Task	Cutoff Score	Old NC[1]	Mild AD[1]	Mod. AD[1]	X^2
MENTAL STATUS					
Mental Status	11.5	.05	.66	1.00	121.3
EPISODIC MEMORY					
Story Retelling - Immediate	8.5	.05	.56	.96	109.2
Story Retelling - Delayed	0.5	.08	.83	1.00	120.2
Word Learning - Free Recall	4.5	.09	.85	1;00	121.5
Word Learning - Total Recall	13.5	.07	.93	.98	133.6
Word Learning - Recognition	42.5	.05	.80	.96	116.8
LINGUISTIC EXPRESSION					
Object Description (nail)	5.5	.08	.37	.82	74.2
Generative Naming (transportation)	6.5	.06	.46	.87	80.5
Confrontation Naming	13.5	.06	.24	.82	85.6
Concept Definition	43.5	.03	.65	1.00	48.3
LINGUISTIC COMPREHENSION					
Following Commands	7.5	.01	.15	.60	69.1
Comparative Questions	5.5	.06	.24	.69	61.8
Repetition	56.5	.05	.32	.79	75.7
Reading Comprehension - Word	7.5	.07	.22	.73	63.6
Reading Comprehension - Sentence	5.5	.13	.33	.73	48.9
VISUOSPATIAL CONSTRUCTION					
Generative Drawing	8.5	.05	.22	.73	75.0
Figure Copying	9.5	.06	.10	.62	59.2

1 = The specified value is the proportion of subjects who fall below the cutoff. (If the value
    is multiplied by 100, it can be converted to a percent.)
2 = 2-sided $p \leq .0005$ for all ABCD subtests.

Adapted from Bayles, K. A. & Tomoeda, C. K. (1993). *Arizona Battery for Communication Disorders of Dementia.* Tucson: Canyonlands Publishing, by permission. Copyright 1993 by Canyonlands Publishing, Inc.

Internal consistency was computed using the data of 50 AD subjects with Cronbach's α for each relevant task. These results are reported in Table 2.3. Most subtests contain dichotomous (correct/incorrect) items, in which case Cronbach's α reduces to the Kuder-Richardson Formula 20 (Allen & Yen, 1979). For Concept Definition, each item is scored on a 0 to 3 scale and for Repetition an item's scale depends on length of phrase; therefore, for this analysis each item score was converted to a common 0 to 15 scale.

From Cronbach's alpha and the sample variance can be computed the standard error of measurement (SEM), which gives an indication of the confidence that can be placed in the measurement process. This quantity is given by

$$SEM = [variance * (1 - \alpha)^{.5}]$$

If performances are normally distributed, then one can be 95 percent confident that the interval of + 1.96* SEM about a patient's measured score covers his or her "true" score. Internal consistency analyses can be somewhat misleading if the task is either too easy or too difficult. For example, the extraordinarily high α for Story Retelling Delayed results from the fact that almost every AD subject missed every item on this task.

TABLE 2.3 Internal Consistency of ABCD Subtests

CONSTRUCT Task	*Items[1]	Dichotomous	Cronbach's Alpha	Standard Error of Measurement
MENTAL STATUS				
Mental Status	13	Yes	.8448	1.34
EPISODIC MEMORY				
Story Retelling - Immediate	17	Yes	.8557	1.51
Story Retelling - Delayed	17 (13)	Yes	.9853	0.27
Word Learning - Free Recall	16 (15)	Yes	.6320	1.10
Word Learning - Total Recall	16	Yes	.8155	1.72
Word Learning - Recognition	48	Yes	.8447	3.03
LINGUISTIC EXPRESSION				
Object Description (nail)	generative[2]	--	--	--
Generative Naming	generative[2]	--	--	--
Confrontation Naming	20	Yes	.8772	1.57
Concept Definition	10	No	.8389	2.07
LINGUISTIC COMPREHENSION				
Following Commands	9 (7)	Yes	.6962	0.88
Comparative Questions	6	Yes	.5017	0.63
Repetition	10	No	.8002	5.30
Reading Comprehension - Word	8	Yes	.6735	0.77
Reading Comprehension - Sentence	7	Yes	.6898	0.97
VISUOSPATIAL CONSTRUCTION				
Generative Drawing	generative[2]	--	--	--
Figure Copying	12	Yes	.9179	0.95

1 = If there was no variation on an item, then it was removed from the analysis and the
 effective number of items is reported parenthetically.
2 = Not calculated.

Adapted from Bayles, K. A. & Tomoeda, C. K. (1993). *Arizona Battery for Communication Disorders of Dementia.* Tucson: Canyonlands Publishing, by permission. Copyright 1993 by Canyonlands Publishing, Inc.

Strengths. The ABCD was designed for use with dementia patients and has shown reliability and validity. Its numerous subtests can be given individually to assess a particular function or collectively to comprehensively evaluate functional communication, memory, and mental status. The Story Retelling–Immediate and Delayed Subtests are exceptionally discriminating of mild dementia, and because they are short and easily administered, they are useful screening tests. The ABCD overall performance score has been found to be superior to performance on the Modified Wisconsin Card Sort Test (Grant & Berg, 1948; Jenkins & Parsons, 1978; Nelson, 1976), the Block Design Subtest of the WAIS-R (Wechsler, 1981), the MMSE, and a test of verbal fluency for discriminating dementia patients from normals (Bayles, Tomoeda, Wood, Cruz, & McGeagh, 1996). The ABCD can be used to determine mental status and calculate baseline abilities of communicative functions, such as the ability to comprehend language, express self, follow commands, read, write, and name, information that is required by OBRA of all long-term care residents. Such information is critical to the development of patient care plans, which must reflect the resident's documented functional abilities.
    The high correspondence between the performance of the UK and US subjects

suggests the potential of the ABCD for cross-cultural use. The high degree of correlation between performance on the ABCD, the MMSE, and GDS rating indicates its appropriateness for quantifying degree of severity until advanced dementia.

The ABCD is not appropriate for use with severely demented individuals, those whose GDS–Functional Assessment Stages (FAST) ratings are 7, because of a floor effect in their performance. Patients who are GDS-FAST 6a through 6d generally are tested with the ABCD, although a floor effect is associated with verbal episodic memory test performance. The overall ABCD scores of these patients ranges from 8 to 12 (best score=25).

Limitations. The ABCD is inappropriate for severe AD patients. Having said that, the point should be made that it is difficult to develop a measure that is both sensitive to mild dementia and appropriate for use with severe late-stage patients. If test items are sufficiently easy as to be answerable by late-stage patients, they are too easy for mild and moderate patients, and a ceiling effect becomes a problem.

An important limitation of the ABCD is that it has been standardized for only literate White subjects who have either AD or PD. However, it has been translated into French and Spanish and is being standardized with French speakers in Canada and Spanish speakers in Puerto Rico, Texas, and Arizona, so normative data for some other ethnic groups should become available.

Another limitation is that the ABCD has not been given to dementia patients with etiologies other than AD and PD. Of value would be performance data from patients with vascular disease, Lewy body disease, Creutzfeld-Jakob disease, and Pick's disease.

Functional Linguistic Communication Inventory (FLCI)

The FLCI (Bayles & Tomoeda, 1994) was designed to quantify the effects of advanced dementia on functional communication and provide clinicians a tool by which to obtain the information required by OBRA about each nursing home resident. The test items are less complex than those on the ABCD; many are dichotomous, allowing the examiner to specify whether the patient can do them.

The 10 FLCI components evaluate the following functions: greeting and naming, question answering, writing, sign comprehension and object-to-picture matching, word reading and comprehension, ability to reminisce, following of commands, pantomime, gesture, and conversation. The test evolved from the longitudinal research of Bayles and Tomoeda on the effects of AD on communicative function. In fact, approximately half of the test items were taken from a research battery used in a 5-year longitudinal study of 91 subjects. The other items were designed to increase the sensitivity of the test to disease effects on what has been termed "functional" communication.

The full complement of test items was administered to 40 AD patients diagnosed according to the NINCDS-ADRDA diagnostic criteria for AD (McKhann et al., 1984). Subjects were recruited through the Tucson chapter of the Alzheimer's Association and the memory disorders clinic at the Arizona Health Sciences Center and from adult care homes, nursing facilities, and day care centers. All subjects spoke English as a first language, could read, and had normal premorbid intelligence as estimated using the regression equation developed by Wilson, Rosenbaum, Brown, Rourke, and Whitman (1978). All subjects oriented to the sound of speech. Although the socioeconomic status of subjects was not controlled, most were from middle-income families, and no subject was destitute. Exclusionary criteria were the same as those for the ABCD standard-ization study.

The severity of dementia was defined with a modified version of FAST (Reisberg, Ferris, & Franssen, 1985), an extension of the GDS (Reisberg et al., 1982) in which later stage patients are further categorized. This scale was modified slightly for use in the FLCI standardization study (see Tables 2.4 and 2.5).

In Table 2.6 is the breakdown of dementia patients according to severity rating and associated score on the MMSE. The performance of these individuals, who varied in severity, is plotted in Figure 2.1, and in Table 2.7 are the means and standard deviations and specification of significant intergroup differences.

These data show that the FLCI is sensitive to differences in patients who are in the advanced stages of AD. Clinicians can compare the performance of their moderate or severe dementia patients to those in the standardization sample, determine functional communication strengths, and predict those functions vulnerable as the disease progresses. Patients who score 0 on the FLCI are those for whom a maintenance rather than restorative/compensatory care program generally is more appropriate.

Validity. The ABCD was administered to those 13 subjects in the sample of 40 whose level of dementia was sufficiently mild to permit test administration. Results were compared with FLCI performance. Pearson product-moment correlation was used to measure the strength and direction of the correlation. A strong positive correlation ($r = .78$) was obtained ($p < .002$).

TABLE 2.4 Functional Assessment Stages (FAST) for Dementia of the Alzheimer's Type (DAT)

Stage	Level of Functioning	Clinical Diagnosis
1	No decrement	Normal adult
2	Subjective deficit in word finding	Normal aged adult
3	Deficit in demanding employment settings	Compatible with incipient DAT
4	Assistance required in complex tasks (handling finances, marketing, or planning dinner for guests)	Mild DAT
5	Assistance required in choosing proper clothing	Moderate DAT
6a	Assistance required in putting on clothing	Moderately severe DAT
6b	Assistance required in bathing properly	
6c	Assistance required with the mechanics of toileting (flushing, wiping, and so on)	
6d	Urinary incontinence	
6e	Fecal incontinence	
7a	Speech ability limited to approximately a half-dozen intelligible words	Severe DAT
7b	Intelligible vocabulary limited to a single word	
7c	Ambulatory ability lost	
7d	Ability to sit up lost	
7e	Ability to smile lost	
7f	Consciousness lost	

From Reisberg, B., Ferris, S. H., & Franssen, E. (1985). An ordinal functional assessment tool for Alzheimer's-type dementia. *Hospital and Community Psychiatry, 36*, 593-595, by permission. Copyright 1985 by the American Psychiatric Association.

TABLE 2.5 Modified FAST Scale Used in the FLCI Standardization Study

Modified FAST Scale	Dementia Severity	Additional Defining Characteristics
4	Mild	Same as GDS and FAST stage 4
5	Moderate	Same as GDS and FAST stage 5
6	Moderately severe	Incontinent of bladder but not bedridden; same as FAST stages 6a through 6d
7	Severe	Incontinent of bladder and bowel but not bedridden; same as FAST stages 6e through 7c
8	Very Severe	Incontinent of bladder and bowel and bedridden; same as FAST stages 7d through 7f

Reprinted from Bayles, K. A. & Tomoeda, C. K. (1993). *Arizona Battery for Communication Disorders of Dementia.* Tucson: Canyonlands Publishing, by permission. Copyright 1993 by Canyonlands Publishing, Inc.

TABLE 2.6 Demographic Characteristics of Subjects in the FLCI Standardization Study

Variable		Modified FAST Stage				
		4	5	6	7	8
Total	$N =$	4	14	10	8	4
Gender						
Male	$N =$	2	5	3	6	0
Female	$N =$	2	9	7	2	4
Age	M	80.98	83.41	79.09	83.13	82.12
	SD	7.61	6.16	6.12	6.70	11.41
Education	M	13.25	12.42	13.11	13.75	14.50
	SD	3.10	2.39	2.26	3.11	3.79
Estimated I.Q.	M	111.87	110.08	110.21	112.60	114.09
	SD	6.72	5.76	5.36	8.62	8.07
MMSE Score	M	20.25	15.21	6.80	1.50	0.00
	SD	2.63	2.89	3.55	1.41	0.00

Reprinted from Bayles, K. A. & Tomoeda, C. K. (1994). *Functional Linguistic Communication Inventory.* Tucson: Canyonlands Publishing, with permission. Copyright 1994 by Canyonlands Publishing, Inc.

Reliability. Half of the subjects in the standardization study were given the FLCI a second time 1 week after the first testing. The degree of association between performance at the two test times was measured by Pearson product-moment correlation and Kendall's τ. Results indicate high test-retest reliability (Bayles & Tomoeda, 1994).

Strengths. The FLCI was designed for use with middle- and late-stage dementia patients and provides data about functional communication of long-term care residents that is required by law. The test is designed to reveal residual strengths of patients that may be used to improve their quality of care and life. Patient performance on the FLCI can serve as a baseline against which the efficacy of various linguistic and environmental inter-ventions can be measured. The FLCI is short, easy to administer, has high test-retest reliability, and differentiates among moderate, moderately severe, severe, and very severe patients in terms of functional communication. Together with the FAST, the

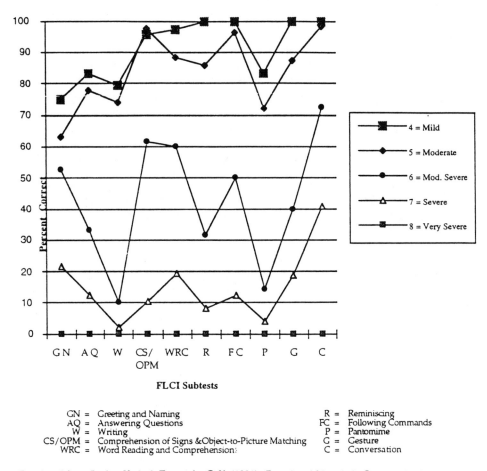

FLCI Subtests

GN	=	Greeting and Naming		R	=	Reminiscing
AQ	=	Answering Questions		FC	=	Following Commands
W	=	Writing		P	=	Pantomime
CS/OPM	=	Comprehension of Signs &Object-to-Picture Matching		G	=	Gesture
WRC	=	Word Reading and Comprehension:		C	=	Conversation

Reprinted from Bayles, K. A. & Tomoeda, C. K. (1994). <u>Functional Linguistic Communication Inventory</u>. Tucson: Canyonlands Publishing, with permission. Copyright 1994 by Canyonlands Publishing, Inc.

Figure 2.1 Performance by severity level of standardization study subjects on FLCI subtests.

FLCI gives the clinician a comprehensive picture of the capacities and limitations of the patient.

Weaknesses. To date, the test has only been administered to a small sample of American, White, AD patients. Lacking are performance data for individuals from other cultural or ethnic groups, and for those who have a different origin associated with their advanced dementia.

Severe Impairment Battery

The purpose of the SIB is to assess severely demented individuals who are unable to complete conventional neuropsychological tests. Authored by Saxton, McGonigle-Gibson, Swihart, Miller, and Boller (1990), the SIB comprises 57 questions that divide

TABLE 2.7 Mean Scores and Standard Deviations for FLCI Subtests and Total FLCI Scores of Standardization Study Subjects Subcategorized According to Severity

FLCI Subtests	Total Score Possible	Significant Intergroup Difference*	Modified FAST Stage				
			4	5	6	7	8
Greeting & Naming	15	c,e,f	11.25	9.50	7.90	3.25	0.00
			(2.6)	(1.7)	(3.0)	(2.3)	(0.0)
Question Answering	12	b,c,d,e,f	10.00	9.36	4.00	1.50	0.00
			(1.2)	(1.5)	(2.0)	(2.1)	(0.0)
Writing	11	b,c,d,e	8.75	8.14	1.10	0.25	0.00
			(0.5)	(2.7)	(1.9)	(0.5)	(0.0)
Comprehension of Signs & Object-to-PictureMatching	6	b,c,d,e,f	5.75 (0.5)	5.86 (0.4)	3.70 (1.6)	0.63 (0.9)	0.00 (0.0)
Word Reading & Comprehension	18	b,c,d,e,f	17.50 (0.6)	15.93 (1.9)	10.80 (2.9)	3.50 (3.3)	0.00 (0-0)
Reminiscing	6	b,c,d,e	6.00	5.14	1.90	0.50	0.00
			(0.0)	(1.1)	(1.7)	(1.1)	(0.0)
Following Commands	2	b,c,d,e,f	2.00	1.93	1.00	0.25	0.00
			(0.0)	(0.3)	(0.8)	(0.5)	(0.0)
Pantomime	9	b,c,d,e	7.50	6.50	1.30	0.38	0.00
			(1.7)	(1.4)	(1.5)	(1.1)	(0.0)
Gesture	4	b,c,d,e	4.00	3.50	1.60	0.75	0.00
			(0.0)	(1.1)	(1.8)	(1.0)	(0.0)
Conversation	4	c,d,e,f	4.00	3.93	2.90	1.63	0.00
			(0.0)	(0.3)	(0.7)	(1.1)	(0.0)
TOTAL SCORE	87	b,c,d,e,f	76.75	69.79	36.20	12.63	0.00
			(5.4)	(7.2)	(9.0)	(8.1)	(0.0)

* Schéffe test with significance level ≤ .05

a = GDS 4 vs. GDS 5	c = GDS 4 vs. GDS 7	e = GDS 5 vs. GDS 7
b = GDS 4 vs. GDS 6	d = GDS 5 vs. GDS 6	f = GDS 6 vs. GDS 7

Reprinted from Bayles, K. A. & Tomoeda, C. K. (1994). *Functional Linguistic Communication Inventory.* Tucson: Canyonlands Publishing, with permission. Copyright 1994 by Canyonlands Publishing, Inc.

into nine subscales: Language, Attention, Orientation, Memory, Praxis, Visuospatial Perception, Construction, Social Skills, and Orienting the Head to Name. Possible scores range from 0 to 152, and credit is given to nonverbal and partially correct answers. Items take the form of one-stage commands and are presented together with gestural cues. They can be repeated to facilitate comprehension. Forty-six of the points can be earned on questions that assess language functions, such as ability to write and copy one's name, repeat, read, and converse. Several items relate to color naming and responsive naming, for example, "What do you call the thing you drink coffee from?"

The SIB was standardized on 41 dementia patients: 31 met the NINCDS-ADRDA criteria for probable and 9 for possible AD. One individual met the criteria for multi-infarct dementia. The mean age of subjects was 72 years, with an average of 11.6 years of education and mean disease duration of 5.7 years. The socioeconomic status of subjects varied. The median annual income of 9 of the subjects was less than $9,000;

10 of the subjects had incomes between \$10,000 and 19,999; 11 subjects had median annual incomes between \$20,000 and 29,999; and 4 had incomes exceeding \$30,000.

All subjects were given a neurological, psychiatric, and physical examination including computed tomographic scans and electroencephalographic recordings. Laboratory studies were used to rule out other conditions that could cause altered mental status. The MMSE scores of standardization subjects ranged from 0 to 13. The subject group was divided into individuals whose MMSE score fell between 0 and 4 and those with MMSE scores between 5 and 9, and correlations of SIB and MMSE scores were calculated. MMSE and SIB scores were not significantly correlated for the more severe group (.20), likely because these subjects' SIB scores ranged from 15 to 114. A significant correlation was obtained for those subjects whose MMSE scores ranged from 5 to 9 (.68; $p < .01$). Information was not provided about the range of SIB scores for the higher scoring subjects.

Reliability. Interrater reliability was shown with high correlation coefficients and low mean score discrepancies. High test-retest reliability also was obtained for a retest interval that averaged 14.3 days. A correlation coefficient of r = .85 ($p < .001$) was obtained for overall score, indicating stability in test performance over time. However, when test-retest correlations were calculated for the individual subscales, Orientation and Construction did not reach significance.

Validity. To show the construct validity of the SIB, the authors correlated performance of the standardization subjects on the SIB to performance on the MMSE. The obtained correlation coefficient was $r = .74$ ($p < .001$).

In 1994, Panisset and colleagues administered the SIB to 69 patients who met the DSM-III criteria for dementia and the NINCDS-ADRDA criteria for AD. Their mean age was 92.9 years, and the mean MMSE score was 10.7 ($SD = 6.14$). Patients were separated into four severity groups according to MMSE scores: 0 to 5, 6 to 11, 12 to 17, and greater than 17. The two lowest MMSE scoring groups were significantly different in their scores on the SIB; however, no SIB differences were found among the subgroups with MMSE scores of 6 to 11, 12 to 17, and greater than 17. Fifteen AD patients whose MMSE scores were less than 6 had SIB scores that ranged from 7 to 81. These researchers concluded that the SIB is more appropriate for AD patients with MMSE scores of less than 12 and that it loses power for higher functioning patients.

The most difficult questions were identified as related to orientation, praxis, and memory. The SIB separates language according to type of stimuli—that is, verbal compared with written—and according to the functions of fluency, naming, comprehension, and repetition.

Strengths. The SIB elicits a range of performance on language and eight other functions in advanced dementia patients. Examiners can obtain a sense of what cognitive functions are particularly impaired and spared. Because the battery evaluates a variety of cognitive functions, performance on the SIB can readily be compared with results of other neuropsychological testing.

Limitations. The SIB is not primarily a test of communicative abilities, and of the questions related to language function, most relate to naming. Certain of the "language" items are of questionable usefulness in assessing language—namely, those in which examinees are asked to name the color of objects and their shape. The standardization sample was relatively small and heterogeneous in terms of origin. Information has yet to be obtained on the performance of patients of different ethnicity. In addition, because the SIB subscales are not equated for difficulty level, it is difficult to make intersubscale comparisons. Finally, the range of SIB scores was large for subjects whose MMSE scores were between 0 and 4.

OTHER COMMUNICATION MEASURES FREQUENTLY ADMINISTERED TO DEMENTIA PATIENTS

Naming Tests

Both confrontation and generative naming tests have been administered to dementia patients. Generative naming, also called verbal fluency, has been assessed by letter and semantic category fluency tests. The most often used confrontation naming test is the Boston (Kaplan, Goodglass, & Weintraub, 1983). The most common letter category naming test is the FAS test, developed by Borkowski, Benton, and Spreen (1967); the most common semantic categories are animals, vegetables, and fruits.

Boston Naming Test (BNT)

Stimuli consist of line drawings of objects that the patient is asked to name. The 60-item version of the BNT is the one most frequently given to dementia patients. Normative data for normal elders provided in the test manual are scanty but other investigators have conducted normative studies. Van Gorp, Satz, Kiersch, and Henry (1986) administered the 60-item version to 78 normal older adults who ranged in age from 59 to 95. Results indicated that confrontation naming declines modestly with age and that performance variability increases. The correlation coefficient obtained between test performance and age was $r = -.33$. The investigators did note that individuals in their sample were well educated and intelligent.

The 85-item experimental version, the 60-item version, and a smaller 15-item version all have been given to AD patients. Huff and colleagues (1986) divided the 85-item version into two forms that correlated in the .71 to .82 range for normal elders and .97 for AD patients. The AD patients' scores were significantly inferior to those of normal subjects. Even the short 15-item form has been found to be sensitive to the presence and severity of dementia (Morris et al., 1989).

Generally, confrontation naming diminishes in proportion to severity of dementia (Martin & Fedio, 1983), and a floor effect in the performance of dementia patients is not present until late in the disease. Some data regarding the naming performance of late-stage patients are available from the standardization study of the FLCI, which has a short, 9-item, confrontation-naming test. The mean performance of GDS-FAST 6a to 6d patients in the standardization study was 1.89 ($SD = 2.2$) out of a possible 9, and .53 ($SD = 1.2$) for 6e through 7c patients.

FAS Test of Verbal Fluency

The FAS test also is known as the Controlled Oral Word Association test and is part of the Neurosensory Center Comprehensive Examination for Aphasia (Benton & Hamsher, 1989). In this test, examinees are asked to generate as many words as possible that begin with the letters, F, A, and S, respectively. They are instructed not to give proper names and numbers. D'Elia, Boone, and Mitrushina (1995) have compiled the norms for this test. When the data from several studies are reviewed, performance variability can be seen to be greater in less well educated individuals. For those normals whose education equals or exceeds 13 years, the mean scores hold well until the mid-70s when they decline. The reliability of the test is high. Snow and colleagues (1988) obtained a reliability coefficient of .70 and .71 for *F* and *S* after one year; however, the coefficient for A was lower.

Many investigators have administered this test or part of it to AD patients, and all have reported their significantly inferior performance compared with normal subjects (Appell, Kertesz, & Fisman, 1982; Bayles, Trosset, Tomoeda, Montgomery, & Wilson, 1993; Becker, Huff, Nebes, Holland, & Boller, 1988; Monsch et al., 1992). Additionally, performance of moderately demented AD patients is significantly inferior to that of mildly demented patients (Bayles, Boone, Tomoeda, Slauson, & Kaszniak, 1989; Martin & Fedio, 1983; Shuttleworth & Huber, 1988). Severely demented patients (GDS-FAST 6a to 7f) are likely to vary in their capacity to respond on this test. Many will score 0; others may produce a few exemplars across the three stimuli. GDS-FAST 7a to 7e patients typically are unable to perform this task.

Semantic Category Naming

Semantic category naming is another type of generative naming test. Examinees are asked to name as many exemplars from a category as possible within one minute. The semantic categories most used are animals, fruits, and vegetables.

Like letter category naming, semantic category naming is very sensitive to mild dementia and is useful for staging dementia until the advanced stage. Semantic category naming performance can be expected to be similar to performance on letter category naming (Bayles, Tomoeda, Kaszniak, & Trosset, 1991), although for some individuals, naming words is easier than category items. Overall, the cognitive demands of both types of generative naming are similar. Monsch and colleagues (1992) observed that when comparing the performance of AD patients with normal control subjects, the sensitivity and specificity of semantic category naming is better than for letter category naming. In a recent study by Azuma and colleagues (1996), performance on generative naming tasks was found to be dependent on the particular categories used. Certain semantic categories were easier than certain letter categories but more difficult than others. These authors concluded that the relative difficulty of fluency tasks must be calculated before conclusions are drawn about the performance of a clinical sample.

Strengths and Limitations of Naming Tests

Both confrontation and generative naming tests are sensitive to dementia. Performance of patients on the tests generally reflects the degree of dementia severity through GDS-FAST stage 6. Both types of tests are short and easily administered. An argument that some clinicians might make regarding confrontation naming is that it does not test "functional" naming—for example, the ability to name people and items of personal relevance to the examinee. A similar argument might be made about the generative naming test in that individuals rarely have to perform the function of naming exemplars in a category. However, the fact that these tests are not functionally oriented does not deny their usefulness for identifying the adverse effect of dementing diseases on the naming and generative skills that underlie normal cognitive functioning nor does it deny the high association between test performance and day-to-day functioning.

VOCABULARY TESTS

Two well-known vocabulary tests have been given to dementia patients, the Vocabulary Subtest of the WAIS-R (Wechsler, 1955, 1981) and the Peabody Picture Vocabulary Test—Revised (PPVT-R) (Dunn & Dunn, 1981).

Vocabulary Subtest of the WAIS-R

This WAIS-R subtest consists of 40 words and takes approximately 20 minutes to administer. The examiner asks, "What does ___ mean?" The test can be discontinued if the examinee misses five consecutive words. One or 2 points are given for each correct definition depending on the accuracy, precision, and aptness of the response.

Scores on this test are highest for adults in middle age, after which a slow decline is observed in the sixth and seventh decades (Wechsler, 1955, 1981). More influential than age on performance is education (Kaufman, Reynolds, & McLean, 1989; Malec, Ivnik, Smith, & Tangalos, 1992). Gender has little, if any, effect. Test-retest correlation coefficients generally range between .78 and .84 (Ryan, Georgemiller, Geisser, & Randall, 1985). Split-half correlations for the various age groups for both forms of the Vocabulary test are high, approximately .95 (Wechsler, 1955, 1981). As might be expected, performance on Vocabulary is highly correlated with performance on the three other verbal tests in the WAIS-R battery, specifically, Information, Comprehension, and Similarities.

Sullivan and colleagues (1989) reported that performance on Vocabulary holds well in early dementia but nonetheless declines (Crawford, 1989). The quality of responses deteriorates as a function of the severity of dementia with answers becoming less precise. Individuals in GDS-FAST stage 6 averaged raw scores of 3, and most more advanced patients were unable to do the task.

Peabody Picture Vocabulary Test–Revised

Vocabulary is an expressive vocabulary test, whereas the PPVT-R is a receptive vocabulary test. It was originally published in 1965 (Dunn, 1965) and comprised 150 items. In 1981, it was revised and contains 175 items. Examinees must point to or give the number of the picture associated with the word spoken by the examiner. There are two equivalent forms. The examiner begins the test at the level appropriate for the subject to ensure that the basal (the highest six consecutive responses) and ceiling (six failures out of eight) scores are achieved without undue effort. Each correct item is given a point, and the total score can be converted to a standard score, percentile rank, stanine, and age equivalent score.

The standardization sample for the original version was 4,012 individuals who ranged in age from 2 to 18 years. The standardization sample for the PPVT-R was 4,200 subjects, of whom 828 were adults between the ages of 19 to 40 years. These individuals were selected from different regions in the United States and represented different occupations. Split-half reliability for the adult group, using the L form only, was .82 (Dunn & Dunn, 1981; Robertson & Eisenberg, 1981). For elderly individuals ranging in age from 60 to 100 years, correlations with WAIS-R Vocabulary were .85 for men and .95 for women (Levine, 1971). Maxwell and Wise (1984) used partial correlation and multiple regression procedures to evaluate the validity of the PPVT as a measure of intelligence and concluded it was valid only as a measure of adult vocabulary.

In a study by Bayles and colleagues (1989), the original form of the PPVT was administered to 21 mild and 37 moderately impaired AD patients, 16 nonfluent aphasia patients, 25 fluent aphasia patients, and 31 normal elders. Both groups of AD patients performed at a level significantly inferior to that of the normal control subjects; the mean score for mild AD subjects was 107.6 (*SD* = 22.09), whereas the mean score for moderate AD subjects was 75.31 (*SD* = 38.65). Variability in performance increased with dementia severity. A significant difference was not observed between the performance of mild AD and aphasia patients (the mean score for nonfluent aphasia patients was 112 (*SD* = 23.0) and 118.8 (*SD* = 25) for fluent aphasia patients). Moderate AD patients were, however, significantly inferior in performance to both groups of aphasia patients. The scores of moderate patients ranged from 1 to 136. Although performance data of GDS-FAST stage 7 subjects on this test are meager, a floor effect in performance can be expected. Also, PPVT performance can reasonably be expected to be inferior to WAIS Vocabulary subtest performance in late-stage patients because the visual perceptual deficits experienced by AD patients will impede review of the four line drawings that must be reviewed for each stimulus item.

MEASURES OF GENERAL LANGUAGE

Two language batteries have been administered to dementia patients, the Western Aphasia Battery (WAB) (Kertesz, 1982) and Community Activities of Daily Living Test (CADL) (Holland, 1980).

Western Aphasia Battery

This battery, generally referred to as the WAB, is modeled after the Boston Diagnostic Aphasia Examination (Goodglass & Kaplan, 1983) and evaluates content, fluency, auditory comprehension, repetition, naming, reading, writing, and calculation. Additionally, the nonverbal skills of drawing, block design, and praxis are tested. A primary purpose of the test is to classify aphasic patients according to their pattern of language dysfunction (Kertesz & Poole, 1974). The four oral language subtests scores are used to produce a value called the "aphasia quotient" (AQ), scores from the nonverbal tests combine to form a "performance quotient," and the aphasia quotient and performance quotient combine to form the "cortical quotient."

In the original standardization study, 150 consecutively examined aphasic patients and 59 normal control subjects were tested (Kertesz, 1982). Patients were admitted to the study if they were considered by a physician or speech pathologist to be aphasic.

Validity and Reliability. The concurrent validity of the WAB was shown by comparing performance on it to performance on the Neurosensory Center Comprehensive Examination for Aphasia (Spreen & Benton, 1977). Kertesz correlated the performance of 20 patients who were tested 1 to 16 days apart on the experimental and commercial versions. The coefficients between the language factors ranged from .85 to .99. The test-retest reliability with a 1-year interval was high (>.90).

In a later study, the WAB was administered to 25 hospitalized AD patients (mean age = 76 years) and a control population of stroke patients (Appell, Kertesz, & Fisman, 1982). The performance of these AD subjects was compared with that of the 21 nonbrain-damaged control subjects from the WAB standardization study. All AD patients were classified as aphasic to some degree, and all speech-language functions were reported to be impaired. The subtest on which AD subjects scored the highest was Word Fluency followed by Repetition, Comprehension, Information, and Naming. Of the four Naming subtests, sentence completion and responsive speech were easiest. When compared with normal subjects, all differences in oral language abilities were significant. The typical milder AD patient had a pattern of retained fluency and articulation, and diminished naming and comprehension. Compared with stroke patients with aphasia, the significant differences were the higher fluency of AD patients and the better comprehension of stroke patients even though the subject groups were matched for AQ. Unfortunately, the severity of dementia of the AD subjects was not described by Kertesz and colleagues, making it difficult to define the relation of dementia severity to test performance. All the subjects were hospitalized, the average length being 13 months, with a range from 1 to 50 months. Kertesz, Appell, and Fisman (1982) followed 20 of the 25 hospitalized AD patients in their 1982 study and 9 others for a year retesting them with the WAB. Their language functioning deteriorated, and a floor effect was observed on the word fluency subtest. Performance on the repetition and yes/no comprehension sections, which were less impaired at the first test time, declined and brought the aphasia quotient down significantly. Also, declines in performance on the nonverbal subtest of construction and calculation were significant.

Communicative Activities of Daily Living

This test, better known as the CADL, involves subjects in role playing as a means to assessing their abilities to manage activities of daily living. Commonly occurring situations are simulated, such as going to the doctor, or shopping for groceries. Like the examinee, the examiner must play a role. Responses are scored on a 3-point scale according to the degree of their communicative effectiveness. A score of 2 indicates satisfactory communication, and a score of 1 is given when the examinee's responses relate to the topic but do not impart the appropriate meaning. There are 68 items that sample 10 categories of behavior.

The test originally was standardized on 130 aphasic subjects and did differentiate among patients with the major types of aphasia. Performance on the CADL was found to be sensitive to age, but not sex or social background.

Fromm and Holland (1989) reported results of an investigation of the performance of 48 AD patients on the CADL whose performance was compared with that of 26 normal elders, 26 Wernicke's aphasia patients, and 15 depressed elders. Mild and moderate AD subjects were significantly impaired on the CADL, and moderately demented AD patients were more impaired than were their mildly demented counterparts. Mild dementia was defined by a score of 20 to 26 on the MMSE and moderate by a score of 13 to 19. The mean proportion correct for the different test categories was calculated, and for moderate AD subjects, they ranged from a low of .57 for sequential relations to a high of .83 for social convention. Clearly, no floor effect was present among moderate patients; performance data for severe patients were not provided. Best preserved were automatic, overlearned communication acts, such as social conventions and speech acts. More affected were tasks that required effortful cognitive processing, such as divergencies, using context, reading, calculating, and sequential relations.

STATE OF THE ART

Clinicians have numerous measures with proven reliability and validity with which to screen and comprehensively document the communicative functioning of dementia patients. Even though a substantive body of data exists on the performance of AD patients, little is known about the performance of other types of dementia patients on these measures. The clinical utility of the measures that were reviewed in this chapter would be increased with information about their suitability for different cultural groups, individuals with different levels of education, and individuals with low socioeconomic status. Most performance data have been gathered on individuals who are White, relatively well educated, and middle class. Data have yet to be provided about how performance on these measures predicts the responsiveness of dementia patients to various types of therapeutic interventions.

REFERENCES

Allen, M. J., & Yen, W. M. (1979). *Introduction to measurement theory.* Monterey, CA: Brooks/Cole.

American Psychiatric Association. (1994). *Diagnostic and statistical manual of mental disorders* (4th ed.). Washington, DC: Author.

Appell, J., Kertesz, A., & Fisman, M. (1982). A study of language functioning in Alzheimer's patients. *Brain and Language, 17,* 73-91.

Armstrong, L., Bayles, K. A., Borthwick, S. E., & Tomoeda, C. K. (1996). Use of the Arizona Battery for Communication Disorders of Dementia in the U.K. *European Journal of Disorders of Communication, 31,* 171-180.

Azuma, T., Bayles, K. A., Cruz, R. F., Tomoeda, C. K., Wood, J. A. McGeagh, A., & Montgomery, E. B. (1996). *Comparing the relative difficulty of letter, semantic, and name fluency tasks for normal elderly and Parkinson's patients.* Manuscript under revision.

Bayles, K. A., Boone, D. R., Tomoeda, C. K., Slauson, T. J., & Kaszniak, A. W. (1989). Differentiating Alzheimer's patients from the normal elderly and stroke patients with aphasia. *Journal of Speech and Hearing Disorders, 54,* 74-87.

Bayles, K. A., & Tomoeda, C. K. (1993). *The Arizona Battery for Communication Disorders.* Tucson: Canyonlands.

Bayles, K. A., & Tomoeda, C. K. (1994). *The Functional Linguistic Communication Inventory.* Tucson: Canyonlands.

Bayles, K. A., Tomoeda, C. K., Kaszniak, A. W., & Trosset, M. W. (1991). Alzheimer's disease effects on semantic memory: Loss of structure or impaired processing. *Journal of Cognitive Neuroscience, 3,* 166-182.

Bayles, K. A., Tomoeda, C. K., Wood, J. A., Cruz, R. F., & McGeagh, A. (1996). Comparison of sensitivity to Alzheimer's dementia of the ABCD and other measures. *Journal of Medical Speech Language Pathology, 4,* 183-194.

Bayles, K. A., Trosset, M. W., Tomoeda, C. K., Montgomery, E. B., & Wilson, J. (1993). Generative naming in Parkinson Disease patients. *Journal of Clinical and Experimental Neuropsychology, 15,* 547-562.

Becker, J. T., Huff, F. J., Nebes, R. D., Holland, A., & Boller, F. (1988). Neuropsychological function in Alzheimer's disease: Pattern of impairment and rates of progression. *Archives of Neurology, 45,* 263-268.

Benton, A. L., & Hamsher, K. S. (1989). *Multilingual Aphasia Examination.* Iowa City: AJA Associates.

Borkowski, J. G., Benton, A. L., & Spreen, O. (1967). Word fluency and brain damage. *Neuropsychologia, 5,* 135-140.

Crawford, J. R. (1989). Estimation of premorbid intelligence: A review of recent developments. In J. R. Crawford & D. M. Parker (Eds.), *Developments in clinical and experimental neuropsychology.* New York: Plenum.

D'Elia, L., Boone, K., & Mitrushina, A. (1995). *Handbook of normative data for neuropsychological assessment.* New York: Oxford University Press.

Dunn, L. M. (1965). *Peabody Picture Vocabulary Test.* Circle Pines, MN: American Guidance Service.

Dunn, L. M., & Dunn, L. M. (1981). *Peabody Picture Vocabulary Test–Revised.* Circle Pines, MN: American Guidance Service.

Folstein, M., Folstein, S., & McHugh, P. (1975). "Mini-Mental State": A practical method for grading the cognitive state of patients for the clinician. *Journal of Psychiatric Research, 12,* 189-198.

Fromm, D., & Holland, A. (1989). Functional communication in Alzheimer's disease. *Journal of Speech and Hearing Disorders, 54,* 535-540.

Goodglass, H., & Kaplan, E. (1983). *Boston Diagnostic Aphasia Examination (BDAE).* Malvern, PA: Lea & Febiger.

Grant, D. A., & Berg, E. A. (1948). A behavioral analysis of degree of reinforcement and ease of shifting to new responses in a Weigl-type card sorting problem. *Journal of Experimental Psychology, 38,* 404-411.

Hamilton, M. (1967). Development of a rating scale for primary depressive illness. *British Journal of Social and Clinical Psychology, 6,* 278-296.

Holland, A. (1980). *Communicative abilities in daily living.* Austin: Pro-Ed.

Huff, J., Collins, C., Corkin, S., & Rosen, T. (1986). Equivalent forms of the Boston Naming Test. *Journal of Clinical and Experimental Neuropsychology, 8,* 556-562.

Jenkins, R. L., & Parsons, O. A. (1978). Cognitive deficits in male alcoholics as measured by a modified Wisconsin Card Sorting Test. *Alcohol Technical Reports, 7,* 76-83.

Kaplan, E., Goodglass, H., & Weintraub, S. (1983). *The Boston Naming Test* (2nd ed.). Malvern, PA: Lea & Febiger.

Kaufman, A., Reynolds, C., & McLean, J. (1989). Age and WAIS-R intelligence in a national sample of adults in the 20 to 74-year age range: A cross-sectional analysis with educational level controlled. *Intelligence, 13,* 235-253.

Kertesz, A. (1982). *Western Aphasia Battery.* New York: Grune & Stratton.

Kertesz, A., & Poole, E. (1974). The aphasia quotient: The taxonomic approach to measurement of aphasic disability. *Canadian Journal of Neurosciences, 1,* 7-16.

Lazarus, L. W., Newton, N., Cohler, B., Lesser, J., & Schweon, C. (1987). Frequency and presentation of depressive symptoms in patients with primary degenerative dementia. *American Journal of Psychiatry, 144,* 41-45.

Levine, N. R. (1971). Validation of the Quick Test for intelligence screening of the elderly. *Psychological Reports, 29,* 167-172.

Malec, J. F., Ivnik, R. J., Smith, G. E., & Tangalos, E. G. (1992). Mayo's older American normative studies: Utility of corrections for age and education for the WAIS-R. *The Clinical Neuropsychologist, 6* (Suppl.), 31-47.

Martin, A., & Fedio, P. (1983). Word production and comprehension in Alzheimer's disease: The breakdown of semantic knowledge. *Brain and Language, 19*, 124-141.

Maxwell, J., & Wise, F. (1984). PPVT IQ validity in adults: A measure of vocabulary, not of intelligence. *Journal of Clinical Psychology, 40*, 1048-1053.

McKhann, G., Drachman, D., Folstein, M., Katzman, R., Price, D., & Stadlan, E. (1984). Clinical diagnosis of Alzheimer's disease: Report of the NINCDS-ADRDA work group under the auspices of the Department of Health and Human Services task force on Alzheimer's disease. *Neurology, 7*, 486-488.

Monsch, A., Bondi, M., Butters, N., Salmon, D., Katzman, & Thal, L. (1992). Comparisons of verbal fluency tasks in the detection of dementia of the Alzheimer's type. *Archives of Neurology, 49*, 1253-1258.

Morris, J. C., Heyman, A., Mohs, R. C., Hughes, J. P., van Belle, G., Fillenbaum, G., Mellits, E. D., Clark, C., & the CERAD Investigators (1989). The Consortium to Establish a Registry for Alzheimer's Disease (CERAD): 1. Clinical and neuropsychological assessment of Alzheimer's disease. *Neurology, 39*, 1159-1165.

Nelson, H. E. (1976). A modified card sorting test sensitive to frontal lobe defects. *Cortex, 12*, 313-324.

Panisset, M., Roudier, M., Saxton, J., & Boller, F. (1994). Severe Impairment Battery: A neuropsychological test for severely demented patients. *Archives of Neurology, 5*, 41-45.

Reisberg, B., Ferris, S. H., de Leon, & Crook, T. (1982). Signs, symptoms, and course of age associated with cognitive decline. In S. Corkin et al. (Eds.), *Alzheimer's disease: A report of progress: Vol. 19. Aging.* New York: Raven .

Reisberg, B., Ferris, S. H., & Franssen, E. (1985). An ordinal functional assessment tool for Alzheimer's-type dementia. *Hospital and Community Psychiatry, 36*, 593-595.

Robertson, G. J., & Eisenberg, J. L. (1981). *Peabody Picture Vocabulary Test–Revised: Technical supplement.* Circle Pines, MN: American Guidance Service.

Rosen, W. G., Terry, R. D., Fuld, P. A., Katzman, R., & Peck, A. (1980). Pathological verification of ischemic score in differentiation of dementias. *Annals of Neurology, 7*, 486-488.

Ryan, J. J., Georgemiller, R. J., Geisser, M. E., & Randall, D. M. (1985). Test-retest stability of the WAIS-R in a clinical sample. *Journal of Clinical Psychology, 41*, 552-556.

Saxton, J., McGonigle-Gibson, K., Swihart, A., Miller, M., & Boller, F. (1990). Assessment of the severely impaired patient: Description and validation of a new neuropsychological test battery. *Psychological Assessment, 2*, 298-303.

Shuttleworth, E., & Huber, S. (1988). The naming disorder of dementia of the Alzheimer's type. *Brain and language, 34*, 222-234.

Snow, W., Tierney, M., & Zorzitto, M. (1988). One-year test-retest of selected neuropsychological tests in older adults. *Journal of Clinical and Experimental Neuropsychology, 10*, 60.

Spreen, O., & Benton, A. L. (1977). *Neurosensory Center Comprehensive Examination for Aphasia.* Victoria, BC: University of Victoria Neuropsychology Laboratory.

Sullivan, E. V., Sagar, H. J., Gabrieli, J. D. E., Corkin, S., & Growdon, J. H. (1989). Different cognitive profiles on standard behavioral tests in Parkinson's disease and Alzheimer's disease. *Journal of Clinical and Experimental Neuropsychology, 11,* 799-820.

Van Gorp, W., Satz, P., Kiersch, M., & Henry, R. (1986). Normative data on the Boston Naming Test for a group of normal older adults. *Journal of Clinical and Experimental Neuropsychology, 8,* 702-705.

Wechsler, D. (1955). *Wechsler Adult Intelligence Scale.* New York: Psychological Corporation.

Wechsler, D. (1981). *Wechsler Adult Intelligence Scale–Revised manual.* New York: Psychological Corporation.

Wilson, R., Rosenbaum, G., Brown, G., Rourke, D., & Whitman, D. (1978). An index of premorbid intelligence. *Journal of Consulting and Clinical Psychology, 46,* 1554-1555.

Chapter 3

Vision and Vision Assessment

Alan R. Morse and Bruce P. Rosenthal

How we see and what that means is an area of profound inquiry. Seeing requires complex interaction and integration of myriad factors, which, together, create an approximation of the reality of our world. Indeed, there is no way to know with certainty that any two people looking at the same thing, in fact *see* the same thing. Although much about visual perception is objective, there always remains a level of subjectivity both about the actual perception, which, indeed, might be physiologically assessed, for example, and its importance in our understanding of our world, which cannot be so finely measured. Moreover, the role of the various components of perception that contribute to vision may vary widely from one individual to another. At the very least, when we talk about vision we need to consider acuity, contrast sensitivity, visual fields and color, including considerations of spectral sensitivity, hue preference, and wavelength discrimination. A thorough discussion of vision also must address and differentiate among sensory, perceptual, and cognitive aspects of vision, recognizing that each influences the other. Although a detailed understanding of the mechanisms of perception and vision are beyond the scope of this article, a basic understanding of the visual system is necessary to understand procedures for screening and evaluation of visual functioning and their limitations.

Vision begins with light entering the eye through the cornea. The cornea and the lens together are the equivalent of a camera lens—their purpose is to focus the entering rays of light on the retina, the *film* of the eye. Focusing is accomplished by changing the shape of the lens through opposing pairs of muscles. The pupil size, which controls the amount of light entering the eye, is also changed by opposing muscle pairs. These mechanical structures all have the purpose of delivering to the retina a clear, properly intense, and focused image for further processing.

At the time the image is received by the retina, no vision has yet occurred, because the signal (the image), has not yet been processed. The retina, which is a part of the brain and connected directly to it by the optic nerve, contains two basic types of cells: *rods*, the most frequent retinal cell, provides the ability to see in dim light and provides coarse vision, and *cones,* which, although less numerous, account for the ability to distinguish colors and see fine detail. The retinal area that provides the greatest visual detail is the central portion, the *fovea,* which is completely devoid of rods. Information from the retinal receptors, the rods and cones, is organized into two distinct streams—the *magnocellular* (m-cell), which relates to visual events of high temporal frequency, such as motion perception, and the *parvocellular* (p-cell), which emphasizes color and fine optical discrimination, and passes through the optic nerve, to the *optic chiasm,* where the nerve fibers from each retina come together, are sorted into left and right visual fields and distributed to the *lateral geniculate nucleus* (LGN). Each LGN receives input from both eyes, but only one half of the visual field—the left LGN receiving right field images and the left LGN receiving images of the right visual field. From the LGN the sorted signals are passed on into the *visual,* or *striate, cortex* of the brain (Wandell, 1995). The information is processed, and vision has occurred. Note that vision has not occurred until the information has been processed. The processing of visual information is, in fact, much more complex. The reliance on multiple cell types in intricate layers with highly differentiated functions transmitting their information along highly specialized channels begins to give us an understanding of why vision is so fragile and susceptible to disturbance, from normal events as well as from pathological processes (Hubel, 1988) (Figure 3.1).

VISION CHANGES ASSOCIATED WITH AGING

The prevalence of visual disability increases with increasing age. The risk of legal blindness—20/200 in the best eye with correction, or visual fields of 20 degrees or less—is nearly 10 times greater for those older than age 65 than for those who are younger (Pizarello, 1987). The four major causes of vision loss—cataracts, glaucoma, macular degeneration, and diabetic retinopathy—all increase in prevalence with aging (Morse & Friedman, 1986). The most common condition associated with aging is a change in the integrity of the crystalline lens of the eye, commonly referred to as cataracts. The lens also yellows, increasing the need for blue light to compensate for increased absorption of that portion of the spectrum (Morse, 1982). There is also a significant increase in the prevalence of glaucoma with advancing age as well as other pathological conditions that may contribute to decreased vision in the elderly including persons in nursing homes. In addition, hypertensive retinopathy, optic atrophy, as well as visual loss or disturbance resulting from cerebral vascular, or transient ischemic, accidents all increase in prevalence with aging. Not surprisingly, the prevalence of corrective lens use increases with aging as well, so that by age 75, almost 95% of the population requires some optical correction to maintain visual function (National Center for Health Statistics, 1978), and more than 25% of the population older than age 85 has severe visual impairment (Nelson, 1987), defined as inability to read newsprint even when wearing corrective lenses. For such patients, therefore, optical correction to near normal vision is not possible. They have vision of less than 20/70 in the best eye with correction and are considered to have *low vision* (Faye, 1994), and present special challenges in both evaluation and work to maximize their usable vision. When measuring visual function we are, in fact, addressing one or more of the individual components that constitute vision. Some of the more common and useful measures are discussed subsequently.

VISUAL ACUITY

Acuity is the most common measure of vision and is a universally accepted longitudinal method of measuring changes in vision. For most patients, acuity is the single most important measure of visual function. Visual acuity is a measurement of the resolution capability of the eye, and with aging, there is a significant difference in acuity as the

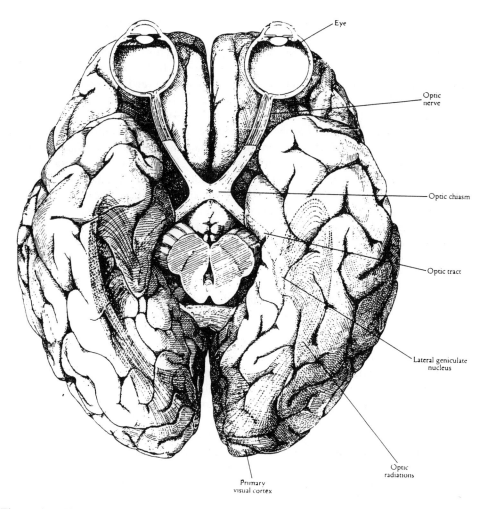

Figure 3.1 The visual pathway, from eyes to primary visual cortex, of a human brain, as seen from below. Information comes to the right halves of the retinas (because the brain is seen upside down) from the opposite half of the environment (the left visual field) and ends up in the right half of the brain. This happens because about half the optic-nerve fibers cross at the chasm, and the rest stay uncrossed. Hence the rules: each hemisphere gets input from both eyes; a given hemisphere gets information from the opposite half of the visual world.

From David H. Hubel (1987). *Eye, Brain, and Vision.* New York: WH Freeman. Copyright © 1988 by Scientific American Library. Reprinted with permission.

target moves from near to distant. Therefore, particularly with older patients, it is important to assess acuity at both near distances, such as those used for reading, and at distances other than for reading. The modern method for measuring resolution capability was first developed by Herman Snellen in 1862 (Johnston, 1991; Newell, 1969). Snellen's recognition system, which is still in use and universally employed in testing visual acuity, requires that letters, numbers, or other shapes must be identified correctly. Snellen's acuity method is also noteworthy because it is based on the concept of the eye being able to resolve detail subtending a minimum angle of resolution (MAR) of 1 minute of arc (1' or 1/60°). The English astronomer Robert Hooke is credited with this concept when he proposed that two stars could be discerned as separate if the angle they subtended at the eye was 1' or greater. This value is known as the threshold angular subtense of "normal vision."

One of the most important aspects of acuity vision testing is consistency in chart construction. The actual letter used in the construction of an eye chart has an overall height of 5 minutes of arc, where each "stroke width" is one fifth of the overall symbol height (see the E later). In a clinical setting, visual acuity measurements are taken to assess and quantify the eyes' ability to resolve varying letter sizes. The resolving power of the eye is also dependent on the eyes' health and integrity (Davidson, 1991). The smallest letter, number, or picture seen on the end chart is then recorded as a fraction where the smallest size letter seen is the numerator of the fraction, and the test distance at which the optotype subtends 5' of overall height is the denominator. The Snellen fraction is recorded as follows:

Snellen acuity=test distance/distance at which optotype
would subtend 5 minutes of arc at the retina

Bailey and Lovie introduced a new concept in visual acuity chart design in 1976 (Bailey & Lovie, 1976). Their chart made use of the geometric progression of letter size and while their charts are designed in minimum angle of resolution (MAR), they noted that a geometric progression of MAR was an arithmetic progression in the logarithm of MAR—hence, the term, logMAR. The Bailey-Lovie chart is based on a progression of letter size by a factor of 1.26×, a factor proposed by others (Ogle, 1953; Westheimer, 1979). Another way of looking at this geometric progression is that each line of letters is 0.1 log units larger than the previous line. Bailey and Lovie's contribution was to ensure that the chart had letters of equal legibility, the same number of letters in each row, and uniform letter and between-row spacing. Ferris further modified the chart with Bailey, and the new NEI Ferris-Bailey chart became the standard for all research by the National Eye Institute (Ferris, Kassoff, Bresnick & Bailey, 1982), and is commonly referred to as the Early Treatment Diabetic Retinopathy Study (ETDRS) chart, in which its use became ubiquitous (Figure 3.2). Each letter on the chart is constructed on a 5 × 5 matrix and subtends 5 minutes of arc in height (each stroke width of the letter subtends 1' as described earlier) at a designated viewing distance. Five letters are placed on each line of the chart while letters are placed equally (one letter width), and lines are spaced proportionally (one letter height). Frequently the examiner will hold up fingers or wave a hand when no response is forthcoming on the visual acuity chart. In many instances, there is no response to the letters presented, perhaps because of impaired cognitive functioning. In such instances, there is no useful information known about that patient's vision.

Because of the importance of vision to patient functioning, extra efforts should be made to obtain some usable information to aid in planning for patient care. Where conventional ETDRS vision testing is not useful, other methods may be used to estimate visual acuity. Use of a pinhole aperture placed in front of the eye, when the patient is

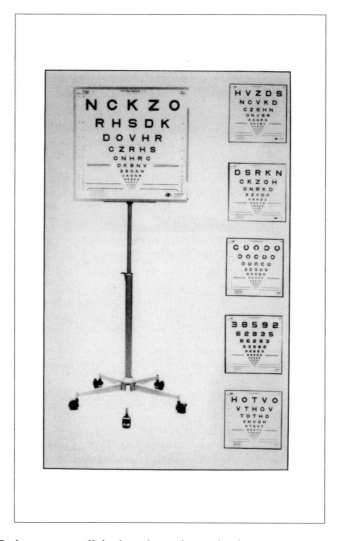

Figure 3.2 Early treatment diabetic retinopathy study chart.

unable to read beyond the 20/30 chart line, is useful in determining whether additional optical correction is useful. If, with the use of a pinhole, a patient is unable to see better, the cause may be pathology such as impaired macular function or cataracts.

Teller Acuity Cards

(Hartmann, 1996; McDonald, Ankrum, & Preston, 1986; McDonald, Dobson, & Sebris, 1985; McDonald, Sebris & Hohn, 1986). Researchers investigating visual acuity in infants found that infants prefer to fixate on high-contrast, bold stripes rather than homogeneous fields of light (Fantz, Ordy, & Udelf, 1962). This led to the development of the Teller Acuity Cards (Figure 3.3). They have been successful in testing children

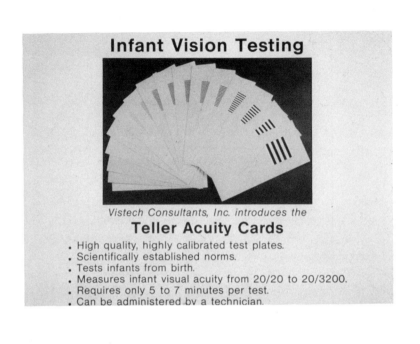

Figure 3.3 Teller Acuity Cards®. Photographed with permission of Vistech Consultants Incorporated.

between the ages of 1 and 12 months. It was shown by Mayer, Fulton, and Rodier (1984) that acuities obtained from grating tests, such as preferential looking, generally yield better visual acuity than recognition visual tests (Scheiman, 1991).

Teller Acuity Cards are a useful proxy to test individuals who are not able to respond to the ETDRS chart, or where patient cooperation is difficult to obtain (Marx, Werner, Cohen-Mansfield, & Hartmann, 1990; Morse, Yatzkan, Rosenthal, Holmes, & Teresi, 1990). Recently Marx, Werner, Friedman, and Cohen-Mansfield (1989) used Teller Acuity Cards with a nursing home population including patients with cognitive impairment. Binocular Teller Acuity Card vision compared with Snellen acuity ($r = .72$), and test-retest reliability was .90. Using a forced-choice preferential looking approach, cards of a known and precise bandwidth are presented to determine the finest grating that can be perceived. The patient will attend to the stripe, if it is able to be perceived, and where it is indistinguishable from the neutral gray stimulus, eye movement will be random. One side of each card is blank, and the other contains a square wave grating (vertical black and white stripes), ranging in steps from 38.0 to .32 cycles/cm. The grating is located to the left or right or an aperture that is located in the middle of the card. Each card is labeled on the back with the grating size (Scheiman, 1991), with bandwidth being correlated with conventional measures of acuity. The stripes cannot be discriminated from the background if the pattern is below an individual's acuity threshold.

To test acuity, the examiner sequentially displays a series of Teller cards, one at a time, each containing a black-and-white grating of a different spatial frequency (stripe width), located on the left or right of the central peephole. Once the examiner is able to get the person's attention, the examiner observes the patient through the peephole and on the basis of the eye movements or visual responsiveness, decides which card contains the finest stripe that the patient can see. Testing continues until the examiner feels confident enough about the responses to make a judgment concerning the finest grating that can be detected. The Teller Acuity Cards have recently been used in studying acuity in patients with dementias. Compared with standard ETDRS acuity testing, the Teller procedure resulted in significantly greater numbers of testable patients among a sample of demented patients where dementia was established using the Reisberg Global Deterioration Scale (Reisberg, Ferris, Deleon, & Crook, 1988). Many patients classified as "untestable" with ETDRS procedures were able TO have their acuity assessed with Teller cards, useful for epidemiological as well as for patient-specific data. Teller Acuity Cards are a useful method of determining acuity in patients who retain the ability to attend, if ever so briefly, to the presentation of a visual stimuli (see Table 3.1).

Variations in the Measurement of Acuity

Although visual acuity is generally considered to be the common denominator of vision testing, responses on visual acuity charts are dependent on many factors. Level of illumination present, at the chart, significantly affects acuity. Test distance also affects performance because it may be difficult for the patient to visually attend to a chart at the standard viewing distance of 20' (6M); for this reason, many charts have been restandardized at closer distances, typically 3 m. The form of the chart characters (i.e., optotypes), the number optotypes per chart line, and whether they are letters, numbers, or symbols used also affects performance. Number charts, rather than letter charts, are easier for most patients because of the more limited choices. Such charts yield higher estimates of acuity than charts using letters (9 choices rather than 26).

Performance on acuity measures is also affected by cognitive state. Cognitive function of the patient may be impaired as a result of aphasia, an impairment of expressive or receptive language skills usually resulting from lesions of the left frontal and temporal lobes (Dixon, Trexler, & Layton, 1993); stroke, which may result in a loss in cognitive functioning as well as visual acuity, visual field, and contrast sensitivity; brain lesions, such as those affecting the angular gyrus, which produces alexia—a

TABLE 3.1 Increase in Testable Vision Using Teller Cards by Dementia Level

Dementia Stage	Total Cases	Assessed with ETDRS (%)	Total n Assessed (%)	Net Increase over ETDRS (% of *n*)
Mild	57	54 (95)	57 (100)	3 (5)
Moderate	57	50 (88)	54 (95)	4 (7)
Severe	81	47 (58)	61 (75)	14 (17)
Very Severe	48	10 (21)	20 (42)	10 (21)
Total	243	161 (66)	192 (79)	31 (13)

From Morse, Rosenthal, & Yatzkan (1993).

visual aphasia in which the patient is unable to understand the meaning of written words—coupled with agraphia, an inability to write— with such patients retaining only recognition of isolated letters or numbers (Higgins, 1984); and dementia, with ability to perform visual tasks at least partly because of the severity or level of the dementia.

CONTRAST SENSITIVITY

The standard visual acuity test measures vision under near-ideal contrast levels (100%) (Waiss & Cohen, 1991). Contrast testing gives some indication of how the patient sees under nonideal conditions and may give a more realistic indication of his or her ability in real-life situations. Visual acuity measures the resolving power of the eye along a single variable (size), whereas contrast sensitivity measures it along two variables (size and contrast).

The most usable contrast information is obtained by generating the patient's contrast sensitivity function curve. There are numerous spatial frequency receptor channels in the visual system, each with a unique contrast threshold (Ginsburg, 1981). The contrast sensitivity curve plots the contrast sensitivity function (inverse of the contrast threshold) versus the spatial frequency (size) of the target. The test is analogous to an audiogram.

Contrast sensitivity can be assessed in a variety of ways. The traditional laboratory research involves sine wave gratings projected onto an oscilloscope. However, this is not practical for clinical use. A quicker assessment of contrast sensitivity can be achieved with the Vistech Contrast Sensitivity Test. (Figure 3.4) The examiner stands with the chart at a distance of 1 M with the best refractive correction (modified for the test distance, i.e., add +1.00 add). The patient is instructed to look at the four bottom patches on the chart while the examiner shows that the patches contain either lines going up and to the left, up and to the right, straight up, or gray. Pointing to each patch, the patient should demonstrate the direction of the lines with the hand. The examiner proceeds to the next line when the patient can no longer identify the correct orientation of the lines in the circle.

The Pelli-Robson chart (Pelli, Robson, & Wilkins, 1988) is another printed clinical contrast sensitivity test widely used in clinical practice. It is composed of 16 3-letter groupings in which each triplet becomes progressively lighter until the observer is no longer able to distinguish the letters from the background. The Vistech findings are measured with a series of gratings at various spatial frequencies and can be plotted on a contrast curve, whereas the Pelli-Robson method yields peak contrast. The Vistech chart has been normed for so-called normal-and low-vision patients, enhancing their usefulness in a population where visual impairment is prevalent, whereas no such norms yet exist for the Pelli-Robson method.

Contrast sensitivity deficiencies in AD patients may result from a loss of M-cells, which have a high degree of sensitivity to contrast (Livingstone & Hubel, 1987). M-cell loss may also help explain deficits in spatial orientation and eye movement, whereas acuity remains relatively unaffected. Optic nerve degeneration in AD may result in acuity deficits as well as loss of some color vision or contrast sensitivity (Mendez, Tomsak, & Remler, 1990; Sadun, Bochert, & DeVita, 1987). Sholtz, Swettenham, Brown, & Mann (1981) found that both blind and demented patients showed reduced amounts of myelin in the visual cortex and suggest that because the degree of myelinazation may be stimulus-dependent, demented patients may have unrecognized visual impairment.

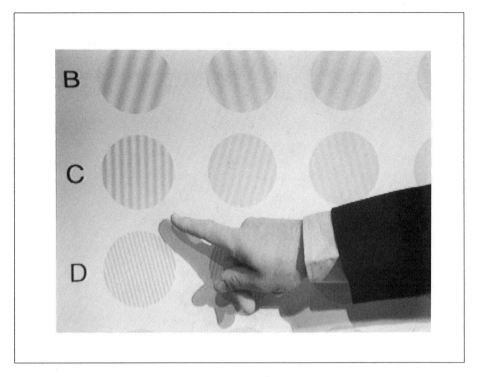

Figure 3.4 Vistech Contrast Sensitivity Test®. Photographed with permission of Vistech Consultants Incorporated.

COLOR VISION ASSESSMENT

Color vision assessment is rarely performed on older individuals, much less those with dementia. In fact, color vision loss in individuals with dementia has only begun to be addressed (Morse, Rosenthal, Yatzkan, & Teresi, 1995). Although the necessity of color vision for normal functioning has been questioned, Jose (1983) suggests that color clues may be beneficial to a patient in terms of mobility. A more important question about color vision loss is whether there are any apparent changes in color vision unique to Alzheimer's disease.

Standard color vision tests include polychromatic plates, such as the Ishihara, in which primary color dots are printed among gray background dots, which increasingly camouflage the patterns and shapes of color. Another approach to determine acquired color vision loss is the Farnsworth Panel D-15 test (Bailey, 1991) (Figure 3.5), which consists of a set of 16 different colored caps (from the Munsell system). There is a reference cap from which the other caps are placed in sequence. Responses are then recorded on a score sheet to represent the arrangement of the caps. Major color confusions or deficiencies are determined by the order in which the caps are placed and the degree of deviance from the correct spectral sequence. For example, major color confusions, such as red-green or yellow-blue, will be apparent by type of errors made.

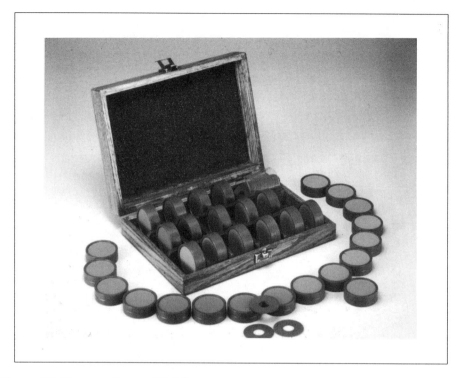

Figure 3.5. Farnsworth panel D-15 test.

The Macbet Easel Lamp is the standard illumination used with the D-15 Panel Test. The Farnsworth includes a holder for the box that contains the caps. As with all vision tests, but especially with tests of color vision, correct and proper illumination has significant effect on test results.

Although the Farnsworth is useful for patients with mild dementia, there is no adequate measure of color vision for patients with advanced dementia.

DARK ADAPTATION AND PHOTOSTRESS

A common complaint among older adults is the increase in time necessary for dark adaptation. Dark adaptometry is a psychophysical method for determining the light sensitivity threshold as a function of time in the dark and evaluates retina function. Including the initial preadaptation phases, dark adaptometry testing usually takes at least 30 minutes to perform and measures return to visual function after time in the dark (Pitman & Yolton, 1986). Photostress evaluates the length of time necessary to resolve fine detail after exposure to bright light (Wolkstein & Carr, 1979). Where a patient does not appear to function well after being in a dark environment, photostress is a clinically useful way of assessing macular function and recovery. The patient is presented with a standard acuity measure. After recording performance, a flashlight is held a few centimeters from the eye for at least 10 seconds, and the patient is retested. Average recovery time to regain normal performance is about 1 minute. Longer times indicate macular dysfunction.

SELF-REPORT MEASURES OF VISION STATUS

Visual acuity is generally measured by asking the patient to identify optotypes of varying sizes and comparing the result against normal (i.e., 20/20) vision. The size of the characters that can be correctly perceived represents the degree of vision. The standard test of acuity is a form of self-report because the findings are those reported by the patient rather than objectively found by the examiner. A standard vision self-report measure, the Amsler Grid (Amsler, 1994; Amsler, 1974; Yanuzzi, 1982), is used to evaluate macular integrity and to detect central vision defects. The grid, approximately 10 cm^2, consists of white horizontal and vertical lines forming squares of 5 mm on a black background. The patient is asked to focus on a small white dot in the center of the grid and then asked to answer a series of questions including whether the central spot is visible, whether the entire grid appears intact, and whether the lines appear straight and parallel. Self-report questionnaires are commonly used to evaluate need for further vision examination and typically ask a series of questions about vision and vision problems. For example, Horowitz, Teresi, and Cassels (1991) developed a 15-item instrument to screen community-based elderly for vision problems; typical items elicit information about whether the person feels that "vision problems make things difficult" or that she or he "cannot see headlines." Eighty percent of all cases were properly classified with a sensitivity of .64 and a positive predictive value (PPV) also of .64, indicating that 64% of those individuals identified by the instrument were ultimately determined to have an actual vision problem, using a cut score of 9, determined to be the most effective balance between PPV and sensitivity. The negative predictive value was .86, thus yielding 14% false negatives.

Response to items on self-report inventories necessarily requires the ability to comprehend both the question and to form an appropriate responsive answer, and to have the ability to respond. Self-report vision measures are inherently limited by the ability of the respondent to comprehend and correctly respond to the items. Other measures, such as the Activities of Daily Vision Scale (Mangione et al., 1992), have been developed to determine cataract-related functional disability. The Comprehensive Assessment and Referral Evaluation (CARE) (Gurland et al., 1977), developed using a community sample of elderly, contains an 11-item self-report Vision subscale; the Cohen's κ coefficients using three raters ranged from .70 to .80 across items. Interrater reliabilities for the scale, estimated using a mixed effects intraclass correlation coefficient, was in the .80s. The α coefficient for the Vision Disorders scale was .80 (Golden, Teresi, & Gurland, 1984). These and other self-report instruments and measures may have widespread utility in a community-based population, but are generally not useful in an institutional population where about 70% to 80% of the patients have some level of impaired cognitive ability, and only about 40% are capable of completing a diagnostic interview (Teresi, Lawton, Ory, & Holmes, 1994). In such settings, brief examination techniques, such as those described earlier, are more appropriate as screening procedures.

OCULAR EFFECTS OF SYSTEMIC MEDICATIONS

Another important, but largely overlooked, factor causing decreased vision is the ocular side effects of common medications. Many medications have an adverse affect on visual function. Some of the ocular functions that may be impaired by medications include visual acuity, visual fields, contrast sensitivity, depth of field, depth of focus, extraocular muscle function, tearing (lacrimation), ocular surface integrity, perceived brightness, pupil size, rate of blinking, and tear film quality (Oliver, 1996).

In practical terms, for example, a patient taking an ophthalmic ointment or taking methylcellulose may have a temporary decrease in contrast sensitivity and a reduction in visual acuity. This can translate into increased difficulty with mobility. Another example of medication interfering with everyday function would be an individual who, as the result of a medication, has an enlarged pupil. This could result in decreased contrast sensitivity, reduced depth of field, blurred vision, and increased brightness or photophobia (light sensitivity). This list of drugs with ocular side effects is lengthy. Among the more common medications affecting acuity are allopurinol, chloramphenicol, chloroquinine, corticosteriods, indomethicin, tetracycline, monoamine oxidase inhibitors, and excess amounts of vitamin A. Frequently prescribed medications affecting pupillary response include amphetamines, antihistimines, anticholinergics, Elavil, and haloperidol. Commonly used medications affecting ocular motility include chlordiazepoxide, diazepam, tetracycline, phenytoin, and vitamin A. Amphetamines, anticholinergics, corticosteriods and tricyclic antidepressants may affect intraocular pressure. In brief, many commonly prescribed medications may alter visual function (Yamamoto, 1980). Therefore, knowledge of which medications are being used is an important part of patient history *before* visual function is assessed.

ASSESSING VISION IN NURSING HOME PATIENTS

The prevalence of *severe* visual impairment increases from 14.3% for those 65 to 74 years of age to 27.5% for those 85 years old and older (National Center for Health Statistics, 1989). Nevertheless, vision examination of nursing home patients is not common; only 5% to 20% of nursing home residents receive routine examinations (Leslie & Greenberg, 1980; Morse, O'Connell, & Finkelstein, 1988; Newell & Walser, 1987; Snyder, Pyrek, & Smith, 1976).

It is essential that subjective and objective methods be readily available to determine the visual status of the nursing home patient. The standard vision assessment in a nursing home, when and if a vision examination is performed, consists of the following.

1. Limited case history
2. Determination of the distance visual acuity using the nonstandardized Snellen chart
3. Determination of the near-visual acuity
4. External and internal (ophthalmoscopy) assessment of the health of the eye
5. Glaucoma screening with a tonometer to determine the intraocular pressure and the presence of glaucoma
6. Refraction to assess the need for corrective lenses for distance viewing and reading

Rarely, if ever, does a nursing home visual evaluation include an assessment of a patient's contrast sensitivity function or an analysis of color vision, despite the usefulness and importance of these vision components.

Nursing home patient populations reflect a high prevalence of dementia which imposes an added challenge in assessing visual function. According to Mendez, Mendez, Martin, Smyth, & Whitehouse (1990), "There are gaps in understanding the extent of complex visual disturbances in Alzheimer's Disease and their clinical consequences." Conventional protocols to assess visual function may be inadequate for patients with dementia. First, cognitive impairments, including deficits in language, comprehension, and memory, can interfere with visual task performance. In addition, basic visual deficits may affect tests of more complex visual functioning (U.S. Department of Health and Human Services). Difficulty in completion of complex visual tasks including construction, figure-ground, visual object, and face recognition are common among Alzheimer's disease patients (Waiss & Cohen, 1991).

Traditional examination procedures emphasize ocular disease. Although acuity measures provide accurate data about visual function under a specific set of controlled conditions, they do not provide an accurate representation of *how* the patient uses visual data. Vision care should be one of the cornerstones of effective care for elderly patients. Although sensory loss is well known as a concomitant of aging, its role as a determinant of patient functioning is too often overlooked. Patients with cognitive impairment suffer from a deficit in processing. How much greater is their impairment a result of a deficit in sensory input? Clearly, vision impairment contributes to excess morbidity in patients with AD and other cognitive impairments; the degree and nature of the contribution remains unclear. Adequate assessment of vision is a first step toward understanding the role played by vision in the functioning of patients with cognitive impairment.

REFERENCES

Amsler, M. (1974). L'examen qualitatif de la fonction maculaire. *Ophthalmologica, 114*, 248-261.

Amsler, M. (1994). Quantitative and qualitative vision. *Transactions of the Ophthalmological Societies of the United Kingdom, 69*, 397-410.

Bailey, I. L., & Lovie, J. K. (1976). New design for visual acuity letter charts. *American Journal of Optometry and Physiological Optics, 53*, 740-745.

Bailey, J. E. (1991). Color vision. In J. B. Eskridge, J. F. Amos, & J. D. Bartlett (Eds.), *Clinical procedures in optometry* (pp.99–120). Philadelphia: J. B. Lippincott.

Davidson, D. W. (1991). Visual Acuity. In J. B. Eskridge, J. F. Amos, & J. D. Bartlett (Eds.), *Clinical procedures in optometry* (p. 17). Philadelphia: J. B. Lippincott.

Dixon, T. M., Trexler, L. E., & Layton, B. S. (1993). Brain injury: Trauma and stroke. In M. G. Eisenberg, R. L. Gluechauf, & H. H. Zaretsky (Eds.), *Medical aspects of disability: A handbook for the rehabilitation professional* (pp.76–91). New York: Springer Publishing Co.

Fantz, R. I., Ordy, J. M., & Udelf, M. S. (1962). Maturation pattern vision in infants during the first six months. *Journal of Comparative Physiology Psychology, 55*, 907-917.

Faye, E. E. (1994). *Clinical low vision* (2nd ed.). Boston: Little, Brown.

Ferris, F., Kassoff, A., Bresnick, G. H., & Bailey, I. (1982). New visual acuity charts for clinical research. *American Journal of Ophthalmology, 94*, 91-96.

Ginsburg, A. P. (1981). Spatial filtering and vision: Implications for normal and abnormal vision. In I. M. Proenza, J. M. Enoch, & A. Jampolsky (Eds.), *Clinical applications of visual psychophysics* (pp. 70-106). Cambridge: Cambridge University Press.

Golden, R. R., Teresi, J. A., & Gurland, B. J. (1984). Development of indicator scales for the Comprehensive Assessment and Referral Evaluation (CARE) interview schedule. *Journal of Gerontology*, *39*(2), 138-146.

Gurland, B. J., Kuriansky, J. B., Sharpe, L. K., Simon, R., Stiller, P., & Birkett, P. (1977). The Comprehensive Assessment and Referral Evaluation (CARE): Rationale, development and reliability. *International Journal of Aging and Human Development*, *8*, 9-42.

Hartmann, E. (1996). Functional vision assessment of vision. In R. G. Cole & B. P. Rosenthal (Eds.), *Functional assessment of vision* (pp. 45–62). St. Louis: C. V. Mosby.

Higgins, D. J. (1984). Postoptic nerve visual pathway. In *Ocular assessment: The manual of diagnosis for office practice* (pp. 511-516). Boston: Butterworths.

Horowitz, A., Teresi, J. A., & Cassels, L. A. (1991). Development of a Vision Screening Questionnaire for older people. *Journal of Gerontological Social Work*, *17*(3/4), 37-56.

Hubel, D. H. (1988). *Eye, brain and vision*. New York: Scientific American Library.

Johnston, A. W. (1991). Making sense of the M, N, and logMAR systems of specifying visual acuity. In B. Rosenthal & R. Cole (Eds.), *A structured approach to low vision care* (p. 394). Philadelphia: J. B. Lippincott.

Jose, R. (Ed.). (1983) *Understanding low vision*. New York: American Foundation for the Blind.

Leslie, W. J., & Greenberg, D. A. (1980). A survey of the prevalence of vision defects and ocular anomolies in 43 Ontario residential and nursing homes. *Canadian Journal of Public Health*, 413-423.

Livingstone, M. S., & Hubel, D. (1987). Psychophysical evidence for separate channels for the perception of form, color, movement and depth. *Journal of Neuroscience*, *7*, 3416-3468.

Mangione, C. M., Phillips, R. S., Seddon, J. M., Lawrence, M. G., Cook, E. F., Dailey, R., & Goldman, L. (1992). Development of the Activities of Daily Vision Scale: A measure of functional vision status. *Medical Care*, *30*, 1111-1126.

Marx, M. S., Werner, P., Cohen-Mansfield, J., & Hartmann, E. E. (1990). Visual acuity estimates in the non-communicative elderly persons. *Investigative Ophthalmology & Visual Science*, *31*(3), 593-596.

Marx, M. S., Werner, P., Friedman, P., & Cohen-Mansfield, J. (1989). Visual acuity estimates in the aged. *Journal of Clinical Visual Science*, *4*, 179-182.

Mayer, D. L., Fulton, A. B., & Rodier, D. (1984). Grating and recognition acuities of pediatric patients. *Ophthalmology*, *91*, 947-953.

McDonald, M. A., Ankrum, C., & Preston, K. (1986). Monocular and binocular acuity estimation in 18- to 36-month olds: Acuity card results. *American Journal of Optometry and Physiological Optics*, *63*, 181-186.

McDonald, M. A., Sebris, S., & Hohn, G. (1986). Monocular acuity in normal infants: The acuity cared procedure. *American Journal of Optometry and Physiological Optics*, *63*, 127-134.

McDonald, M., Dobson, V., & Sebris, S. (1985). The acuity card procedure: A rapid test of infant acuity. *Investigative Ophthalmology & Visual Science*, *26*, 1158-1162.

Mendez, M. F., Mendez, M. A., Martin, R., Smyth, K. A., & Whitehouse, P. J. (1990). Complex visual disturbances in Alzheimer's dementia. *Neurology*, *40*, 439-443.

Mendez, M. F., Tomsak, R. L., & Remler, B. (1990). Disorders of the visual system in Alzheimer's disease. *Journal of Neuro-Ophthalmology, 10*(1), 62-69.

Morse, A. R. (1982). Vision problems and vision care in nursing homes In R. G. Cole & B. P. Rosenthal (Eds.) *Problems in Optometry:Patient and Practice Management in Low Vision, 4*(1), 125-132.

Morse, A. R., & Friedman, D. (1986). Vision rehabilitation and aging. *Journal of Visual Impairment and Blindness, 6*, 803-804.

Morse, A. R., O'Connell, J. J., & Finkelstein, H. (1988). Assessing vision in nursing home residents. *Journal of Vision Rehabilitation, 2*(4), 1-10.

Morse, A. R., Rosenthal, B., & Yatzkan, E. (1993). *Vision assessment, vision loss and dementia.* Paper presented at the annual meeting of the Association for Research in Vision and Ophthalmolgy, Sarasota, FL.

Morse, A. R., Rosenthal, B., Yatzkan, E. S., & Teresi, J. A. (1995, November 16). Color vision in patients with dementia. Paper presented at the Gerontological Society of America, Los Angeles.

Morse, A. R., Yatzkan, E. S., Rosenthal, B., Holmes, D., & Teresi, J. A. (1990, November 22). *Methodological issues in assessing vision in patients with dementia.* Paper presented at the annual meeting of the Gerontological Society of America, New Orleans.

National Center for Health Statistics. (1978). Nursing home residents utilization health status and care received: National Nursing Home Survey.

National Center for Health Statistics. (1989). The National Nursing Home Survey: 1985 summary for the United States (DHHS Publication No. [PHS] 89-1758). In *Vital and health statistics series 13.* Washington, DC: U.S. Government Printing Office.

Nelson, K. A. (1987). Visual impairment among elderly Americans: Statistics in transition. *Journal of Visual Impairment and Blindness, 81,* 331-334.

Newell, F. W. (1969). *Ophthamology principles and concepts* (2nd Ed., p. 136). St. Louis: C. V. Mosby.

Newell, S. W., & Walser, J. J. (1987). Nursing Home Glaucoma and Acuity Screening Results in Western Oklahoma. *Annals of Ophthamology, 17,* 186-189.

Ogle, K. N. (1953). On the problem of an international nomenclature for designating visual acuity. *American Journal of Ophthalmology, 36,* 909-921.

Oliver, G. E. (1996). Pharmaceutical effects on the management of the low vision patient. In R. G. Cole & B. P. Rosenthal (Eds.), *Remediation and management of low vision.* (pp. 123–138). St. Louis: C. V. Mosby.

Pelli, D. G., Robson, J. G., & Wilkins, A. J. (1988). The design of a new letter chart for measuring contrast sensitivity. *Journal of Clinical Visual Science, 2,* 187-199.

Pitman, J. R., & Yolton, R. L. (1986). Introduction to special tests for the assessment of vision in elderly patients. In A. A. Rosenbloom & M. W. Morgan (Eds.), *Vision and Aging: General and Clinical Perspectives* (pp. 222-223). New York: Professional Press Books, Fairchild Publications.

Pizarello, L. D. (1987). The dimensions of the problem of eye disease among the elderly. *Ophthalmology, 94*(9), 1191-1195.

Reisberg, B., Ferris, S. H., Deleon, M. J., & Crook, T. (1988). Global deterioration scale. *Psychopharmacology Bulletin, 24*(4), 661-663.

Sadun, A. A., Bochert, M., & DeVita, E. (1987). Assessment of visual impairment in patients with Alzheimer's disease. *American Journal of Ophthalmology, 104,* 110-120.

Scheiman, M. (1991). Pediatric visual acuity. In J. B. Eskridge, J. F. Amos, & J. D. Bartlett (Eds.), *Clinical Procedures in Optometry* (pp. 641-644). Philadelphia: J. B. Lippincott.

Sholtz, C. L., Swettenham, K., Brown, A., & Mann, D. M. (1981). A histoquantitative study of the stiat cortex and laternal geniculate body in normal, blind and demented subjects. *Neuropathology and Applied Neurobiology, 7*, 103-114.

Snyder, L. H., Pyrek, J., & Smith, K. C. (1976). Vision and mental function of the elderly. *The Gerontologist, 16*(6), 491-495.

Teresi, J. A., Lawton, P., Ory, M., & Holmes, D. (1994). Measurement issues in chronic care populations: Dementia special care units. *Journal of Alzheimer's Disease & Related Disorders, 8*(Suppl. 1), S144-S183.

U.S. Department of Health and Human Services ([PHS] 86-1582). *Estimates from the National Health Interview Survey, United States, 1983, 10*(154).

Waiss, B. W., & Cohen, J. M. (1991, September). Glare and contrast sensitivity for low vision practitioners. In *A structured approach to low vision care* (Vol. 3, pp. 443-446). Philadelphia: J. B. Lippincott.

Wandell, B. (1995). *Foundations of vision.* Sunderland, MA: Sinauer.

Westheimer, G. (1979). Scaling of visual acuity measurement. *Archives of Ophthalmology, 97*, 327-330.

Wolkstein, M., & Carr, R. (1979). Macula function tests. In Yannuzzi, Gittler & Shatz (Eds.), *The Macula: A comprehensive test and atlas* (pp. 14-24). Baltimore: Williams & Wilkens.

Yamamoto, G. K. (1980). Ocular drug toxicity. In D. Pavan-Langston (Ed.), *Manual of ocular diagnosis and therapy* (pp. 415–431). Boston: Little, Brown.

Yanuzzi, L. A. (1982). A modified Amsler grid. A self-assessment test for patients with macular disease. *Ophthalmology, 89*, 157-159.

Chapter 4

Measurement of Behavioral Disturbance in Chronic Care Populations

Pierre N. Tariot, Anton Porsteinsson, Linda Teri, and Myron F. Weiner

DEFINITION OF CONSTRUCTS

The purpose of this chapter is to review the assessment of behavioral change in the chronic care population. To set the stage for such an undertaking, some preliminary comments and definitions are in order, recognizing that the totality of an individual's behavior will be difficult to define, and any definition must be acknowledged as somewhat arbitrary. At the first level of resolution, "behavior" could refer to all of what a person says and does, resulting from complex interactions among subject, social, and environmental factors. At the next level of resolution, we can focus more specifically on the chronic care population, where several relevant domains can be identified. These domains might include, for instance, cognition, functional performance, social performance, medical status, neurological status, biological status, environmental factors, and "quality of life," in addition to behavior.

The term *behavior,* even within this framework, still reflects a broad concept that is multidetermined, pleomorphic, and dynamic. One way to sharpen it further would be to use clinically discernible phenomena to help define the constructs. Contextually, this is a particularly salient approach, because our charge is to survey the different means available to characterize and quantify clinical phenomena in chronic care populations.

It then follows to identify the most common clinical phenomena in the chronic care setting. The nursing home is one setting that offers itself as a useful paradigm. In the nursing home, dementias, other organic mental disorders, depression, schizophrenia, and mental retardation and developmental disabilities are the most common neuropsychiatric diagnoses, covering 90% of patients (Rovner, Kafonek, Filipp, Lucas, & Folstein, 1986; Tariot, Podgorski, Blazina, & Leibovici, 1993). These diagnoses are associated with a host of behavioral changes, however measured. For instance, 90% of nursing home patients were shown to have at least one behavioral problem, and roughly 50% had four or more (Rovner et al., 1986; Tariot et al., 1993). Therefore, it is reasonable for the present purposes to focus on behavioral changes associated with the dementias as the paradigm for construct definition because such changes are so prevalent in the long-term care setting and so frequently complicated by behavioral symptomatology.

At first, behavior problems associated with dementia can appear confusing because they vary considerably over time and among individuals. Several investigators have begun to characterize these changes and to identify clusters of signs and symptoms that frequently co-occur in individuals with dementia (Burns, Jacoby, & Levy, 1990; Reisberg, Franssen, Sclan, Kluger, & Ferris, 1989; Tariot et al., 1995b; Teri, Larson, & Reifler, 1988; Wragg & Jeste, 1989). These include delusions, hallucinations, depressive features, anxious features, agitation, and apathy and withdrawal (Tariot & Blazina, 1994). Constructs, such as this, which are useful clinically but require more empirical research before being considered as well defined, have individual components. For instance, depressive features could include sad affect, tearfulness, subjective reports of low mood, guilty or self-deprecatory ideation, pessimism, preoccupation with death, suicidality, and certain vegetative features. The authors will, therefore, use these clinically identifiable behavioral syndromes as a schematic framework with which to organize our review of behavioral assessment tools. The measures will be deemed adequate to the extent that they address all of these domains including addressing in a relevant way the particular components constituting these domains. Although the present proposal is schematic and an oversimplification, it nonetheless offers a logical means to organize a survey of the literature.

METHODOLOGICAL ISSUES

Instrument development studies vary widely in patient selection and in important clinical characteristics, such as diagnoses and diagnostic ascertainment, prior psychiatric history, stage of illness, and gender. There are also important differences in sample size, design (e.g., cross-sectional versus longitudinal, retrospective versus prospective case control versus population based), criteria used for characterizing behavior, reliability, type of analysis, time frame of relevance, setting, characteristics of interviewers, and source of information (Tariot & Blazina, 1994; Teri & Logsdon, 1995). The literature is understandably heterogeneous. These methodological issues will not be reviewed here but should be borne in mind when reviewing the original studies.

The first objective of a behavioral rating is to determine if and how often a particular behavior has occurred. Appraisals of severity, which have their place, are more subjective and less reliable. This basic measurement issue is important in assessing all behavioral rating scales. Existing instruments can be judged by a variety of other important psychometric criteria, many of which were reviewed by Teri and Logsdon (1995). Not every rating scale of relevance has ideal psychometric properties. Conversely, depending on the purpose for which a scale is used, one or another of these criteria may be of particular importance. In general, those with clear constructs, established reliability, demonstrated validity and sensitivity, and practical features suitable for the intended purpose will be the most logical choices.

Bearing these criteria in mind, the authors have selected several instruments that may be of potential interest for rating behavior in the chronic care population. Many of these have been reviewed or referenced elsewhere (Tariot et al., 1995b; Teri & Logsdon, 1995; Weiner et al., 1996). In the following section, the authors present a group of behavior rating instruments of interest because of their particular strengths, grouped according to source of information. The authors largely ignore instruments that do not address multiple domains (e.g., those that address depression only, which are reviewed in chapter 6 by Katz and Parmelee). The major exception is the authors' inclusion of instruments that address agitation. These are presented in the third section because agitated behaviors are so common in the population and because there is a plethora of such instruments. The authors conclude the chapter with a more detailed presentation of six instruments that are especially well suited to this clinical problem, and offer an interesting spectrum of attributes and weaknesses illustrating the current state of methodology. The scales are presented alphabetically in each section.

OVERVIEW OF GENERAL BEHAVIORAL MEASURES OF INTEREST

Caregiver (Family or Professional) as Informant

Behavioral Pathology in Alzheimer's Disease Rating Scale (BEHAVE-AD) (Reisberg et al., 1987). This empirically derived scale was based originally on a retrospective chart review of outpatients with Alzheimer's-type dementia. It has been applied subsequently in several longitudinal and cross-sectional studies of patients with dementia (e.g., Patterson et al., 1990; Reisberg, Franssen, Sclan, Kluger, & Ferris, 1989; Sclan, Saillon, Franssen, Hugonot-Diener, & Saillon, 1996) including nursing home patients. The scale consists of 25 items grouped into seven domains: paranoia/delusions, hallucinations, activity disturbance, aggression, sleep/wake cycle disturbance, affective disturbance, and anxiety/phobic symptoms. A 2-week interval is rated. Scoring is based on severity, not frequency. Severity scores in some cases vary on the basis of item content (e.g., type of delusion), in some cases on the basis of caregiver response. This clinically appealing approach to scoring may create some psychometric instability. The scale is completed based on interview of a caregiver by a clinician, but it can also be completed by a caregiver with proper training. It takes approximately 25 to 35 minutes to complete. The domains covered are relevant for purposes of this review, although there is less emphasis on agitated behaviors and apathy compared with some other scales. There are some encouraging reliability data available concerning severity ratings, with κ ranging from 0.62 to 1.00 in study samples ranging in size from 20 to 140 subjects (Patterson et al., 1990; Sclan, Saillon, Franssen, Hugonot-Diener, & Saillon, 1996). One of the first comprehensive scales, it is as a foundation for others, such as the Columbia University Scale for Psychopathology in Alzheimer's Disease (CUSPAD) (Devenand et al., 1992) and the CERAD Behavior Rating Scale for Dementia (Tariot et al., 1995b), and for structured interviews for the Clinical Global Impression of Change (Reisberg, Ferris, Tarossian, Kluger, Monterio, 1992).

Behavioral Symptoms Scale for Dementia (Devenand, Miller, Richards, Marder, & Bell, 1992). This scale was based on interviews with caregivers of 106 outpatients diagnosed with dementia of the Alzheimer type. It consists of 30 items intended to capture five domains and "other clinical features": disinhibition, catastrophic reaction, apathy/indifference, sundowning, and denial; it also has a general item. An interviewer conducts a structured interview of an informant based on events over 1 week. The items are rated in some cases according to frequency, and in others according to severity; one is rated according to caregiver response. The severity levels lack clear guidelines. The proposed factors blend constructs that could arguably be separated (e.g., crying and verbal aggression are included in the disinhibition factor). Some constructs that are relevant to this review (i.e., hallucinations, delusions, vegetative features, and physical aggression) are not included in the scale. Interrater and intraclass correlation coefficients range from 0.40 to 0.90 and 0.76 to 0.95 for global scores of the five domains.

Caretaker Obstreporous Behavior Rating Scale (Drachman, Swearer, O'Donnell, Mitchell, & Maloon, 1992). This instrument was developed based on studies of both outpatients (*n*=31) and nursing home patients (*n*=36) with several types of dementia. It is a caregiver-based interview consisting of 39 items addressing four constructs: aggression/assaultiveness, disordered ideas/personality, mechanical/motor abnormalities, and vegetative disorders. It was one of the first scales to address vegetative features more rigorously by including continence, sleep disorders, changes in sexuality, weight change, appetitive change, and altered pain tolerance. The time window is 3 months. Each behavior is rated according to frequency (with clear guidelines) and severity (based on degree of disruption); scoring ranges vary by item. A total of 12 summary scores is produced reflecting what domains were affected, how many behaviors were rated, and how frequent and disruptive the behaviors were. Potentially important domains, such as depression, anxiety, and illusions, are not captured by the scale. Test-retest correlations of the summary scores ranged from 0.44 to 0.65, with interrater reliability correlations for summary scores 0.30 to 0.99.

CUSPAD (Devanand, Miller, Richards, Marder, & Bell, 1992). This is one of several instruments partially based on the BEHAVE-AD (Reisberg et al., 1987). It was also based on observations in 91 outpatients with probable Alzheimer's disease, and by design emphasizes psychotic features. It includes items relevant to other domains. It consists of a rater interview of a caregiver, lasting about 20 minutes, examining 28 items pertaining to a 1-month interval. Some items are rated according to frequency and some according to severity. It has particularly good operational definitions of psychotic features. Because it offers little detail on agitation or depression and does not address anxiety or vegetative features, it would generally be reserved for screening primarily psychotic symptoms in this population. Interrater reliability between a psychiatrist and trained lay interviewer was high (κ 0.74 to 1.00). It was used as one of the springboards in the development of the CERAD Behavior Rating Scale for Dementia.

Dementia Behavior Disturbance Scale (Baumgarten, Becker, & Gauthier, 1990). This scale was developed based on observations of 96 outpatients with mixed types of dementias, addressing behaviors likely to cause stress to caregivers regardless of orgin. It ordinarily entails interview of a caregiver, although this scale can be self-administered by the caregiver. The authors suggest that it measures a single construct, caregiver burden, although it appears to reflect multiple constructs. It consists of 28 items rated on a Likert-type scale with five possible responses corresponding to the frequency of behavior in the preceding week. These include, for instance, changes in sleep, continence, and eating, purposeless activities, and repetitive questioning. Depression, anxiety, hallucinations, delusions, illusions, and apathy/withdrawal are not addressed despite the fact that these could also be distressing to caregivers. Preliminary psychometrics are encouraging but not extensive. Specifically, the average Cronbach's α internal consistency coefficients for items in two samples (*n*=46 and 50) were 0.83 and 0.84, respectively. Pearson's correlation coefficient for test-retest (after 2 weeks) was 0.71.

Dysfunctional Behavior Rating Instrument (DBRI) (Molloy, McIllroy, Guyatt, & Lever, 1991). The DBRI was developed based on a study of 184 cognitively impaired older subjects (45 to 90 years), many of whom presumably had dementia. A rater interviews the caregiver, or it can be self-administered by the caregiver, addressing 25 items over a several-week period. Each item is scored according to clearly defined frequency guidelines and less clearly defined severity ratings addressing "how much of a problem" the behavior represents. The items, which are not collapsed into factors or constructs, address the following: repetitive verbalizations, uncooperativeness, anger, withdrawal, aggression (undefined), fear of being left alone, hiding things, suspiciousness, temper outbursts (undefined), delusions, hallucinations, agitation (undefined), crying, frustration (undefined), wandering and wanting to leave, being up at night, changing one's mind, and embarrassing behavior. Domains, such as anxiety, illusions, some forms of agitation, apathy, and other vegetative features, are not included. Despite potential concern about variance resulting from lack of item definition in some cases, and ambiguous definitions of severity, reliability has been reported as good; an intraclass correlation of 0.75 was found for successive administration of the instrument at 3-week intervals, with more variable estimates of validity.

Nursing Home Behavior Problem Scale (Ray, Taylor, Lichtenstein, & Meador, 1992). This instrument was developed to rapidly assess disruptive behaviors in the nursing home and was studied in more than 500 nursing home residents from 6 nursing homes, irrespective of diagnosis. Behaviors identified were those associated with the use of antipsychotic medications or physical restraints. A nurse or aide completes a 29-item checklist assessing frequency of behaviors over a 3-day period (although the frequency guidelines are not specified). It can be completed in less than 5 minutes. Six subscales are derived: uncooperative/aggressive, irrational/restless, annoying, inappropriate, dangerous, and sleep disturbance. It does not cover several domains of relevance to the present survey. It correlates reasonably well with other relevant instruments, such as the CMAI (Cohen-Mansfield, 1986), and, as expected, high scores were correlated with use of restraints and antipsychotics. Interrater reliability correlations ranged from 0.75 to 0.83 among a total of 553 subjects from 6 sites. Its clinical utility is uncertain at this point, although it has been used in one study of the effect of an intervention to decrease behavioral problems.

Combined Subject and Caregiver Interview

Alzheimer's Disease Assessment Scale (ADAS) (Rosen, Mohs, & Davis, 1984). The ADAS was developed to address the most common clinical symptoms encountered in 31 patients proven by biopsy to have Alzheimer's disease. The major emphasis of this scale is cognitive function, and the cognitive portion of the instrument is used widely in therapeutic studies in Alzheimer's disease. Ten other questions assess behavioral and emotional changes, based on an interview of both an informant and the patient: tearfulness, depressed mood, impaired concentration, cooperativeness, delusions, hallucinations, pacing, motor activities, tremor, and appetite: Spearman rank order for interrater reliability was 0.65 to 0.99. Several domains of potential relevance to the present survey are not addressed (e.g., anxious features, sleep/wake disturbance).

Behavioral and Emotional Activities Manifested in Dementia (BEAM-D) (Sinha et al., 1992). The BEAM-D was developed to assess the efficacy of pharmacotherapeutic interventions for behavioral problems in dementia. It was based on identification of "the most common troublesome and disruptive behaviors that cause anxiety and concern for the caregivers" among 45 patients with dementia, 16 of whom were in nursing homes. It mixes observation and interview of patient and caregiver; the time frame is 1 week. There are observed target behaviors: hostility/aggression, destruction of property, disruption, uncooperative, noncompliance, attention seeking, and sexually inappropriate behaviors; and "inferred" behaviors: depression, delusions, hallucinations, anxiety, appropriateness/stability of affect, increased/decreased appetite, and insomnia. The items are rated according to severity and frequency in a mixed fashion, and some include caregiver impact as well. Mean interrater reliability of items was 0.90. The anchors for some items are ambiguous (e.g., "inconsiderate" or "unconcerned") and frequency guidelines are clear for some items (e.g., "three or fewer instances"), but not others ("several occasions," "frequently," or "consistently"). The domains assessed by this scale fit well with the schematic in the present review, although the methodological issues may limit the scale's utility.

Dementia Signs and Symptoms Scale (Loreck, Bylsma, & Folstein, 1994).
This relatively new scale was based on review of other existing scales used for study of behavioral symptoms in patients with and without dementia, and also on the clinical experience of the authors. It was piloted on a mixed population of 56 patients with dementia of the Alzheimer type, 20 with Huntington's disease, and 19 older subjects with anxiety and depressive disorders, as well as 13 normal controls. It consists of 43 items clustering in five factors that assess anxiety, mania, depression, "behavior," and delusions/hallucinations. A trained clinician interviews the caregiver and patient, assessing behaviors over 1 month. Some items are assessed according to frequency and some according to severity. Severity ratings include an assessment of caregiver impact. Interrater reliability was 0.92 to 0.99 for four raters.

Subject Interview Only

Neurobehavioral Rating Scale (NRS) (Levin et al., 1987). This scale was originally based on a study of patients with mixed neuropsychiatric disorders. It builds on one of the most frequently used behavior rating scales, the Brief Psychiatric Rating Scale (BPRS) (Overall & Gorham, 1962), and extends the domains of the BPRS with the addition of cognitive/neurological changes, which are not directly pertinent to the scope of this review. It has been successfully applied to patients with dementia (Sultzer, Berisford, & Gunay, 1995). Twenty-eight items are assessed by a skilled clinician, each with a clear descriptor, collapsing into six factors: cognition/insight, agitation/disinhibition, behavioral retardation, anxiety/depression, verbal output disturbance, and psychosis. The correlation coefficient in the first report (n=15) for the NRS total was 0.93 (Sultzer, Berisford, & Gunay, 1995). Other studies using the instrument have addressed its validity and applicability to other dementia diagnoses (Sultzer, Levin, Mahler, High, & Cummings, 1992, 1993). It would provide sensitive, reliable assessment by a trained clinician of cognitive, neurological, and behavioral disturbances in this population. Although not in wide use, it is under active study.

Agitation Measures

Brief Agitation Rating Scale (Finkel, Lyons, & Anderson, 1993). This is a reduced version of the Cohen-Mansfield Agitation Inventory (Cohen-Mansfield, 1986), consisting of only 10 items. As it is intended only to assess agitation, it omits many of the other domains of interest for this review.

Cohen-Mansfield Agitation Inventory (CMAI) (Cohen-Mansfield, 1986).
This instrument was derived empirically from observation of nursing home patients,

some of whom had dementia. The study on which this is based is widely regarded as one of the most comprehensive of its kind. The scale is administered by a rater, not necessarily a clinician, to a qualified caregiver informant regarding behaviors observed over a 2-week period. There are 29 items falling into four factors: aggressive, physical nonaggressive, verbal agitation, and hiding/hoarding. Frequency is assessed on a 7-point scale. Interrater agreement ranged from 0.88 to 0.92. This often-cited and widely used instrument is probably the most commonly used measurement for agitated behaviors. It does not address other clinically relevant domains and as a consequence would not be used as a general behavioral scale.

Discomfort Scale for Advanced Alzheimer Patients (Hurley, Volicer, Hanrahan, 1992). This scale assesses clinical phenomena presumed to reflect distress in severely impaired dementia patients. It is based on nursing staff observations of nine observable manifestations of (presumed) discomfort, such as noisy breathing or negative vocalization. It combines assessments of frequency and severity. It does not address several domains of relevance for this survey but may be of use for assessing comfort in advanced patients.

Disruptive Behavior Rating Scales (Mungas, Weiler, Franzi, Henry, 1989). The scale was based on a study of 16 nursing home patients with dementia. It includes 21 items assessed over a 7-day period, all of which address only the domains of physical aggression, verbal aggression, agitation, and wandering. It does not include other domains of potential relevance. Scoring mixes frequency as well as consequences. The psychometric foundation is limited in extent.

Pittsburgh Agitation Scale (Rosen et al., 1994). This was developed for use in inpatients with dementia. It assesses severity of four domains over an 8-hour time frame: aberrant vocalization, motor agitation, aggressiveness, and resistance to care. It is completed by a nurse and takes less than 1 minute to administer. Severity is assessed according to whether the behavior is disruptive, unsafe, or interferes with routine. It omits many domains of potential interest.

Rating Scale for Aggressive Behavior in the Elderly (RAGE) (Patel & Hope, 1992). This 21-item scale was developed to measure aggressive behavior in psychogeriatric inpatients. By design, it does not address numerous other domains and would not be useful for general screening, but offers a detailed look at aggressive behaviors.

Ryden Aggression Scale (Ryden, 1988). This scale also assesses aggression only. It is worthy of mention as it was one of the first of its kind and offers assessment of sexually aggressive behaviors.

A Detailed Look at Six Scales

The following six scales were selected because they have a sound basis for application in chronic care populations and offer a reasonable spectrum of attributes from which to compare and contrast unique strengths and weaknesses for specific purposes to which a scale might be applied. These key methodological attributes are summarized in Table 4.1, providing an overview of domains addressed, samples on which each instrument was originally based, source of information, rater characteristics, time to administer, number of items, and type of measurement. Table 4.1, which in essence summarizes standards by which behavioral instruments can be assessed, provides a bird's-eye view;

the text provides more detail. The scales are presented in alphabetical order; all but the first use the caregiver as informant.

Brief Psychiatric Rating Scale (BPRS) (Overall & Gorham, 1962, 1988).
The BPRS was initially developed to provide rapid, reliable assessment of psychophar-macologic treatment effects in general adult psychiatric inpatients. It originally con-sisted of 16 items but was modified in 1965 to include two additional items. Each of the 18 items addresses a specific construct, based on primary factors chosen from the more extended inpatient Multidimensional Psychiatric Scale (Lorr, Klett, McNair, & Lasky, 1962; Overall & Gorham, 1988). These are "somewhat global, clinically familiar, symptom and behavior constructs that span much of the range of manifest psychopa-thology" (Rhoades & Overall, 1988). Familiarity with the full range of behavioral phenomena of interest is a prerequisite for BPRS raters to recognize mild symptoms as well as gauge the severity of more intense symptoms. The rating constructs represent a process of abstraction and synthesis that models clinical judgment and decision making, and takes advantage of clinical experience. Five factors have been identified in a geropsychiatric population including depression, agitation, cognitive dysfunction, psychotic distortion, and hostile/suspicious (Overall & Beller, 1984). The authors are not aware of specific factor analyses having been performed in dementia subgroups, something that would probably further enhance the value of this instrument.

The BPRS has been widely used to document treatment effects of clinical trials in many populations, including the elderly, and has also been used as a primary or secondary measure of psychopathological state in more descriptive studies of patients with dementia (Frederiksen, Tariot, & DeJonghe, 1996; Hedlund & Vieweg, 1980; Rhoades & Overall, 1988; Tariot et al., 1987, 1995; Tariot, Podgorski, Blazina, & Leibovici, 1993). Interrater reliability was originally reported as ranging from 0.56 to 0.87 (Overall & Gorham, 1962). There has been considerable subsequent evidence regarding its reliability, validity, utility, and sensitivity to change (Hedlund & Vieweg, 1980).

The instrument would probably be most useful as a flexible, reliable, sensitive, and simple general indicator of level of psychopathology and change in level of psychopa-thology. To a lesser extent, it can provide a profile. It provides data comparable with many other data sets. There is not a specific training manual, but various versions of structured or semistructured interviews have been offered over the years (Tarell & Schulz, 1988). Because it relies on clinical experience and judgment, interpersonal and communication skills, and synthesis of information, it requires a trained clinician to apply it reliably. This requirement is both a strength and a weakness: relatively sophisticated personnel are required, but it may model clinical reasoning. It is intended to be a present-state interview, thereby missing behaviors that occur outside the interview, and it ignores the potentially useful information available from caregivers. Some investigators further modify the BPRS to incorporate caregiver information, which might increase the sensitivity but would probably decrease its reliability.

The CERAD Behavior Rating Scale for Dementia (BRSD) (Tariot et al., 1995b). The BRSD resulted from a multicenter research initiative to develop a standardized technique for reliably and comprehensively characterizing psychopathol-ogy in demented patients. The intent was to develop a scale that sampled a range of behaviors sufficiently wide to be useful for most patients with dementia, with differing severity of dementia; composed of well-anchored, homogeneously scaled items; that could be administered by interviewers without extensive psychiatric training. The item pool was based on a formal review of literature regarding behavior change in dementia,

TABLE 4.1 Summary of Six Selected Rating Scales Strengths and Weaknesses

	Anxious features	Depressive features	Delusions	Hallucinations	Illusions	Physically disruptive	Verbal aggression	Physical aggression
BPRS	2	2	2	2	0	1	2	2
BRSD	3	3	3	3	2	2	2	2
MOSES	3	3	0	0	0	2	2	2
NPI	3	3	3	3	1	2	3	3
PGDRS	1	0	1	1	0	2	2	2
RMBPC	3	3	1	1	1	3	3	3

	Study Sample	Source of Information	Rater	Administrative Time	# items	Frequency
BPRS	Numerous dementia samples including nursing home	Patient interview	Trained clinician	30-40"	18	N
BRSD	AD outpatients, nursing home patients	Caregiver interview	Technician	30"	48	Y
MOSES	Many elderly chronically ill	Caregiver questionnaire	NA	20-30"	40	Some
NPI	Outpatients with dementia	Caregiver interview	Technician	15-45"	12 screen 92 f/u	Y
PGDRS	Numerous studies in	Caregiver questionnaire	NA	5-10"	16	Y
RMBPC	AD outpatients	Caregiver questionnaire	NA	15-20"	24	Y

Footnote: Adequacy of assessment of each domain is arbitrarily rated from 0 (none) to 3 (comprehensive) based on number and clarity of items.
BPRS = Brief Psychiatric Rating Scale
BRSD = CERAD Behavior Rating Scale for Dementia
MOSES = Multidimensional Observation Scale for Elderly Subjects
NPI = Neuropsychiatric Inventory
PGDRS = Psychogeriatric Dependency Rating Scale
RMBPC = Revised Memory and Behavior Problems Checklist

review of existing scales, and the clinical experience of the CERAD Behavioral Pathology Committee. It used the Behavioral Pathology in Alzheimer's Disease Rating Scale (Reisberg, Borenstein, Salob, Ferris, & Franssen, 1987), the Columbia University Scale for Psychopathology in Alzheimer's Disease (Devenand, Miller, Richards, Marder, & Bell, 1992), and the Cornell Scale for Depression in Dementia (Alexopoulos, Abrams, Young, & Shamoian, 1988) as its foundations. The original scale had 51 items reflecting a wide range of behaviors. The subsequent revision of the scale has 48 items. It is administered to a knowledgeable informant because of the concerns about the reliability of patients as informants. The scale is completed by a trained interviewer who can question the informant, supplement items with appropriate examples, and make overall judgments about the validity of the informant's response. Items are scaled by frequency of occurrence because of concern that severity judgments would be more difficult to anchor and, hence, less reliable. Behaviors occurring only within a limited period (the previous month) are rated, although provision is made for noting occurrence of behaviors before the last month but since the illness began. Rating training is afforded via a training manual and video demonstration tape: clinical expertise is not required.

The original 51-item scale was applied to 303 subjects with dementia of the Alzheimer type who had undergone standardized clinical evaluations by the Consortium to Establish a Registry for Alzheimer's Disease. About 7% of these subjects resided in long-term care settings. Interrater reliability was high, with item κ ranging from .77 to 1.0. Preliminary factor analysis indicated that 8 factors could be mapped onto clinically relevant domains: depressive features, psychotic features, defective self regulation, irritability/aggression, vegetative features, apathy, aggression, and affective lability.

The subjects in this study were primarily mildly–moderately and severely demented. Within the severity range available, there were generally more behavioral changes in the more severely dementia patients, but this issue needs to be addressed further. While establishing validity of this scale was not the primary objective of the study, preliminary analyses indicated convergence between the BRSD and a separate global estimate of behavioral change.

Based on this study, the instrument was modified and shortened slightly, to 48 items. A follow-up study of the revised version has been performed in more than 700 patients with dementia including a large proportion who had more severe dementia. The fundamental psychometric properties of the scale stood up well. Factor analysis indicated 6 clinically interpretable factors for more severely impaired patients, and five for the less severely impaired patients, which overlap with those found in the preliminary study. A scoring manual and norms for scoring are available (Mack J, 1996, personal communication). The scale has been used in several multicenter studies performed by the Alzheimer's Disease Cooperative Study. It has also been used successfully as an outcome measure in a study in agitated demented nursing home patients (Tariot, 1996, unpublished observation). Further studies are under way to perform cluster analysis and address test/retest reliability, change in the BRSD over time, and the relationship of change in this instrument to change in other commonly used scales. Some of these studies are examining the advantage of increasing the range of possible frequency endorsements, which may increase the sensitivity of the instrument in assessing clinical change. The major advantage of the instrument is that it is comprehensive, was developed according to sound psychometric principles, has a rapidly expanding psychometric foundation, and is reliable and easy to use. The major disadvantage is its length. For that reason, the authors are developing a 17-item short version.

Multidimensional Observation Scale for Elderly Subjects (MOSES) (Helmes, Csapo, & Short, 1987).

The MOSES was developed to provide a standardized, objective measure of the physical needs and intellectual functioning of elderly residents of long-term care facilities. This, in turn, would assist in decision making regarding institutional needs, clinical change, program evaluation, and any other research requiring valid and reliable assessment tools (Helmes, Csapo, & Short, 1987). It was developed in the context of a longitudinal research program and was based on empirical factor analyses of earlier instruments to identify major areas of functioning that made theoretical sense. Clear anchor descriptors are included, and scaling is homogeneous. The result of the development process was a 40-item scale assessing five areas of functioning with eight items each: self-care functioning, disoriented behavior, depressed/anxious mood, irritable behavior, and withdrawn behavior. The original study was performed in 2,542 individuals, not all of whom had a dementia. For purposes of this review, the domains addressing other than disturbed behavior will be ignored.

This scale is a self-administered questionnaire for the caregiver having the most frequent day-to-day contact with the patient. Behaviors are rated over the past week. Most items are based on frequency assessment, although some also according to severity. The psychometric foundation of this instrument is solid, with high levels of interreliability (0.58 to 0.97) and internal consistency (0.8). The instrument is sensitive to change over time, easy to use, and simply worded. Neither subjective judgment nor direct observation is required. Perhaps its major drawback, as Table 4.1 indicates, is that certain domains are excluded, such as psychosis and vegetative features. Conversely, the MOSES captures positive or adaptive behaviors that other instruments do not. The MOSES has a firm place in the repertoire of behavioral scales in this setting.

Neuropsychiatric Inventory (NPI) (Cummings, Mega, Gray, Rosenberg-Thompson, & Carusi, 1994).

The NPI was developed to assess a wide range of behaviors encountered in dementia patients, to provide a means of distinguishing frequency and severity of behavioral changes, and to facilitate rapid behavioral assessment through the use of screening questions (Cummings, Mega, Gray, Rosenberg-Thompson, & Carusi, 1994). The original subjects were 40 outpatients with different types of dementias, and 40 normal controls. The constructs were selected after comprehensive review of the literature and pilot work in patients with dementias. The domains are as follows: delusions, hallucinations, agitation, depression, anxiety, euphoria, apathy, disinhibition, irritability, aberrant motor behavior, night time behaviors, and appetite and eating changes.

To minimize the time required to assess multiple domains, the NPI incorporates screening questions providing an overview of each specific behavioral domain. If the behavior is present, the domain is then explored with up to eight further questions, providing more detailed information. If the behavioral domain in question is absent, the follow-up questions are ignored. The follow-up questions address both frequency (clearly anchored) and severity (not as clearly anchored: "mild, moderate, marked") as well as caregiver distress. This yields four scores for each domain: frequency, severity, total (frequency times severity), and caregiver distress. Information is obtained from a structured interview of a qualified informant with a total of up to 92 questions. This process can take from 10 to 35 minutes, depending on the complexity of the patient's behavioral syndrome. A training manual and videotape are available at cost (UCLA Neuropsychiatric Institute, 740 Westwood Plaza, Los Angeles, CA 90024). The time window is arbitrarily determined by the needs of the study. Published interrater agreement for the target domains ranges from 89.4% to 100%.

The NPI has several potential advantages. It provides clear language and is easy to use. The frequency scoring is clear, although the severity is less well anchored. It provides comprehensive coverage of the domains of interest. The novel use of screening questions reduces the time required for administration in simple cases, although not for more complex cases. The definition of domains is more detailed than most other instruments, and the instrument covers some domains not covered by other instruments, such as euphoria (not often seen in dementia), and disinhibition and lability. The NPI is still early in development so its value is not yet firmly established. Its applicability to severely impaired patients, or those in the nursing home, is not yet known. There are unpublished data showing its utility as an outcome measure (Kaufer, Cummings, & Christine, 1996), and it is being used as a secondary measure in several multicenter studies, including in the nursing home, meaning that it will have a greater psychometric foundation presently.

Psychogeriatric Dependency Rating Scale (PDGRS) (Wilkinson & Graham-White, 1980). The PGDRS is a structured standardized observer rating scale for the evaluation of several domains pertinent to elderly institutionalized patients: physical function, orientation, and behavior. The behavioral subscale, which is separate, is the focus of this review. The instrument consists of 16 clearly anchored items that are rated accorded to frequency, intended to capture the time-demanding characteristics of the behaviors in question. The scale is self-administered by an institutional staff member most familiar with the subject. It can also be administered as a structured interview. Interrater reliability was originally reported to range from 0.71 to 0.87, and its validity measured by its ability to predict organic diagnosis (0.71) and mortality (0.40) (Wilkinson & Graham-White, 1980). This has been supported by extensive subsequent work (Deutsch, Bylsma, Rovner, Steele, & Folstein, 1991; Frederiksen, Tariot, & DeJonghe, 1996; Morriss, Rovner, & German, 1995; Rovner, Kafonek, Filipp, Lucas, & Folstein, 1986; Tariot, Podgorski, Blazina, & Leibovici, 1993). It has also been shown to be sensitive to change in clinical conditions of nursing home patients over time and as a result of interventions (Burton, Rovner, German, Brant, & Clark, 1995; Tariot et al., unpublished observations).

The major advantage of the instrument is that it is brief, with simple and clear instructions for scoring. It was developed specifically for use in nursing home populations, not necessarily restricted to dementias, although certainly applicable for dementia patients as well. The major disadvantage is that it omits several domains of interest (see Table 4.1) and does not offer any level of detail. Scoring is based on examination of individual items, use of an overall total frequency score, or use of the number of behaviors present. There is no widely accepted factor analysis, although Morriss, Rovner, and German (1995) performed factor analysis on 451 nursing home residents at admission and identified four factors: antisocial behavior problems, motor activity behavior problems, difficult communication, and demanding behavior. It remains to be seen if these factors are robust in further studies.

Revised Memory and Behavior Problems Checklist (RMBPC) (Teri et al., 1992). This is a 24-item, caregiver-report measure based on the Memory and Behavior

Problems Checklist (Zarit, Orr, & Zarit, 1986), developed to assess behaviors in community-residing patients with dementia). It was based on data obtained from 201 geriatric patients and their caregivers. It is a self-administered questionnaire, on which the caregiver rates the frequency of each behavior problem during the past week and the caregiver's reaction to each behavior. It is easy to complete in 15 to 20 minutes and easy to score. Factor analysis confirmed three first-order factors: memory-related problems, depressive features, and disruptive behaviors. Although the memory-related items, such as repeated questions, do not strictly fit the construct of this review, the depressive and disruptive items do. Nine items address depressive or anxious features, and eight address disruptive behaviors including arguing, awakening the caregiver, verbal and physical aggression, embarrassing behavior, and verbal disruption. Internal consistency is reported as good, with mean coefficients of 0.75 for frequency ratings and 0.87 for reaction ratings. Delusions, hallucinations, illusions, most vegetative features, and apathetic features are not assessed by this checklist, probably related to the deliberate focus on observable as well as conceptually relevant and potentially modifiable behaviors, using objective frequency criteria. The RMBPC is currently being used in a series of longitudinal investigations and treatment outcome studies.

Wagner, Teri, and Orr-Rainey (1995a, 1995b), created a version of the RMBPC suited to nursing home use, the Memory and Behavioral Problem Checklist–Nursing Home (MBPC-NH). Items from the RMBPC that were not applicable to nursing home residents were omitted (e.g., unable to shop, clean house, and handle money). Another change was that informants rated behaviors that occur frequently (defined as two to three times per week) in a dichotomous yes/no fashion rather than a Likert scale. Finally, items relevant to a wide range of memory, emotional and functional problems, such as those found in the nursing home, were added (e.g., unable to follow verbal direction, or appears sad or depressed).

The item descriptors are simple and clear, and examples of frequency are provided. All items are based on observation or questioning of the patient. The 41 items have been grouped into four categories: memory, emotional problems, functional problems, and other problems. For purposes of this review, the functional and memory problems will not be considered. The empirically derived groupings could arguably be made differently, for instance, based on syndromal considerations, but given the lack of data on syndromal characteristics in a nursing home population, an empirical categorization may be best.

This newly revised scale has a limited psychometric foundation in its current form, although its predecessors are well grounded, and preliminary results regarding reliability ($\alpha = 0.82$) are encouraging (Wagner, Teri, & Orr-Rainey, 1995). It provides a rapid and apparently reliable screening survey of virtually all of the domains of interest. The person completing the questionnaire must have a 10th-grade reading ability, which may limit its utility somewhat. Future studies will clarify whether factors emerge that map onto the domains proposed as the organizing principle for this review. Because the RMBPC and the MBPC-NH are closely related and there are more psychometric data regarding the former, the RMBPC is included in Table 4.1.

CONCLUSION

There are a wide variety of behavioral tools to choose from, each with relative advantages and disadvantages. Some are widely used for specific purposes, and have a well-established psychometric foundation, but miss domains of interest, such as the

CMAI. For the most comprehensive assessment of the domains relevant for this review, the CERAD, BRSD, and NPI may be the best choices. However, they are incompletely developed from a psychometric perspective. The simplest instrument, with extensive nursing home use, is the PGDRS; its major weakness is that it is short on detail. The MBPC–NH and the MOSES are intermediate in this regard. Both have extensive psychometric foundations cover domains outside of the purview of the article, such as cognition and functional status, and the MOSES captures positive, adaptive behaviors. The MOSES was also incorporated into the core battery of the Special Care Unit Collaborative Study (Ory, 1994). The BPRS is probably best reserved for applications where a sensitive, reliable, general measure of psychopathology is needed to assess change, usually as a result of an intervention.

This article makes an important point: assessing behavior objectively is an important undertaking in attempting to improve our understanding of the welfare of chronically ill patients. The recent proliferation of behavioral assessment measures underscores the need for continued scrutiny of the methods employed in their development. This article offers an overview of some of the standards that should be applied to existing instruments as well as those to come and offers more detailed profiling of specific choices.

REFERENCES

Alexopoulos, G. S., Abrams, R. C., Young, R. C., & Shamoian, C. A. (1988). Cornell scale for depression in dementia. *Biological Psychiatry, 23*, 271-284.

Baumgarten, M., Becker, R., & Gauthier, S. (1990). Validity and reliability of the Dementia Behavior Disturbance Scale. *Journal of American Geriatrics Society, 38*, 221-226.

Burns, A., Jacoby, R., & Levy, R. (1990). Psychiatric phenomena in Alzheimer's disease. *British Journal of Psychiatry, 157*, 72-94.

Burton, L. C., Rovner, B. W., German, P. S., Brant, L. J., & Clark, R. D. (1995). Neuroleptic use and behavioral disturbance in nursing homes: A 1-year study. *International Psychogeriatrics, 7*, 535-545.

Cohen-Mansfield, J. (1986). Agitated behaviors in the elderly: 2. Preliminary results in the cognitively deteriorated. *Journal of American Geriatrics Society, 34*, 722-732.

Cummings, J. L., Mega, M., Gray, K., Rosenberg-Thompson, S., & Carusi, D. A. (1994). The neuropsychiatric inventory: Comprehensive assessment of psychopathology in dementia. *Neurology, 44*, 2308-2314.

Deutsch, L. H., Bylsma, F. W., Rovner, B. W., Steele, C., & Folstein, M. F. (1991). Psychosis and physical aggression in probable Alzheimer's disease. *American Journal of Psychiatry, 148*, 1159-1163.

Devanand, D. P., Miller, L., Richards, M., Marder, K., Bell, K., & et al. (1992). The Columbia University Scale for Psychopathology in Alzheimer's Disease. *Archives of Neurology, 49*, 371-376.

Drachman, D. A., Swearer, J. M., O'Donnell, B. F., Mitchell, A. L., & Maloon, A. (1992). The Caretaker Obstreperous-Behavior Rating Assessment (COBRA) Scale. *Journal of American Geriatrics Society, 40*, 463-470.

Finkel, S. I., Lyon, J. S., & Anderson, R. L. (1993). A Brief Agitation Rating Scale (BARS) for nursing home elderly. *Journal of American Geriatrics Society, 41*, 50-52.

Frederiksen, K., Tariot, P., & DeJonghe, E. (1996). Minimun Data Set Plus (MDS+) scores compared with scores from five rating scales. *Journal of American Geriatrics Society, 44*, 305-309.

Helmes, E., Csapo, K. G., & Short, J. A. (1987). Standardization and validation of the Multidimensional Observation Scale for Elderly Subjects (MOSES). *Journal of Gerontology, 42*, 395-405.

Hedlund, J. L., & Vieweg, B. W. (1980). The Brief Psychiatric Rating Scale (BRRS): A comprehensive review. *Journal of Operational Psychiatry, 11*, 48-65.

Hurley, A., Volicer, B., & Hanrahan, P. (1992). Assessment of discomfort in advanced Alzheimer patients. *Research in Nursing and Health, 15*, 369-377.

Kaufer, D. I., Cummings, J. L., & Christine, D. (1996). Effect of Tracrine on behavioral symptoms in Alzheimer's disease: An open-label study. *Journal of Geriatrics, Psychiatry, and Neurology, 9*, 1-6.

Levin, H. S., High, W. M., Goethe, K. E., Sisson, R. A., Overall, J. E., & Rhoade, H. M., Eisenberg, H. M., Kalisky, Z., Gary, H.E. (1987). The Neurobehavioral Rating Scale: Assessment of the behavioral sequalae of head injury by the clinician. *Journal of Neurology, Neurosurgery, Psychiatry, 50*, 183-193.

Loreck, D. J., Bylsma, F. W., & Folstein, M. F. (1994). A new scale for comprehensive assessment of psychopathology in Alzheimer's disease. *American Journal of Geriatric Psychiatry, 2*, 60-74.

Lorr, M., Klett, C. J., McNair, D. M., & Lasky, J. J. (1962). *Inpatient Multidimensional Psychiatric Scale, Manual.* Palo Alto, CA: Consulting Psychologists Press.

Molloy, D. W., McIlroy, W. E., Guyatt, G. H., & Lever, J. A. (1991). Validity and reliability of the Dysfunctional Behaviour Rating Instrument. *Acta Psychiatrica Scandinavica, 84*, 103-106.

Morriss, R. K., Rovner, B. W., & German, P. S. (1995). Clinical and psychosocial variables associated with different types of behaviour problem in new nursing home admissions. *International Journal of Geriatric Psychiatry, 10*, 547-555.

Mungas, D., Weiler, P., Franzi, C., & Henry, R. (1989). Assessment of disruptive behavior associated with dementia: The Disruptive Behavior Rating Scales. *Journal of Geriatrics, Psychiatry, and Neurology, 2*, 196-202.

Ory, M. (1994). Dementia special care: The development of a National Research Initiative. *Alzheimer's Disease and Associated Disorders, 8*(Suppl. 1), S389-S404.

Overall, J. E., & Beller, S. A. (1984). The Brief Psychiatric Rating Scale in geropsychiatric research: 1. Factor structure on an inpatient unit. *Journal of Gerontology, 39*, 187-193.

Overall, J. E., & Gorham, D. R. (1962). The Brief Psychiatric Rating Scale. *Psychological reports, 10*, 799-812.

Overall, J. E., & Gorham, D. R. (1988). The Brief Psychiatric Rating Scale (BPRS): Recent developments in ascertainment and scaling. *Psychopharmacology Bulletin, 24*, 97-98.

Patel, V., & Hope, R. A. (1992). A Rating Scale for Aggressive Behavior in the Elderly-the RAGE. *Psychological Medicine, 22*, 211-221.

Patterson, M., Schnell, A., Martin, R., Mendez, M., Smyth, K., & Whitehouse, P. J. (1990). Assessment of behavioral and affective symptoms in Alzheimer's disease. *Journal of Geriatric Psychiatry and Neurology, 3*, 21-30.

Ray, W., Taylor, J., Lichtenstein, M., & Meador, K. (1992). The nursing home behavior problem scale. *Journal of Gerontology*, M9-M16.

Reisberg, B., Borenstein, J., Salob, S. P., Ferris, S. H., Franssen, E., & Georgotas, A. (1987). Behavioral symptoms in Alzheimer's disease: Phenomenology and treatment. *Journal of Clinical Psychiatry, 48*, 9-15.

Reisberg, B., Franssen, E., Sclan, S. G., Kluger, A., & Ferri, S. H. (1989). Stage specific incidence of potentially remediable behavioral symptoms in aging and Alzheimer's disease: A study of 120 patients using the BEHAVE-AD. *Bulletin of Clinical Neurosciences, 54,* 95-112.

Reisberg, B., Ferris, S. H., Tarossian, C., Kluger, A., & Monteiro, I. (1992). Pharmacologic treatment of Alzheimer's disease: A methodologic critique based upon current knowledge of symptomatology and relevance for drug trials. *International Psychogeriatrics* (Suppl. 1), 9-42.

Rhoades, H. M., & Overall, E. (1988). The semistructured BPRS interview and rating guide. *Psychopharmacology Bulletin, 24,* 101-104.

Rosen, J., Burgio, L., Kollar, M., Cain, M., Allison, M., Fogleman, M., Michael, M., & Zubneko, G. (1994). The Pittsburgh Agitation Scale: A user-friendly instrument for rating agitation in dementia patients. *American Journal of Geriatric Psychiatry, 2,* 52-59.

Rosen, W. G., Mohs, R. C., & Davis, K. L. (1984). A new rating scale for Alzheimer's disease. *American Journal of Psychiatry, 141,* 1356-1364.

Rovner, B. W., Kafonek, S., Filipp, L., Lucas, M. J., & Folstein, M. F. (1986). Prevalence of mental illness in a community nursing home. *American Journal of Psychiatry, 143,* 1446-1449.

Ryden, M. (1988). Aggressive behaviors in persons with dementia who live in the community. *Alzheimer's Disease Related Disorders, 2,* 342-355.

Sclan, S. G., Saillon, A., Franssen, E., Hugonot-Diener, I., Saillon, A., & et al. (in press). The Behavior Pathology in Alzheimer's Disease Rating Scale (BEHAVE-AD): Reliability and analysis of symptom category scores. *International Psychogeriatrics.*

Sinha, D., Zemlan, F. P., Nelson, S., Beinenfeld, D., Thienhaus, O., & et al. (1992). A new scale for assessing behavioral agitation in dementia. *Psychiatry Research, 41,* 73-88.

Sultzer, D. L., Berisord, M. A., & Gunay, I. (1995). The Neurobehavioral Rating Scale: Reliability in patients with dementia. *Journal of Psychiatric Research, 29,* 185-191.

Sultzer, D. L., Levin, H. S., Mahler, M. E., High, W. M., & Cummings, J. L. (1992). Assessment of cognitive, psychiatric, and behavioral disturbances in patients with dementia: The Neurobehavioral Rating Scale. *Journal of American Geriatrics Society, 40,* 549-555.

Sultzer, D. L., Levin, H. S., Mahler, M. E., High, W. M., & Cummings, J. L. (1993). A comparison of psychiatric symptoms in vascular dementia and Alzheimer's disease. *American Journal of Psychiatry, 150,* 1806-1812.

Tarell, J. D., & Schulz, S. C. (1988). Nursing assessment using the BPRS: A structured interview. *Psychopharmacology Bulletin, 24,* 105-111.

Tariot, P. N., & Blazina, L. (1994). The psychopathology of dementia. In J. C. Morris (Ed.), *Handbook of dementing illnesses* (pp. 461-475). New York: Dekker.

Tariot, P. N., Cohen, R. M., Sunderland, T., Newhouse, P., Yount, D., Mellow, A., Weingartner, H., Mueller, E. A., & Murphy, D. L. (1987). L-deprenyl in Alzheimer's disease: Preliminary evidence for behavioral change with MAO-B inhibition. *Archives of General Psychiatry, 44,* 427-433.

Tariot, P. N., Frederiksen, K., Erb, R., Leibovici, A., Podgorski, C. A., Asnis, J., & Cox, C. (1995). Lack of carbamazephine toxicity in frail nursing home patients: A controlled study. *Journal of American Geriatrics Society, 43,* 1026-1029.

Tariot, P. N., Mack, J. L., Patterson, M. B., Edland, S. D., Weiner, M. F., Fillenbaum, G., Blazina, L., Teri, L., Rubin, E., Mortimer, J. A., Stern, Y., & the CERAD Behavioral Pathology Committee. (1995). The Behavior Rating Scale for dementia of the consotium to establish a registry for Alzheimer's disease. *American Journal of Psychiatry, 152,* 1349-1357.

Tariot, P. N., Podgorski, C. A., Blazina, L., & Leibovici, A. (1993). Mental disorders in the nursing home: Another perspective. *American Journal of Psychiatry, 150,* 1063-1069.

Teri, L., Larson, E. B., & Reifler, B. V. (1988). Behavioral disturbance in dementia of the Alzheimer's type. *Journal of American Geriatrics Society, 36,* 1-6.

Teri, L., Truax, P., Logsdon, R., Uomoto, J., Zarit, S., & Vitaliano, P. (1992). Assessment of behavioral problems in dementia: The revised memory and behavior problems checklist. *Psychology of Aging, 7,* 622-631.

Teri, L., & Logsdon, R. G. (1995). Methodologic issues regarding outcome measure for clinical drug trials of psychiatric complications in dementia. *Journal of Geriatrics, Psychiatry, and Neurology, 8*(Suppl.), S8-S17.

Wagner, A. W., Teri, L., & Orr-Rainey, N. (1995). Behavior problems among dementia residents in special care units: Changes over time. *Journal of American Geriatrics Society, 43,* 784-787.

Wagner, A. W., Teri, L., & Orr-Rainey, N. (1995). Behavior problems among dementia residents in Special care units: Changes over time. *Alzheimer's Disease and Associated Disorders, 9,* 121-127.

Weiner, M. F., Koss, E., Wild, K. V., Folks, D. G., Tariot, P., Luszcynska, H., & Whitehouse, P. (1996). Measures of psychiatric symptoms in Alzheimer's patients: A review. *Alzheimer's Disease and Associated Disorders, 10,* 20-30.

Wilkinson, I., & Graham-White, J. (1980). Psychogeriatric Dependency Rating Scale (PGDRS): A method of assessment for use by nurses. *British Journal of Psychiatry, 137,* 558-565.

Wragg, R. E., & Jeste, D. V. (1989). Overview of depression and psychosis in Alzheimer's disease. *American Journal of Psychiatry, 146,* 577-587.

Zarit, S. H., Orr, N. H., & Zarit, J. (1986). Subjective burden of husbands and wives as caregivers: A longitudinal study. *The Gerontologist, 26,* 260-266.

Chapter 5

Assessing Personality in Chronic Care Populations

Robert C. Abrams

In this chapter, measurement issues relevant to the personality functioning of patients in chronic care are reviewed. The studies on which this review is based are relatively recent and limited in number, but may have important implications for both scientists and caregivers. The text is divided into two main sections. The first section covers the measurement of personality in dementia, which relies on various trait dimensions, and the second section deals with the assessment of personality dysfunction in geriatric depression, which largely involves clinical personality disorder nosology. For the purposes of this review, personality *traits* are defined as the long-standing, characteristic ways in which a person perceives and relates to himself and others; personality *disorders* are enduring patterns of dysfunctional behavior that pervade multiple facets of a person's life.

MEASUREMENT OF PERSONALITY IN DEMENTIA

Nature of the Construct

A small but influential literature concerned with the progression of personality changes in dementia has emerged since the late 1980s. Most of these articles have reported on patients with Alzheimer's disease, although some also included multiinfarct or other dementias. Virtually all of the studies in this area have used the same basic format: Caregiver or relative ratings of subjects' premorbid and postonset personality traits. However, what differs from study to study is the selection of personality assessment instrument, with the result that the traits evaluated also vary, and the overall directions of the field can be difficult to distinguish.

It is helpful to organize this literature into three groups according to the content of personality assessment. The first group of studies based personality assessment on the 11 personality items of the Blessed Dementia Scale (Blessed et al., 1968), and then used factor analysis and further combinations of factors to produce sets of clinically related behaviors (Bozzola et al., 1992; Rubin, Morris, & Berg, 1987; Rubin, Morris, Storandt, & Berg, 1987); the second group of studies relied on an inventory originally applied by

Acknowledgment. This study was supported by NIMH grants K07-MH01025-04, P20-MH49762, and RO-MH51842.

Brooks and McKinlay (1983) to patients with head injury (Cummings et al., 1990; Petry et al., 1988, 1989); and the third group used the NEO-PI (Costa & McRae, 1985) (Chatterjee et al., 1992; Siegler et al., 1991, 1994; Strauss et al., 1993; Strauss & Pasupathi, 1994; Welleford et al., 1995).

Several other instruments that include some assessment of personality do not fit conveniently into this organization because their content is focused mainly on the behavioral symptoms of dementing disorders, or their coverage of personality traits is not comprehensive. Examples of instruments measuring mostly behavior include the Caretaker Obstreperous–Behavior Rating Assessment Scale (Drachman et al., 1992); the Behavioral Pathology in Alzheimer's Disease Rating Scale (Behave-AD) (Reisberg & Ferris, 1985; Reisberg et al., 1987); the Cohen-Mansfield Agitation Inventory (Cohen-Mansfield, 1986); and a behavioral symptomatology scale designed for Alzheimer patients by Kumar et al. (1988). The scales for irritability, aggression, and apathy used by Burns et al. (1990) overlap partially with personality domains. Psychiatric assessments designed for general populations but sometimes used for demented clients, such as the Brief Psychiatric Rating Scale (Overall & Gorham, 1988), also include some coverage of personality traits.

What are the domains of personality assessed by these instruments? The investigators using factor analysis of Blessed Dementia Scale personality items, for example, Rubin et al. (1987), proposed four clinically recognizable groups of traits: passive, agitated, self-centered, and suspicious. Similarly, investigators using the Brooks and McKinlay inventory, for example, Petry et al. (1988), organized traits into three clinical categories: passive, coarsened, and immature. The NEO-PI, based on the five factors of neuroticism, extraversion, openness, conscientiousness, and agreeableness, includes traits covered by the other instruments, but the factors are somewhat less identifiable clinically. Conversely, an advantage of the five-factor model is that the dimensions represent more fully the scope of normal personality and in the absence of disease are relatively stable over the adult age range (Costa & McCrae, 1989); thus, personality change in dementia can be comprehensively evaluated using the NEO-PI and is likely to be associated with the dementing process.

However, there remains doubt about whether the passivity, withdrawal, loss of interest, lability, and immaturity of emotional responses seen in dementia should be viewed as "personality" phenomena rather than simply behavioral manifestations of central nervous system dysfunction. Changes in intellectual functioning, mood, and behavior can all be subsumed under the rubric of dementing syndromes; agitation and irritability, in particular, seem to be symptomatic expressions of dementia. However, Cummings et al. (1990) argue persuasively that changes in the manner of emotional expression, ways of relating to others, enthusiasm, and maturity all reflect alterations in long-standing behavioral style and can thus be conceptualized as personality changes.

Another possible problem is that none of the three major trait schemes fully capture the aspects of personality mentioned by Cummings et al. (1990). They are essentially measures of temperament on which comprehensive theories of personality are built and for which there is some normative and reliability data. However, the trait schemes alone do not satisfactorily describe what changes about the demented person's inner experience or interactions with others. Thus, there is room for the creation of new dimensions.

What would be the content of the new dimensions? There are numerous possibilities. To elaborate one, Crowell et al. (1990), who analyzed criteria for DSM-III-R personality disorders according to Epstein's Cognitive-Experiential Self-Theory (Epstein, 1991), suggested that individuals consciously or unconsciously hold particular views of the world and assumptions about themselves ("self-postulates"); these idiosyncratic self-postulates strongly influence their coping styles, and pathological coping styles in turn constitute personality disorders. Although the intent of Crowell et al. (1990) was to find a theoretical basis for personality disorder comorbidity, other applications may be possible. Demented patients can also manifest self-postulates and coping styles, and these could be assessed systematically by staff members in chronic care settings. Even nonverbal dementia patients have characteristic coping styles and may retain consistent strategies of approaching the world. Thus, caregiver observations might be directed toward assessment of personality disorder equivalents, or at least toward clinically richer categories than arrived at through single dimensions or factor analysis. However, extensive work would be needed to establish convergent validity for this or any other scheme.

Personality Change in Dementia: Preliminary Findings

In senile dementia of the Alzheimer type (SDAT), the most frequent early personality change using the Blessed and Brooks and McKinlay schemes is an increase in passivity, including loss of interest in hobbies and activities, loss of spontaneity, and general disengagement (Petry et al., 1988; Rubin, Morris, & Berg, 1987). As the illness progresses, agitated and self-centered behaviors also become apparent (Rubin, Morris, & Berg, 1987). Based on the NEO-PI, there is an early SDAT profile of increased neuroticism and reduced extraversion and conscientiousness compared with premorbid baseline (Chatterjee et al., 1992); these trends continue as the disease progresses, along with smaller decreases in openness and agreeableness (Siegler et al., 1994; Welleford et al., 1995). The increased neuroticism has been interpreted to be consistent with the negative emotionality seen in Alzheimer patients, the reduced extraversion with decreased social functioning, and the reduced conscientiousness with intellectual decline (Strauss & Pasupathi, 1994). Early SDAT may also be associated with more anxiety and dysphoria than more advanced stages, when patients' awareness of the illness seems to recede (Chatterjee et al., 1992; Siegler et al., 1991). In multiinfarct dementia (MID), patients at a comparable phase of illness may show greater maturity and control than individuals with SDAT (Cummings et al., 1990), but over time both SDAT and MID patients show deterioration in social functioning and loss of integrity of the personality.

Personality changes do not seem to have a simple linear relationship to the severity of cognitive impairment. The presence of personality changes at a mild stage of SDAT does not necessarily imply a more rapid progression of dementia (Rubin, Morris, & Berg, 1987), whereas only one personality dimension of the Brooks and McKinlay scheme, excitability, correlated significantly with severity of intellectual impairment (Petry et al., 1988). Moreover, the personality changes associated with dementia bear no particular relationship to premorbid personality style. There is no evidence to support the popular belief that dementia exacerbates premorbid personality patterns. Rather, the consistency of the reported personality changes suggests that they reflect structural and functional deficits resulting from the disease process itself (Petry et al., 1988; Siegler et al., 1991). The lack of an obvious relationship between premorbid traits and personality functioning in SDAT does not, however, preclude the possibility that premorbid personality traits influence the expression of other psychiatric symptoms after the dementia is established. For example, in their sample of SDAT patients, Chatterjee et al. (1992) found associations between paranoid delusions and premorbid hostility and between hallucinations and premorbid openness. It is not known whether higher premorbid neuroticism predisposes to depressive symptoms in dementia.

Biological Correlates

It is intriguing to speculate on a biological basis for the personality changes described in dementia. The notion that personality dimensions in normal adults have a biological underpinning was proposed by Eysenck (1967). Cloninger (1987) subsequently marshaled evidence that the fundamental trait dimensions of novelty seeking, harm avoidance, and reward dependence are mediated by dopamine, serotonin, and norepinephrine neurotransmitter systems, respectively. The recently reported association of novelty seeking with polymorphism of the dopamine D4 receptor gene appears not to be affected by age despite the reduction with aging of novelty seeking in normative data (Benjamin et al., 1996; Ebstein et al., 1996); as a result of the interest generated by these reports, novelty seeking is likely to become a focus of research seeking to clarify the relative contributions of genes and aging to personality. A possible explanation is that the putative genetic predisposition to novelty seeking may be modified in some individuals by changes in dopamine metabolism or by factors associated with aging.

In SDAT, acetylcholine, norepinephrine, and serotonin neurotransmitter are systematically affected (Gottfries, 1990), which may to some degree account for the uniformity of the personality changes in that disorder. Conversely, personality changes may also be theoretically explained on a structural basis. Because plaques and neurofibrillary tangles tend to affect bilateral medial temporal lobes early in the disease, some of the personality changes of mild SDAT would be expected to be similar to the changes in personality and affect regulation associated with other lesions in this region. For example, remote affect, hyper-religiosity and other behaviors are seen in temporal lobe dysfunction (Miller et al., 1994). The Kluver-Bucy syndrome, described in monkeys after removal of the anterior temporal lobes and amygdala, involves hyperorality, hypersexuality, and placidity (Kluver & Bucy, 1939). Other behaviors might signal frontal lobe involvement later in the course of the dementia. In MID, or vascular dementia, involvement of brainstem and reticular-activating system may account for the overall slowness of mental processing (Mahler & Cummings, 1991). Also, vascular disease involving connections between basal ganglia and cortex, thought to be related to a particular constellation of "vascular" depressive symptoms, may likewise affect personality functioning; patients with "vascular" depression may have a syndrome consisting of deficits in cognitive and executive functions, psychomotor retardation, and impaired activities of daily living, with a relative absence of depressive ideation (Alexopoulos et al., 1996).

Methodological Issues: Problem of Informants

The central methodological problem across all investigations of personality in dementia is the lack of a valid and reliable paradigm for direct assessment of the subjects. Because dementia by definition involves impairments in memory and judgment, self-report cannot be used. Instead, researchers have had no option other than the use of information given by informants. An element of variability is thereby introduced, depending on whether the informants are related or unrelated, and, if related, whether they are spouses, children, or siblings of the subject. For example, unrelated informants frequently cannot provide information on premorbid personality, and they would be more likely to offer objective cross-sectional reports of behavior. In contrast, relative informants should be able to provide information on what the subject was like before the onset of illness, but their observations on the differences in behavior between past and present may be biased by how they are related to the subject, the quality of that relationship, or by their feelings about the illness. For example, Petry et al. (1988) found that SDAT patients were reported by their spouses to have been happier, more social, and more easy going before the onset of dementia than normal subjects were thought to be by their spouses before retirement. Probably the patient's current debilitated state encouraged a distortion of spouses' retrospective memories. In addition, caregivers' own personality traits may color their perceptions and reactions to clients, and influence their levels of stress. Welleford et al. (1995) administered the NEO-PI to Alzheimer patients as well as to their caregiver informants, and found that patient concientiousness and caregiver neuroticism both contributed to caregivers' burden. Depression and other psychiatric syndromes among dementia caregivers have been receiving attention recently (Morris et al., 1988), although informants' mental state has not been explicitly considered in the analysis of the data reviewed here.

Overall, there has probably been more experience using the NEO-PI than other instruments in the collection of informant data on personality traits in demented subjects. Initially standardized using a general adult population rather than college students, the NEO-PI has also been standardized for both self-report and informant formats, with significant concordance between the two found in normal adults (Costa & McCrae, 1988). Also, there is at least initial evidence of interobserver reliability and stability in dementia studies. In an SDAT sample, significant agreement using the NEO-PI was found between the observations of primary caregivers and another informant (Strauss et al., 1993). In that study, intraclass correlations between the two raters for retrospective assessment of premorbid personality ranged from .51 to .60 (except for conscientiousness, which had much lower agreement, with ICC = .24); intraclass correlations between the two raters for assessment of current personality ranged similarly from .48 to .67, with only conscientiousness, which measures adherence to tasks and may be especially sensitive to context, again showing low agreement (.23). The authors argued that this level of interrater agreement provides a measure of validity as well as reliability because the two raters knew the subjects in different settings and situations (Strauss et al., 1993). Also in SDAT patients, caregiver reports of premorbid personality traits on the NEO-PI provided on separate occasions one year apart did not differ significantly (Strauss & Pasupathi, 1994). Nevertheless, the reliability of informant personality data on demented subjects cannot at this stage be confidently assumed.

Methodological issues in this area of research are not confined to the use of informants. Several potentially important confounds have not yet been addressed in the literature. These include the co-occurrence or prior history of major psychiatric illness other than dementia; the use of psychotropic medications; and the demographic, cultural and clinical heterogeneity of samples. Most important is the need for prospective research of sufficient size and duration to establish findings firmly.

Clinical Implications

Personality change is one of the most distressing aspects of dementing illness; the expression of personality traits is a defining feature of one's individuality and humanity, and change in these dimensions has been described by family members as a kind of death (Petry et al., 1988). It is perhaps fortunate that in the inexorable progression of Alzheimer's disease, the patient's own awareness of these changes appears to be less acute than that of other people. However, the contribution of personality change in dementia patients to caregiver depression remains unknown.

Overwhelmingly, the clinical importance of personality changes in dementia results from the difficulties in day-to-day management posed by agitation, aggression, lability, withdrawal, and other behaviors. There is little doubt that these features of the illness are important contributors to the need for institutionalization (Strauss & Pasupathi, 1994) and to the stress and burden of those in close continual contact with the patient (Welleford et al., 1995).

Greater knowledge about the disease-specific progression of personality changes is likely to prove clinically important in several additional ways. First, the nature, direction, and chronology of personality changes may assist in the differential diagnosis of the dementias; in frontal lobe dementias, for example, personality changes may precede prominent intellectual deficits and provide the first clinical evidence of the disorder (Miller et al., 1994). Personality changes may also herald the various stages of the Alzheimer's dementia and facilitate their recognition. Second, knowledge about personality change could inform the development of interventions that could be empirically tested; even before such interventions are developed, caregiver stress and anger at the patient might be minimized by knowing what behaviors to expect and how they are related to the disease process. In this spirit, Deutsch and Rovner (1991) recommend that institutional and family caregivers keep a log of disturbing behaviors to enhance appreciation of the predictability of such events, examine the impact of their interventions, and limit the reaction of helplessness. Third, a more sophisticated understanding of personality psychopathology in dementia could help caregivers and clinicians identify target symptoms that might be amenable to pharmacological intervention (e.g., psychosis-driven symptoms that might respond to antipsychotic medication, affective lability that might respond to mood-stabilizing agents, or depressive symptoms that could be relieved with antidepressants). Of these areas, the phenomenon of depression in primary dementia deserves separate consideration.

Depression, Dementia, and Personality Traits

Both major depression and subsyndromal depressive symptoms occur frequently in the setting of primary dementia (Alexopoulos & Abrams, 1991) and can be difficult to distinguish from personality and behavioral changes. Loss of interest, for example, may be understood as a depressive, cognitive, or personality phenomenon. The Cornell Scale for Depression in Dementia (Alexopoulos et al., 1988) relies on the usually rapid onset or acuity of the loss of interest in depression to distinguish it from the more insidious loss of interest secondary to cognitive impairment or amotivational personality. Similarly, the agitation of demented patients who have comorbid depression may also be more acute and have a distinctive anguished quality (picking at the self, pulling hair, or wringing hands, frequently accompanied by mood-congruent verbal expressions). In some cases in which the clinical context is not sufficiently clear to untangle the depressive, cognitive, and personality features, empirical trials of antidepressant medication may be warranted.

PERSONALITY DISORDERS IN CHRONIC CARE

Cognitively intact elderly individuals are also found in chronic care settings, frequently because they have severe or treatment-resistant depression syndromes. The NEO-PI and other instruments have been used in these patients, and some trait profiles may be particularly associated with suicide (P. Duberstein, personal communication). However, in depressed elderly populations, personality is more frequently assessed according to clinical syndromes, usually the Axis II personality disorders using the Diagnostic and Statistical Manual of Mental Disorders (DSM) criteria (American Psychiatric Association, 1994). In a recent meta-analysis of the literature undertaken to determine the prevalence of personality disorder in the older than 50 years population, an overall rate of 10% was found (Abrams & Horowitz, 1996). Obsessive-compulsive, dependent, and personality disorder not otherwise specified were the most frequent diagnoses. As expected, the highest rates of personality disorder were among patients with a history of major depression, most of whom were assessed for Axis II criteria after treatment for the acute depressive episode; these rates were comparable with those reported in younger adult depressives (Pfohl et al., 1984; Shea et al., 1987).

Assessing Personality Disorders in Elderly Patients: Methodological Issues

Methodological problems abound in this area. Until recently, there was lingering doubt about whether elderly people can legitimately have personality disorders (Abrams, 1991). For example, in the DSM-III introductory notes to Axis II, personality disorders are described as becoming "attenuated" by middle age (American Psychiatric Association, 1980). The diagnostic criteria, particularly for borderline and antisocial disorders, have been thought to be age biased (Fogel & Westlake, 1990). Also, because symptoms are required to be present more or less continuously from adolescence through adulthood, the investigator must ask elderly subjects or informants to provide information over a lengthy time frame; in practice, it can be difficult to obtain detailed information of this nature. (The restrictive time-frame requirement was relaxed for the "organic personality syndrome" and its DSM-IV successor, "personality change due to a general medical syndrome," but only because a specific organic etiology was required).

Contamination of personality disorder assessment by the effects of residual depression poses another difficulty. Depressed patients may accentuate negative aspects of their lives including accounts of their personality psychopathology (Reich et al., 1987). For this reason, personality disorder assessment is usually deferred until resolution of the acute affective episode. The state-trait confound has not been systematically investigated in elderly subjects, but it may prove important even in treated patients because incomplete remissions and chronicity of depression are frequent in this age group (National Institutes of Health Consensus Conference, 1992).

Despite these problems, however, research in geriatric personality disorders has been facilitated by the development of instruments, such as the Personality Disorder

Examination (PDE) (Loranger, 1988), which yield both dimensional scores and categorical personality disorder diagnoses. Associations among continuous variables can thus be examined. The dimensional scores also permit inclusion of the many cases of subthreshold personality disorder seen in geriatric and chronic care populations. The PDE is a semistructured interview designed for administration by experienced clinicians; this feature permits the clarification of potential confounds between personality and depression symptoms through the use of clinical judgment in the scoring.

Significance of Personality Disorder Symptoms in Geriatric Depression

Associations have been reported between personality disorder and chronicity of affective symptoms (Devanand et al., 1994), suicide (Loebel, 1990), and poor outcome in short-term psychotherapy for depression (Thompson et al., 1994). However, the effect of personality disorder symptoms on long-term outcomes of major depression in the elderly has not been established. Partly because geriatric depression is characterized by chronicity or frequent relapses, and because personality disorders are not optimally assessed during periods of acute depression, attention has turned to personality disorder symptoms during the period of remission from depression.

For example, preliminary data suggest that instrumental activities of daily living (IADL) and interpersonal functioning may be areas in which personality disorder symptoms influence the quality of the recovery from geriatric depression (Abrams et al., 1996). IADL performance in remitted depressives was inversely correlated with overall personality disorder symptoms and particularly with the avoidant and dependent disorders (Abrams et al., 1996); the recovered elderly depressives with long-standing avoidant and dependent behaviors appeared to exaggerate obstacles in their approach to routine daily tasks, and thus experienced more disability after the acute phase of depression. With respect to interpersonal functioning, a similar picture emerged. Both sociability (active participation in social exchanges) and presence of a satisfying relationship (a measure of intimacy) were inversely correlated with overall personality disorder symptoms and particularly with the paranoid, schizoid, schizotypal, and narcissistic disorders.

Because remission from major depression is often incomplete, and residual depressive symptoms can also contribute to disability and poor interpersonal functioning (National Institute of Health Consensus Conference, 1992), clarifying the true source of effects is necessary. In the study cited previously, the associations between personality disorder symptoms and disability or poor interpersonal functioning were overwhelmed by high levels of residual depression. In contrast, at lower levels of depression personality disorder symptoms were predictive, both alone and in interaction with depression, of impaired functioning after remission (Abrams et al., 1996). Thus, with geriatric depression now appreciated as a persistently disabling illness (Alexopoulos & Chester, 1992), the contribution of personality disorder to long-term functioning is expected to be increasingly a subject of interest to clinicians.

CONCLUSION

Personality assessment in chronic care is becoming recognized as an important area of inquiry. In dementia, personality changes represent a loss of the patient's core identity and are responsible for considerable distress among family members if not among the patients themselves; yet personality changes in dementia may also serve as useful diagnostic and clinical markers, and provide targets for the development of pharmacological and environmental interventions. Further experience is needed using established dimensions, whereas newer approaches focusing more broadly on character would provide additional insight. In the absence of novel approaches or paradigms, however, the assessment of personality traits in demented subjects unavoidably requires informant data. At the present time, the NEO-PI has the strongest claims to interobserver reliability, stability, and convergent validity of informant assessments of personality in dementia patients; for this reason, the NEO-PI is emerging as the standard instrument of the new field.

Among the cognitively intact elders in chronic care, including those with depression syndromes, the personality assessment involves personality disorders as well as trait dimensions. Personality disorders are important as potential predictors of disability and social functioning in recovered elderly depressives. To minimize the possibility that a report of personality disorder, in fact, represents residual depression, it is recommended that the personality disorder assessment be undertaken only by experienced clinicians and at a time when depression symptoms are as completely remitted as possible. Most useful in research are instruments, such as the PDE, which do not rely entirely on self-report but allow for clinical judgment, and which yield dimensional data as well as categorical personality disorder diagnoses. Finally, in the cognitively intact group, personality assessment may be advanced by creative efforts to develop an age-sensitive personality disorder nosology.

REFERENCES

Abrams, R. C. (1991). The aging personality. (Editorial). *International Journal of Geriatric Psychiatry, 6,* 1-3.

Abrams, R. C. & Horowitz, S. V. (1996). Personality disorders after age 50: A meta-analysis. *Journal of Personality Disorders, 10,* 271-281.

Abrams, R., Spielman, L., Horowitz, S., Klausner, E., & Alexopoulos, G. (1996). Personality, ADL, and sociability in elderly depressives. In *Abstracts of the Ninth Annual Meeting and Symposium, American Association for Geriatric Psychiatry, Tucson, Arizona* (p. 19). Bethesda, MD: American Association for General Psychiatry.

Alexopoulos, G. S., & Abrams, R. C. (1991). Depression in Alzheimer's disease. *The Psychiatric Clinics of North America, 14,* 327-340.

Alexopoulos, G. S., Abrams, R. C., Young, R. C., & Shamoian, C. A. (1988). Cornell Scale for Depression in Dementia. *Biological Psychiatry, 23,* 271-284.

Alexopoulos, G. S., & Chester, J. G. (1992). Outcomes of geriatric depression. *Clinics in Geriatric Medicine, 8,* 363-376.

Alexopoulos, G. S., Meyers, B. S., Young, R. C., Kakuma, T., Charlson, M. E., & Silbersweig, D. A. (1996). The clinical presentation of vascular depression. In *New Research Abstracts, Annual Meeting of the American Psychiatric Association, New York* (p. 205). Washington, DC: American Psychiatric Association.

American Psychiatric Association (1980). *Diagnostic and statistical manual of mental disorders* (3rd ed.). Washington, DC: Author.

American Psychiatric Association (1994). *Diagnostic and statistical manual of mental disorders* (4th ed.). Washington, DC: Author.

Benjamin, J., Li, L., Patterson, C., Greenberg, B. D., Murphy, D. L., & Harner, D. H. (1996). Population and familial association between the D4 dopamine receptor gene and measures of novelty seeking. *Nature Genetics, 12,* 81-84.

Blessed, G., Tomlinson, B. E., & Roth, M. (1968). The association between quantitative measures of dementia and of senile change in the cerebral grey matter of elderly subjects. *British Journal of Psychiatry, 114,* 797-811.

Bozzola, F. G., Gorelick, P. B., & Freels, S. (1992). Personality changes in Alzheimer's disease. *Archives of Neurology, 49,* 297-300.

Brooks, D. N., & McKinlay, W. (1983). Personality and behavioural change after severe blunt head injury—a relative's view. *Journal of Neurology, Neurosurgery, and Psychiatry, 46,* 336-344.

Burns, A., Folstein, S., Brandt, J., & Folstein, M. (1990). Clinical assessment of irritability, aggression, and apathy in Huntington and Alzheimer disease. *The Journal of Nervous and Mental Disease, 178,* 20-26.

Chatterjee, A., Strauss, M. E., Smyth, K. A., & Whitehouse, P. J. (1992). Personality changes in Alzheimer's disease. *Archives of Neurology, 49,* 486-491.

Cloninger, C. R. (1987). A systematic method for clinical description and classification of personality variants. *Archives of General Psychiatry, 44,* 573-588.

Cohen-Mansfield, J. (1986). Agitated behaviors in the elderly: 2. Preliminary results in the cognitively deteriorated. *Journal of the American Geriatrics Society, 34,* 722-727.

Costa, P. T., & McCrae, R. R. (1985). *The NEO-Personality Inventory Manual.* Odessa, FL: Psychological Assessment Resources.

Costa, P. T., & McCrae, R. R. (1988). Personality in adulthood: A six-year longitudinal study of self-reports and spouse ratings on the NEO-PI personality inventory. *Journal of Personality and Social Psychology, 54,* 853-863.

Costa, P. T., & McCrae, R. R. (1989). Personality continuity and the changes of adult life. In M. Storandt, & G. VandenBos (Eds.), *The adult years: Continuity and change*: Vol. 8. *The Master Lectures*). Washington, DC: American Psychological Association.

Crowell J. A., Waters, E., & Kring, A. (1990, November 8-10). *The psychosocial etiologies of personality disorders: What is the answer like?* Paper presented at the National Institute of Mental Health Conference on Personality Disorders, Williamsburg, VA.

Cummings, J. L., Petry, S., Dian, L., Shapira, J., & Hill, M. A. (1990). Organic personality disorder in dementia syndromes: An inventory approach. *The Journal of Neuropsychiatry and Clinical Neurosciences, 2,* 261-267.

Deutsch, L. H., & Rovner, B. W. (1991). Agitation and other noncognitive abnormalities in Alzheimer's disease. *The Psychiatric Clinics of North America, 14*(2), 341-351.

Devanand, D. P., Nobler, M. S., Singer, T., Kiersky, J. E., Turret, N., Roose, S. P., & Sackeim, H. A. (1994). Is dysthymia a different disorder in the elderly? *American Journal of Psychiatry, 151,* 1592-1599.

Drachman, D. A., Swearer, J. M., O'Donnell, B. F., Mitchell, A. L., & Maloon, A. The Caretaker Obstreperous-Behavior Rating Assessment (COBRA) Scale. *Journal of the American Geriatrics Society, 40,* 463-470.

Ebstein, R. P., Novick, O., Umansky, R., Priel, B., Osher, Y., Blaine, D., Bennett, E. R., Nemanov, L., Katz, M., & Belmaker, R. H. (1996). Dopamine D4 receptor (D4DR) exon III polymorphism associated with the human personality trait of novelty seeking. *Nature Genetics, 12,* 78-80.

Epstein, S. (1991). *Cognitive-experiential self-theory: Implications for developmental psychology* (pp. 79-123) (Minnesota Symposium in Child Psychology). Newark, NJ: Erlbaum.

Eysenck, H. J. (1967). *The biological basis of personality.* Springfield, IL.: Charles C Thomas.

Fogel, B. S., & Westlake, R. (1990). Personality disorder diagnoses and age in inpatients with major depression. *Journal of Clinical Psychiatry, 51,* 232-235.

Gottfries, C. G. (1990). Neurochemical aspects of dementia disorders. *Dementia, 1,* 56-64.

Kluver, H., & Bucy, P. C. (1939). Preliminary analysis of functions of the temporal lobes in monkeys. *Archives of Neurology and Psychiatry, 42,* 547-554.

Kumar, A., Koss, E., Metzler, D., Moore, A., & Friedland, R. P. (1988). Behavioral symptomatology in dementia of the Alzheimer type. *Alzheimer Disease and Associated Disorders, 2,* 363-365.

Loebel, J. P. (1990). Completed suicide in the elderly. In *Abstracts of the Third Annual Meeting and Symposium, American Association for Geriatric Psychiatry, San Diego, California* (p.2). Bethesda, MD: American Association for Geriatric Psychiatry.

Loranger, A. W. (1988). *The Personality Disorder Examination (PDE) manual.* Yonkers, NY: DV Communications.

Mahler, M. E., & Cummings, J. L. (1991). Behavioral neurology of multi-infarct dementia. *Alzheimer Disease and Associated Disorders, 5,* 122-130.

Miller, B. L., Chang, L., Oropilla, G., & Mena, I. (1994). Alzheimer's disease and frontal lobe dementias. In C. E. Coffey & J. L. Cummings (Eds.), *Textbook of geriatric neuropsychiatry* (pp. 390-404). Washington, DC: American Psychiatric Press.

Morris, R. G., Morris, L. W., & Britton, P. G. (1988). Factors affecting the emotional well-being of the caregivers of dementia sufferers. *British Journal of Psychiatry, 153,* 147-156.

National Institutes of Health. Consensus Conference. (1992). Diagnosis and treatment of depression in late life. *Journal of the American Medical Association, 268,* 1018-1024.

Overall, J. E., & Gorham, D. R. (1988). Introduction: The Brief Psychiatric Rating Scale (BPRS): Recent developments in ascertainment and scaling. *Psychopharmacological Bulletin, 24,* 97-99.

Petry, S., Cummings, J. L., Hill, M. A., & Shapira, J. (1988). Personality alterations in dementia of the Alzheimer type. *Archives of Neurology, 45,* 1187-1190.

Petry, S., Cummings, J. L., Hill, M.A., & Shapira, J. (1989). Personality alterations in dementia of the Alzheimer type: A three-year follow-up study. *Journal of Geriatric Psychiatry and Neurology, 2,* 203-207.

Reich, J. H., Noyes, R., Hirschfeld, R. M. A., Coryell, W., & O'Gorman, T. (1987). State and personality in depressed and panic patients. *American Journal of Psychiatry, 144,* 181-187.

Reisberg, B., Borenstein, B., Salob, S. P., Ferris, S. H., Franssen, E., & Gengotas, A. (1987). Behavioral symptoms in Alzheimer's disease: Phenomenology and treatment. *Journal of Clinical Psychiatry, 48*(Suppl), 9-15.

Reisberg, B., & Ferris, S. H. (1985). A clinical rating scale for symptoms of psychosis in Alzheimer's disease. *Psychopharmacological Bulletin, 21*, 101-104.

Rubin, E. H., Morris, J. C., & Berg, L. (1987). The progression of personality changes in Senile dementia of the Alzheimer's type. *Journal of the American Geriatrics Society, 35*, 721-725.

Rubin, E. H., Morris, J. C., Storandt, M., & Berg, L. (1987). Behavioral changes in patients with mild senile dementia of the Alzheimer's type. *Psychiatry Research, 21*, 55-62.

Siegler, I. C., Dawson, D. V., & Welsh K. A. (1994). Caregiver ratings of personality change in Alzheimer's disease patients: A replication. *Psychology and Aging, 9*, 464-466.

Siegler, I. C., Welsh, K. A., Dawson, D. V., Fillenbaum, G. G., Earl, N. L., Kaplan, B. B., & Clark, C. M. (1991). Ratings of personality change in patients being evaluated for memory disorders. *Alzheimer Disease and Associated Disorders, 5*, 240-250.

Strauss, M. E., & Pasupathi, M. (1994). Primary caregivers' descriptions of Alzheimer patients' personality traits: Temporal stability and sensitivity to change. *Alzheimer Disease and Associated Disorders, 8*, 166-176.

Strauss, M. E., Pasupathi, M., & Chatterjee, A. (1993). Concordance between observers in descriptions of personality change in Alzheimer's disease. *Psychology and Aging, 8*, 475-480.

Thompson, L. W., Gallagher, D., & Czirr, R. (1988). Personality disorder and outcome in the treatment of late-life depression. *Journal of Geriatric Psychiatry, 21*, 133-146.

Welleford, E. A., Harkins, S. W., & Taylor, J. R. (1995). Personality change in dementia of the Alzheimer's type: Relations to caregiver personality and burden. *Experimental Aging Research, 21*, 295-314.

Chapter 6

Assessment of Depression in Patients With Dementia

Ira R. Katz and Patricia Parmelee

The authors' understanding of the interrelationships between depression and dementia has evolved significantly over the past generation, reflecting the growth and maturation of knowledge. The work of Roth (1955) and Post (1962), begun at a time when the mental disorders of late life were thought to be amorphous and unidimensional, showed that dementia and depression were separable and distinct disorders. The difficulties in distinguishing between the disorders, however, was emphasized by Kiloh (1961), who wrote about "pseudodementias" that could occur in depression as well as other psychiatric disorders. This line of thinking was extended and refined by investigators who emphasized the principle that "pseudodementia" was a misnomer and that major depression could be associated with reversible but real cognitive deficits (Caine, 1981; Starkstein et al., 1989). Reifler and colleagues (Reifler, Larson, & Hanley, 1982; Reifler, Larson, Teri, & Poulsen, 1986) took a different view, noting that dementia and depression were not mutually exclusive states, but, instead, that depression frequently existed as a comorbidity, component, or complication of the syndrome of dementia. With this conceptual restructuring, the focus of both clinicians and investigators moved from "either/or" (i.e., is it depression or dementia?) to "and/or" (i.e., whether or not the patient has a dementing illness, is there a significant degree of depression?). More recently, the authors' understanding of the interactions between dementia and depression has evolved further as evidence has accumulated that depression with reversible cognitive impairment may be a prodrome for dementia rather than a separate and distinct disorder (Alexopoulos, Meyers, Young, Mattis, & Kakuma, 1993), and questions have been raised about whether depression may be a risk factor for irreversible dementia (Agbayewa, 1986; Jorm et al., 1991; Speck et al., 1995).

This review deals with one component of this complex issue, the measurement of depression occurring in association with the irreversible dementias of late life. An estimate of the importance of this problem can be derived from clinical and epidemiological studies that have shown frequencies of depressed mood in patients with Alzheimer's disease (AD), ranging from 0% to 87%, with a median of 41%, and of depressive disorders from 0% to 86%, with a median of 19% (Wragg & Jeste, 1989). The methods used to identify relevant articles included searches of both the Medline and

Acknowledgment. This study was supported, in part, by Clinical Research Center grant MH P30 52129 from the National Institute of Mental Health.

Psychlit databases. Medline was searched for *dementia* (exploded) and *depression or depressive disorders* for the period from 1962 through early 1996. Psychlit was searched for the keywords *depression and dementia* and *depression and Alzheimer's disease*. Abstracts identified through these broad-band searches were scanned online to select for articles with primary data on the issues of measurement and validity. Where relevant, additional articles were identified through review of the literature cited in primary sources.

Although the term *depression* can refer to an affect, a mood, or one or more syndromes, the authors are concerned here with the depressive syndromes that occur in patients with dementia. These states may be viewed from two distinct perspectives, assuming either that they are similar to the depressive disorders that occur among cognitively intact patients or that they may have unique features. The literature borrows, in large part, from advances in the study of late life depression as it is observed in other patient populations. From a practical viewpoint, this approach may best ensure that appropriate individuals with dementia and depression are able to benefit from treatments (psychosocial and somatic) derived from those developed for the treatment of primary depression. There have, however, been suggestions that the affective disorders associated with dementia may have distinctive features. Thus, affective lability as well as depression is recognized among individuals with dementia (and is often considered to be more common in vascular disease). Moreover, Roth (as quoted by Greenwald, 1995) summarized clinical experience with these disorders stating

> There were (dementia) cases which had shown at some stage of the illness a sustained depressive-symptom complex. . . . There is, however, another type of affective change associated with the organic psychoses (dementias) of old age. . . . The mood change is short lived and shallow . . . depressive ideas are fragmentary and transient . . . what interpretation is placed upon the incidence of affective symptoms . . . must depend on whether a distinction is maintained between ill-sustained, atypical depressive symptoms and a depressive symptom-complex. (p. 21)

Although the literature reviewed here demonstrates that current approaches to diagnosis and measurement have acceptable reliability and validity, Roth's concerns remain, in large part, unanswered. Suggestions that depressive disorders are more likely to be self-limited in patients with dementia are supported by finding high placebo response rates in a carefully designed study of drug treatment (Reifler et al., 1989) and by suggestions (Forsell, Jorm, & Winblad, 1994) that there may be a more favorable prognosis for depression in patients with versus those without coexisting dementia. Thus, it is important to recognize that the answer to several questions about the measurement of depression in dementia will require further understanding of the underlying psychopathology.

AVAILABLE INSTRUMENTS

Diagnostic Methods

Although the third edition of the *Diagnostic and Statistical Manual of Mental Disorders* (DSM-III; American Psychiatric Association, 1980) specifically excluded the diagnosis of a major depressive episode when it is judged to be "due to an Organic Mental Disorder," the current edition (DSM-IV; American Psychiatric Association, 1994) is consistent with the clinical reality that major depression can coexist with irreversible dementia. Nevertheless, considerable problems remain when one attempts to apply DSM-IV criteria to patients with Alzheimer's disease and related disorders (ADRD). These include the need to modify diagnostic algorithms because "diminished ability to think or concentrate" cannot serve as a criterion for a depressive diagnosis, and because other symptoms (e.g., loss of interest) can be ambiguous as well as questions about methods for the ascertainment of symptoms that require the recall of recent experiences. Despite these potential problems, Rosen and Zubenko (1991) showed that it was possible to achieve high levels of interrater reliability (κ=0.86) in the diagnosis of major depression among patients with dementia. Although procedures were not presented, this must have required extensive "local conventions" regarding the operations used for ascertaining the presence or absence of symptoms and for deriving syndromal diagnoses from data on individual symptoms. The investigators for this study must have developed explicit algorithms for evaluating and interpreting clinical findings at both the symptom and syndrome levels; it is unfortunate that these were not presented.

Structured approaches to assessing symptoms using information derived from both interview/observation of patients and caregiver reports should, in principle, improve the reliability of the diagnosis of depression in patients with cognitive impairment. Copeland et al., 1976) developed a standardized semistructured interview, the Geriatric Mental State Schedule, for use in older individuals. More recently, a structured instrument, the Cambridge Mental Disorders of the Elderly Examination (CAMDEX), was developed in the UK (Roth et al., 1986) and has been validated in several studies conducted in the United States (Hendrie et al., 1988) and other countries. It includes a cognitive examination, a face-to-face interview conducted with subjects who are able to pass simple cognitive screening questions, systematic observations on the patients appearance and behavior, and a structured interview with a relative or caregiver. The CAMDEX was used to investigate the prevalence and symptomatology of depression in patients with dementia by both Logie et al. (1992) who discussed the differential sensitivity to depressive symptoms of patient interviews, informant interviews, and observer ratings, and by Ballard, Cassidy, Bannister, & Mohan (1993) who proposed operational criteria for use of the CAMDEX for the diagnosis of depressive illness occurring in association with dementia. Although limitations in the caregiver interview may preclude the use of the CAMDEX for the diagnosis of depression among patients with advanced dementia, it appears to be an important advance toward increasing the reliability of diagnoses among those with mild to moderate degrees of cognitive impairment.

Rating Scales

Several instruments using distinct approaches for the ascertainment of information have been used to rate severity of depressive symptoms in populations of older individuals with dementia. Among these, the 8-item Depressive Sign Scale of Katona and Aldridge (1985) relies on the direct observation of subjects' behavior by trained raters; interrater reliability is high (r>.98). The Dementia Mood Assessment Scale of Sunderland et al. (1988) consists of 17 items rated on the basis of both direct observation and a semistructured interview with patients; interrater reliability is high (κ=0.74 for "core raters" and 0.69 for others). The Behavioral Rating Scale for Dementia of the

Consortium to Establish a Registry for Alzheimer's Disease (CERAD; Tariot, Mack, Patterson, & Edland, 1995) and the Columbia University Scale for Psychopathology in Alzheimer's Disease (CUSPAD; Devanand, et al., 1992) are two instruments designed for rating the intensity of a wide variety of psychotic, affective, and behavioral symptoms in patients with dementia on the basis of interviews with caregivers. Depression-related factors on the CERAD instrument include depressive features (7 items), vegetative features (4 items), apathy (4 items), and irritability/agitation (4 items); the depression subscale of the CUSPAD consisted of 6 items. Interrater reliability on individual items for both of these scales were high ($\kappa \geq 0.77$, and 0.74, respectively).

Although each of the instruments appears promising, the rating scales that have been studied most intensively include a self-rating instrument, the Geriatric Depression Scale (GDS; Yesavage, Brink, & Rose, 1983), and two closely related interviewer administered instruments, the Hamilton Rating Scale for Depression (HamD; Hamilton, 1960), and the Cornell Scale for Depression in Dementia (CS; Alexopoulos, Abrams, Young, & Shamoian, 1988).

Self-Rating of Depression. The earliest use of standardized self-report depression rating scales in patients with dementia was that of Miller (1980), who found significant correlations in patients with "senile brain disease" between examiner rating of depression on the HamD and self-ratings with the Beck Depression Inventory and an Adjective Checklist for Depression ($r=.69$ and $.75$, respectively). More recently, Gottlieb, Gur, and Gur (1988) determined that the concurrent validity of self-reports using the Zung scale was reasonable in patients with AD of low severity (Global Deterioration Scale stage 3 or 4), where the correlation with the interview-administered HamD was 0.49, whereas in a high-severity group (Global Deterioration Scale ≥ 5), it was only -.13. There has also been experience with the use of the Hospital Anxiety and Depression Scale (Wands et al., 1990) in patients with early dementia. However, the self-rating instrument that has been most extensively studied has been the GDS, available in 30- and 15-item versions with yes/no responses to questions dealing primarily with the affective and ideational (rather than somatic or vegetative) components of depression. The mode of administration varies between settings and studies; some investigators (Burke, Houston, Boust, & Roccaforte, 1989; Burke, Nitcher, Roccaforte, & Wengel, 1982; Burke, Roccaforte, & Wengel, 1991; Maixner, Burke, & Roccaforte, 1995; Feher, Larrabee, & Crook, 1992) ask impaired subjects to complete written test forms, offering assistance only when subjects cannot do so, whereas others administer the test verbally (Parmelee, Katz, & Lawton, 1989; Parmelee, Lawton, & Katz, 1989). Although Kafonek et al. (1989) raised questions about sensitivity of the GDS as a screening tool for depression among long term care patients, Lichtenberg, Steiner, Marcopulos, and Tabscott (1992) found that the sensitivity and specificity of the (30 item) instrument for detection of a geriatric psychiatrist's diagnosis of "depression" in dementia patients in a long-term care hospital were 82% and 86%, respectively. Burke et al. (1989, 1991) found decreased areas under the curve (AUC) in receiver-operating characteristic (ROC) curves in patients with dementia compared with those who were cognitively intact for both the 30- and 15-item tests relative to chart review diagnoses of major depression. Christensen and Dysken (1990) suggested that these findings could result from errors, primarily underrecognition, in clinical diagnoses. Consistent with this suggestion, Burke et al. (1992) and Maixner et al. (1995) subsequently reported two studies, indicating that the AUC for ROC curves for the GDS was comparable in intact versus demented patients when diagnoses of major depression were made prospectively by geriatric psychiatrists. Parmelee and coworkers (Parmelee et al., 1989a, 1989b) studied the psychometric properties of the GDS in intact and impaired residential care subjects (defined by scores on the Memory-Information-Concentration Test of Blessed, Tomlinson, and Roth [1968] > 10) and found that the internal reliability (α=.91 to .92 in intact and .90 to .92 in demented patients) and concurrent validity (correlation with research staff observational ratings using the Raskin scale were .73 in intact and .68 to .71 in impaired patients; for care staff rating, they were .35 and .37, respectively) were comparable in the two groups. One-year test-retest reliability was .86 in both cognitively intact and impaired residents. Two other studies evaluated the associations between GDS and interviewer-administered ratings of depression. Ott and Fogel (1992) reported high correlations with CS ratings in patients with mild dementia (r=.77 for those with MMSE $\geq$ 22) but noted that the correlation deteriorated in patients with greater impairment; they also reported a decrease in the correlation between scales for patients with impaired insight into their cognitive deficits. Fehrer et al. (1992) studied a sample of patients with probable AD; they note that in regression analyses, GDS scores are predicted by HamD scores with increases in those with greater memory deficits and decreases in those with impaired self-awareness of cognitive impairment. In summary, the available literature supports the use of the GDS in patients with mild to moderate dementia. However, there has been limited systematic research to establish the lower limits of cognitive status for which it remains reliable.

Interviewer-Administered Scales. Developed to rate symptoms of major depression through information gathered in a semistructured interview, the HamD has become the "gold standard" among outcome measures for treatment studies in depression. Despite concerns about the ambiguity of somatic symptoms in the elderly, it has proved reliable and valid with geriatric patient populations. Furthermore, as discussed earlier, it showed concurrent validity versus self-ratings in the earliest research on depressions occurring in patients with dementia. More recently, Lazarus, Newton, Cohler, Lesser, and Schweon (1987) found a correlation of .73 between HamD scores and ratings of depression on a depression subscale derived from the Sandoz Clinical Assessment-Geriatric (SCAG) scale. Correlations found by Gottlieb et al. (1988) with the Zung scale were discussed previously; those with the Brief Psychiatric Rating Scale were .89 in AD patients of low and .57 in those of higher severity. However, Fischer, Simanyi, and Danielczyk (1990) found that HamD scores were significantly related to SCAG ratings of depressed mood in control subjects (r=.57), but that they were unrelated in patients with multiinfarct dementia (r=.09) and marginally related in those with AD (r=.28). Lichtenberg et al. (1992) found sensitivity of only 9%, with a specificity of 92% for HamD, using a cutoff >17 against a geriatric psychiatrist's diagnosis of "depression." Gottlieb et al. (1988) found that they could achieve high interrater reliability for the HamD (κ > .99). However, because it was developed for use in cognitively intact patients, there must be concerns about the reliability of ratings on items that require recall of memory about symptoms, and about those where symptoms of depression and dementia may overlap. Dealing with the former problem requires information from collateral sources, and with the latter, operationalized algorithms for evaluating individual symptoms. Thus, optimizing the reliability of HamD among patients with dementia requires extensive "local conventions" about the ascertainment of data and ratings on individual items. Frequently, however, research reports have not documented the conventions used, and it is, therefore, difficult to determine exactly what is being measured and how ratings are made.

The CS was introduced by Alexopoulos et al. (1988a) to address these concerns. Although the investigators state that items were selected after reviewing the literature on the phenomenology of depression both in demented and nondemented patients, the CS is, in fact, highly similar in item content to the HamD. Seventeen of 21 items in the HamD can be mapped against CS, and 17 of 19 items on the CS, against HamD items. In addition, the procedures for ascertainment were modified to provide for deriving information from interviews with caregivers as well as direct observations and interviews with patients, and several items were redefined to facilitate the distinction between symptoms characteristic of depression from those resulting from dementia. In cognitively intact patients (controls, depressives, and those with other psychiatric disorders) the CS had high internal (Kuder-Richardson coefficient=.98) and interrater reliabilities (κ=.74); it was able to distinguish diagnostic groups as well as the HamD (Alexopoulos, Abrams, Young, & Shamoian 1988). In patients with dementia, internal and interrater reliability remained high (α=.84, κ=.67). Concurrent validity was assessed by evaluating the correlation between ratings and depressive diagnoses rank ordered by severity (r=.83 for the CS; r=.54 for HamD) (Alexopoulos, Abrams, & Young, 1988). Subsequent work by other investigators has confirmed the utility of the scale. The correlations of CS scores with GDS reported by Maixner et al. (1995) are discussed earlier. Patterson et al. (1990) studied a sample of AD patients and spousal controls and found kappa values for individual items ranging from .48 to 1.0. Vida, Des Rosiers, Carrier, and Gauthier (1994) found AUC for ROC curves for the CS and HamD of .91 and .87, respectively, versus Research Diagnostic Criteria diagnoses of major depression in patients with probable AD; they report point-biserial correlations of .68 and .62, respectively. Finally, Logsdon and Teri (1995) found a correlation coefficient of .60 of the CS with HamD scores derived from Schedule of Affective Disorders and Schizophrenia interviews with caregivers. Correlations with surrogate measures of depression completed by caregivers on the Beck Depression Inventory (BDI), GDS, and Center for Epidemiological Studies–Depression were .46, .36, and .46, respectively, for CS and .44, .32, and .48, respectively, for HamD scores (all p<.05). Note, however, that in the latter studies, where HamD and CS had similar performance characteristics, the procedures for ascertainment on the HamD were modified to include caregiver interviews.

POTENTIAL CONFOUNDS

Ascertainment

Most, but not all, studies report that the frequency of depressive symptoms is greater in caregiver reports than in interviews with subjects or direct observations of their behavior. Mackenzie, Robiner, and Knopman (1989) found that 14% of a sample of patients with AD met DSM-III criteria for major depression on the basis of data derived from patient interviews, but 50% met diagnostic criteria on the basis of data derived from caregiver reports. Rubin and Kinscherf (1989), however, reported that the frequency of individual depressive symptoms in patients with mild AD were similar whether they were evaluated through subject interviews or reports from collateral sources (usually close relatives). Teri and Wagner (1991) compared HamD scores for patients with AD with or without depression with information derived from the patient only, from caregivers only, and on the basis of a clinician's judgment that incorporated information from both sources. In the total sample, mean ratings were 5.0 for patient data, 7.6 for caregiver data, and 8.2 for clinician judgment (with all differences significant); for those with coexisting major depression, mean scores were 9.0, 15.2, and 15.5, respectively (with significant differences between patient data and other scores). In this study, the level of dementia was not found to affect the relative sensitivity of the methods. Gilley et al. (1995) further probed these issues by evaluating the relationships between HamD scores derived from interviews with subjects versus reports from collaterals living with them in three groups, patients with AD, those with Parkinsonism, and older patients without neurological disease. Correlations between ratings in the three groups were .29, .92, and .85, respectively. The discrepancies between ratings in patients with AD could have reflected a low rate of symptoms reported by patients, but it could also have reflected a lower level of diagnostic accuracy among AD patients.

In a response to the findings of Mackenzie et al. (1989), Schulz and Williamson (1990) suggested that the apparent differences between patient and caregiver reports of the prevalence of depression in patients with dementia could be due to overreporting of depression by caregivers as a consequence of their own depression. This hypothesis has subsequently been tested by several investigators. Moye, Robiner, and Mackenzie (1993) confirmed that caregivers reported patients' depressive symptoms more frequently than the patients themselves and noted that caregiver reports were not affected by either the patient's level of impairment or the caregiver's scores on the BDI. Teri and Truax (1994) evaluated the hypothesis that caregivers with depression would overreport depressive symptoms in a study in which caregivers were asked to complete modified HamD ratings of their own impaired relative and videotapes of simulated patients; they found significant but modest correlations ($r=.27$) between the caregivers' own HamD scores and their ratings of their relatives, but no association of caregiver depression with videotape ratings. They noted that all caregivers meeting criteria for major depressive disorder reported patient symptoms severe enough to suggest a depressive illness; however, a high proportion of nondepressed caregivers (61%) also reported patient depression. Cummings, Ross, Absher, Gornbein, & Hadjiaghai (1995) tested for a relationship between HamD for demented patients derived from caregiver reports and the caregivers' own scores on the BDI, and found a nonsignificant correlation ($r=.17$).

These findings suggest that discrepancies between patient- and caregiver-derived information in the apparent frequencies of depression coexisting with ADRD are relatively consistent. Available data do not, however, support the hypothesis that this can be explained by overreporting on the part of caregivers because of their own depression. An alternative hypothesis, initially suggested by Merriam, Aronson, Gaston, Wey, & Katz (1988) is that increased variability in mood and associated symptoms of depression in demented patients could lead to both overreporting of depression in caregiver reports and underrecognition by clinicians in interviews and direct observations of behavior that sampled behavior during limited periods.

Ambiguity of Symptoms

Greenwald (1995) and Greenwald et al. (1989) reviewed findings demonstrating that neurovegetative symptoms similar to those that occur in depression can occur in uncomplicated ADRD and proposed criteria for use in the diagnosis of patients with major depression coexisting with severer degrees of dementia. Lazarus et al. (1987) emphasized the principle that most of the depressions occurring in patients with AD were mild or minor, and suggested that case identification should emphasize affective and ideational (rather than somatic or vegetative) symptoms. The major questions regarding the overlap between symptoms of depression and those associated with the underlying dementias, however, deal with the symptoms, such as apathy, passivity, and decreased initiative. Forsell, Jorm, Fratiglioni, Grut, and Winblad (1993) conducted a principal component analysis (with Varimax rotation) of DSM-III-R criterion symptoms for major depression and reported that a motivation disturbance factor (loss of interest, psychomotor change, loss of energy, and thinking/concentration disturbance) accounted for 29% of variance, whereas a mood disturbance factor (dysphoria, appetite disturbance, guilt, and thoughts of death/suicide) accounted for 15% of variance. Although many subjects (34%) complained of sleep disturbance, these symptoms were apparently nonspecific and did not load on either factor. They report that motivation factor scores increased linearly with the severity of dementia, whereas mood symptoms showed a quadratic trend (inverted *U*), with a peak among those with mild dementia. As part of a series of studies on apathy, Marin, Firinciogullari, and Biedrzycki (1993, 1994) developed an Apathy Evaluation Scale (AES) and applied it in several clinical populations. They report (Marin et al., 1993) that the HamD items most associated with apathy are diminished work/interest, psychomotor retardation/agitation, energy, and lack of insight, and that the association between measures of apathy and other symptoms of depression could be attributed to the occurrence of both affective and motivational symptoms in those with major depression. Marin et al. (1994) noted that the correlation between HamD and their AES scores was .54 in patients with probable AD, relative to .64 in those with (primary) major depression, .49 in patients with left hemisphere stroke, .20 (not significant) with right hemisphere stroke, and .26 (not significant) in well elderly. There were significant differences between groups in the frequency of patients with high levels of apathy, with the highest rates in those with AD; similarly, the highest rates of a specific "apathy syndrome" characterized by high levels of apathy and low levels of depression were in those with AD. Thus, despite the significant correlations between HamD and AES scores, these investigators conclude that most of the apathy observed in AD is unrelated to depression. This conclusion has been supported by studies by Galynker, Roane, Miner, Feinberg, and Watts (1995), who used measures of negative symptoms "borrowed" from schizophrenia research and found that they were not significantly related to HamD scores in a sample of patients with Alzheimer's disease and normal controls, and by those of Rubin, Kinscherf, Grant, and Storandt (1991) who studied disturbances of personality in AD and found high levels of passivity, even early in the disease.

To summarize, the hypothesis to be drawn from this literature must be that most of the depression seen in mild to moderate dementia should, in fact, be considered to be a disorder of mood and affect. Emphasizing motivational or vegetative symptoms in an attempt to increase sensitivity for the detection of mild to moderate depressions in mild to moderate dementia is likely to lead to decreased specificity.

CURRENT TRENDS

The authors have noted at several points that assessments of depression among individuals with ADRD are subject to error at several junctures. Particularly when elders' communication skills are impaired, raters may find themselves in the delicate situation of trying to infer an internal state without any clear cues from the individual. Even when persons retain verbal abilities, questions arise about the validity of self-report measures—most of which ask for summary assessments over a period of days or weeks—among individuals who may not be able to recall their last meal. The hypothesis set forward by Merriam et al. (1988) that dementia patients may be more variable in mood and other symptoms of depression raises similar questions about the reliability and validity of standard, one-occasion assessment approaches.

An alternative that seems increasingly viable is to use multiple repeated measures of affect and behavior to develop a "profile" of depressive signs and symptoms over days or even weeks. Research with cognitively intact long-term care residents (Lawton, Parmelee, Katz, & Nesselroade, 1996) suggests that there are differential, clearly identifiable patters of daily variation in positive and negative affect that characterize persons with major, minor, or no depression. Recent findings from Alzheimer's special care units further suggest that it is possible to assess current positive and negative affect in patients with dementia. For example, Lawton, van Haitsma, and Klapper (1996) found that simple observational assessments of six affect states (three positive, three negative) correlated well with self-reports (among those individuals able to provide them), staff ratings of on-unit behavior, and families' assessments of individuals' preimpairment personality. These findings are exciting in their implication that one may, in fact, be able to infer the internal states of cognitively impaired older persons from current overt responses to situational cues.

Thus, repeated assessments of simple self-report or behavioral evidence of mood may prove a useful way of accumulating evidence about the current states of older persons. When such assessments are conducted in parallel with more standard assessments, they may begin to provide additional assurance about the validity of information about depressive states gleaned from various sources, the symptoms that characterize depressive disorders among persons with dementing illnesses, and the association of mood disorders with functional status and other aspects of quality of life.

CONCLUSIONS

To summarize, depression is a frequent concomitant of dementia, but it remains unclear whether it should be considered a comorbidity, component, or complication of cognitive disorders. There also remains some controversy about the comparability of depressive syndromes observed among dementia patients versus cognitively intact older persons. Nonetheless, depression does appear to be a source of excess disability even among dementia patients.

Of nondiagnostic methods, the Geriatric Depression Scale (GDS) seems to offer the best available assessment approach. Self-ratings of depression with the GDS appear to be reliable and valid in mild to moderate dementia, although this may depend on methods of administration. The robustness of the GDS with these populations is encouraging. In principle, performance of this instrument and findings based on it, in patients with mild to moderate dementia could serve as anchor points in the development of scales for use in patients with severer dementia. Non self–reports appear to be of variable utility. DSM diagnoses and Hamilton/Cornell Scales have reasonable reliability and validity even with moderately to severely impaired older persons. However, achieving consistently acceptable psychometric and diagnostic performance requires standardization and formalization of modes of ascertainment. Caregiver reports, particularly those of family caregivers, yield higher rates of depression than do interviews with patients or direct observation of behavior. However, at this point, it is unclear how much of this difference is due to biased reporting, and how much to caregivers' richer understanding because they are able to observe impaired elders' behavior more often and more intensively.

There are questions about the extent to which vegetative and motivational symptoms should be included in diagnoses and measures of depression. However, preliminary evidence suggests that the kind of motivational disturbances commonly associated with depression among intact individuals—lethargy, loss of interest, and decreased ability to experience pleasure—may be misleading among patients with Alzheimer's disease. This differentiation is dependent on the stage of dementia, with vegetative and motivational disturbances becoming more common in later states of disease. Thus, emphasis on these symptoms in an attempt to identify depression in mild to moderate dementia is likely to lead to overdiagnosis in more impaired persons. As in other areas of continuing controversy outlined in this article, future advances will likely depend on innovative approaches to operationalization and assessment of mood. One particularly promising avenue is use of multiple repeated measures of depression-related signs and generalized affect. Even when self-report is not possible, use of these methods by trained observers is likely to yield new insights into the nature and dynamics of depression among older persons with dementia.

REFERENCES

Agbayewa, M. O. (1986). Earlier psychiatric morbidity in patients with Alzheimer's disease. *Journal of the American Geriatrics Society, 34,* 561-564.

Alexopoulos, G. S., Abrams, R. C., Young, R. C., & Shamoian, C. A. Cornell scale for depression in dementia. *Biological Psychiatry, 23,* 271-284.

Alexopoulos, G. S., Abrams, R. C., Young, R. C., & Shamoian, C. A. Use of the Cornell scale in nondemented patients. *Journal of the American Geriatrics Society, 36,* 230-236.

Alexopoulos, G. S., Meyers, B. S., Young, R. C., Mattis, S., & Kakuma, T. (1993). The course of geriatric depression with "reversible dementia": A controlled study. *American Journal of Psychiatry, 150,* 1693-1699.

American Psychiatric Association. (1980). *Diagnostic and Statistical Manual for Mental Disorders* (3rd ed.). Washington, DC: Author.

American Psychiatric Association. (1994). *Diagnostic and Statistical Manual for Mental Disorders* (4th ed.). Washington, DC: Author.

Ballard, C. G., Cassidy, G., Bannister, C., & Mohan, R. N. C. Prevalence, symptom profile, and aetiology of depression in dementia sufferers. *Journal of Affective Disorders, 29,* 1-6.

Blessed, G., Tomlinson, B. E., & Roth, M. The association between quantitative measures of dementia and of senile change in the cerebral gray matter of elderly subjects. *British Journal of Psychiatry, 114,* 797-811.

Burke, W. J., Houston, M. J., Boust, S. J., & Roccaforte, W. H. (1989). Use of the Geriatric Depression Scale in dementia of the Alzheimer type. *Journal of the American Geriatrics Sociery, 37,* 856-860.

Burke W. J., Nitcher, R. L., Roccaforte, W. H., & Wengel, S. P. (1992). A prospective evaluation of the Geriatric Depression Scale in an outpatient geriatric assessment center. *Journal of the American Geriatric Society, 40,* 1227-1230.

Burke W. J., Roccaforte, W. H., & Wengel, S. P. (1991). The short form of the Geriatric Depression Scale: A comparison with the 30-item form. *Journal of Geriatric Psychiatry and Neurology, 4,* 173-178.

Caine, E. D. (1981). Pseudodementia: Current concepts and future directions. *Archives of General Psychiatry, 38,* 1359-1364.

Christensen, K. J., & Dysken, M. W. (1990). The Geriatric Depression Scale in Alzheimer's disease [letter to the editor]. *Journal of the American Geriatrics Society, 38,* 724-725.

Copeland, J. R. M., Kelleher, M. J., Kellett, J. M., Gourlay, A. J., Gurland, B. J., Fleiss, J. L., & Sharpe, L. (1976). A semistructured clinical interview for the assessment of diagnosis and mental state in the elderly: the Geriatric Mental State Schedule. *Psychological Medicine, 6,* 439-449.

Cummings, J. L., Ross, W., Absher, J., Gornbein, J., & Hadjiaghai, L. (1995). Depressive symptoms in Alzheimer disease: Assessment and determinants. *Alzheimer's Disease and Associated Disorders, 2,* 87-93.

Devanand, D. P., Miller, L., Richards, M., Marder, K., Bell, K., Mayeux, R., & Stern, Y. (1992). The Columbia University Scale for Psychopathology in Alzheimer's disease. *Archives of Neurology, 49,* 371-376.

Feher, E. P., Larrabee, G. J., & Crook, T. H., III. (1992). Factors attenuating the validity of the Geriatric Depression Scale in a dementia population. *Journal of the American Geriatrics Society, 40,* 906-909.

Fischer, P., Simanyi, M., & Danielczyk, W. (1990). Depression in dementia of the Alzheimer type and in multi-infarct dementia. *American Journal of Psychiatry, 147,* 1484-1487.

Forsell, Y., Jorm, A. F., Fratiglioni, L., Grut, M., & Winblad, B. (1993). Application of DSM-III-R criteria for major depressive episode to elderly subjects with and without dementia. *American Journal of Psychiatry, 150,* 1199-1202.

Forsell, Y., Jorm, A. F., & Winblad, B. (1994). Outcome of depression in demented and non-demented elderly: Observations from a three-year follow-up in a community-based study. *International Journal of Geriatric Psychiatry, 9,* 5-10.

Galynker, I. L., Roane, D. M., Miner, C. R., Feinberg, T. E., & Watts, P. (1995). Negative symptoms in patients with Alzheimer's disease. *American Journal of Geriatric Psychiatry, 3,* 52-59.

Gilley, D. W., Wilson, R. S., Fleischman, D. A., Harrison, D. W., Goetz, C. G., & Tanner, C. M. (1995). Impact of Alzheimer's-type dementia and information source on the assessment of depression. *Psychological Assessment, 7,* 42-48.

Gottlieb, G. L., Gur, R. E., & Gur, R. C. (1988). Reliability of psychiatric scales in patients with dementia of the Alzheimer type. *American Journal of Psychiatry, 145,* 857-860.

Greenwald, B. S. (1995). Depression in Alzheimer's disease and related dementias. In B. A. Lawlor (Ed.), *Behavioral complications in Alzheimer's disease* (pp. 19-53). Washington, DC: American Psychiatric Press.

Greenwald, B. S., Kramer-Ginsberg, E., Marin, D. B., Laitman, L. B., Hermann, C. K., Mohs, R. C., & Davis, K. L. (1989). Dementia with coexistent major depression. *American Journal of Psychiatry, 146*, 1472-1478.

Hamilton, M. (1960). A rating scale for depression. *Journal of Neurology, Neurosurgery and Psychiatry, 23*, 56-62.

Hendrie, H. C., Hall, K. S., Brittain, H. M., Austrom, M. G., Farlow, M., Parker, J., & Kane, M. (1988). The CAMDEX: A standardized instrument for the diagnosis of mental disorder in the elderly: A replication with a US sample. *Journal of the American Geriatrics Society, 36*, 402-408.

Jorm, A. F., van Duijn, C. M., Chandra, V., Fratiglioni, L., Graves, A. B., Heyman, A., Kokmen, E., Kondo, K., Mortimer, J. A., Rocca, W. A., Shalat, S. L., Soininen, H., Hofman, A., for the EURODEM Risk Factors Research Group. (1991). Psychiatric history and related exposures as risk factors for Alzheimer's disease: A collaborative re-analysis of case-control studies. EURODEM Risk Factors Research Group. *International Journal of Epidemiology, 20*(Suppl.) 2:S43-S47.

Kafonek, S., Ettinger, W. H., Roca, R., Kittner, S., Taylor, N., & German, P. S. (1989). Instruments for screening for depression and dementia in a long-term care facility. *Journal of the American Geriatrics Society, 37*, 29-34.

Katona, C. L. E., & Aldridge, C. R. (1985). The dexamethasone suppression test and depressive signs in dementia. *Journal of Affective Disorders, 8*, 83-89.

Kiloh, L. (1961). Pseudodementia. *Acta Psychiatrica Scandinavica, 37*, 336-351.

Lawton, M. P., van Haitsma, K., & Klapper, J. (1996). Observed affect in nursing home residents with Alzheimer's disease. *Journal of Gerontology, Psychological Sciences, 51*, P3-14.

Lawton, M. P., Parmelee, P. A., Katz, I. R., & Nesselroade, J. (1996). Affective states in depressed and nondepressed older people. *Journal of Gerontology, Psychological Sciences, 51*, 309-316.

Lazarus, L. W., Newton, N., Cohler, B., Lesser, J., & Schweon, C. (1987). Frequency and presentation of depressive symptoms in patients with primary degenerative dementia. *American Journal of Psychiatry, 144*, 41-45.

Lichtenberg, P. A., Steiner, D. A., Marcopulos, B. A., & Tabscott, J. A. (1992). Comparison of the Hamilton Depression Rating Scale and the Geriatric Depression Scale: Detection of depression in dementia patients. *Psychological Reports, 70*, 515-521.

Logie, S. A., Murphy, B., Brooks, D. N., Wylie, S., Barron, E. T., & McCulloch, J. (1992). The diagnosis of depression in patients with dementia: Use of the Cambridge Mental Disorders of the Elderly Examination. *International Journal of Geriatric Psychiatry, 7*, 363-368.

Logsdon, R. G., & Teri, L. (1995). Depression in Alzheimer's disease patients: Caregivers as surrogate reporters. *Journal of the American Geriatrics Society, 43*, 150-155.

Mackenzie, T. B., Robiner, W. N., & Knopman, D. S. (1989). Differences between patient and family assessments of depression in Alzheimer's disease. *American Journal of Psychiatry, 146*, 1174-1178.

Maixner, S. M., Burke, W. J., Roccaforte, W. H., Wengel, S. P., & Potter, J. F. (1995). A comparison of two depression scales in a geriatric assessment clinic. *American Journal of Geriatric Psychiatry, 3*, 60-67.

Marin, R. S., Firinciogullari, S., & Biedrzycki, R. C. (1994). Group differences in the relationship between apathy and depression. *Journal of Nervous and Mental Disease, 182*, 235-239.

Marin, R. S., Firinciogullari, S., & Biedrzycki, R. C. (1993). The sources of convergence between measures of apathy and depression. *Journal of Affective Disorders, 28*, 117-124.

Merriam, A. E., Aronson, M. K., Gaston, P., Wey, S. L., & Katz, I. (1988). The psychiatric symptoms of Alzheimer's disease. *Journal of the American Geriatrics Society, 36*, 7-12.

Miller, N. E. (1980). The measurement of mood in senile brain disease: Examiner ratings and self-reports. In: J. O. Cole & J. E. Barrett (Eds.), *Psychopathology in the aged* (pp. 97-122). New York: Raven Press.

Moye, J., Robiner, W. N., & Mackenzie, T. B. (1993). Depression in Alzheimer patients: Discrepancies between patient and caregiver reports. *Alzheimer's Disease and Associated Disorders, 7*, 187-201.

Ott, B. R., & Fogel, B. S. (1992). Measurement of depression in dementia: Self vs clinician rating. *International Journal of Geriatric Psychiatry, 7*, 899-904.

Parmelee, P. A., Katz, I. R., & Lawton, M. P. (1989a). Depression among institutionalized aged: Assessment and prevalence estimation. *Journal of Gerontology, 44*, M22-M29.

Parmelee, P. A., Lawton, M. P., & Katz, I. R. (1989b). Psychometric properties of the Geriatric Depression Scale among the institutionalized aged. Psychological Assessment: *A Journal of Consulting and Clinical Psychology, 1*, 331-338.

Patterson, M. B., Schnell, A. H., Martin, R. J., Mendez, M. F., Smyth, K. A., & Whitehouse, P. J. (1990). Assessment of behavioral and affective symptoms in Alzheimer's disease. *Journal of Geriatric Psychiatry and Neurology, 3*, 21-30.

Post, F. *The significance of affective symptoms in old age* (Maudsley Monograph No. 10). London: Oxford University Press.

Reifler, B. V., Larson, E., & Hanley, R. (1982). Coexistence of cognitive impairment and depression in geriatric outpatients. *American Journal of Psychiatry, 139*, 623-626.

Reifler, B. V., Larson, E., Teri, L., & Poulsen, M. (1986). Dementia of the Alzheimer's type and depression. *Journal of the American Geriatrics Society, 34*, 855-859.

Rosen, J., & Zubenko, G. (1991). Emergence of psychosis and depression in the longitudinal evaluation of Alzheimer's disease. *Biological Psychiatry, 29*, 224-232.

Roth, M. (1995). The natural history of mental disorders in old age. *Journal of Mental Science, 101*, 281-301.

Roth, M., Tym, E., Mountjoy, C. Q., Huppert, F. A., Hendrie, H., Verma, S., & Goddard, R. (1986). CAMDEX A standardized instrument for the diagnosis of mental disorder in the elderly with special reference to the early detection of dementia. *British Journal of Psychiatry, 49*, 698-709.

Rubin, E. H., & Kinscherf, D. A. (1989). Psychopathology of very mild dementia of the Alzheimer type. *American Journal of Psychiatry, 146*, 1017-1021.

Rubin, E. H., Kinscherf, D. A., Grant, E. A., & Storandt, M. The influence of major depression on clinical and psychometric assessment of senile dementia of the Alzheimer type. *American Journal of Psychiatry, 148*, 1164-1171.

Schulz, R., & Williamson, G. (1990). Biases in family assessments of depression in patients with Alzheimer's disease (letters). *American Journal of Psychiatry, 147,* 377-378.

Speck, C. E., Kukull, W. A., Brenner, D. E., Bowen, J. D., McCormick, W. C., Teri, L., Pfanschmidt, M. L., Thompson, J. D., & Larson, E. B. (1995). History of depression as a risk factor for Alzheimer's disease. *Epidemiology, 6,* 366-369.

Starkstein, S. E., Rabins, P. V., Berthier, M. L., Cohen, B. J., Folstein, M. F., & Robinson, R. G. (1989). Dementia of depression among patients with neurological disorders and functional depression. *Journal of Neuropsychiatry and Clinical Neurosciences, 1,* 263-268.

Sunderland, T., Alterman, I. S., Yount, D., Hill, J. L., Tariot, P. N., Newhouse, P. A., Mueller, E. A, Mellow, A. M., & Cohen, R. M. (1988) .A new scale for the assessment of depressed mood in dementia patients. *American Journal of Psychiatry, 145,* 955-959.

Tariot, P. N., Mack, J. L., Patterson, M. B., & Edland, S. D. (1995). The Behavior Rating Scale for Dementia of the Consortium to Establish a Registry for Alzheimer's Disease. *American Journal of Psychiatry, 152,* 1349-1357.

Teri, L., & Truax, P. (1994). Assessment of depression in dementia patients: association of caregiver mood with depression ratings. *Gerontologist, 34,* 231-234.

Teri, L., & Wagner, A. W. (1991). Assessment of depression in patients with Alzheimer's disease: Concordance among informants. *Psychology and Aging, 6,* 280-285.

Vida, S., Des Rosiers, P., Carrier, L., & Gauthier, S. (1994). Depression in Alzheimer's disease: Receiver operating characteristic analysis of the Cornell Scale for depression in dementia and the Hamilton Depression Scale. *Journal of Geriatric Psychiatry and Neurology, 7,* 159-162.

Wands, K., Mersky, H., Hachinski, V. C., Fisman, M., Fox, H., & Boniferro, M. (1990). A questionnaire investigation of anxiety and depression in early dementia. *Journal of the American Geriatrics Sociery, 38,* 535-538.

Wragg, R. E., & Jeste, D. (1989). Overview of depression and psychosis in Alzheimer's disease. *American Journal of Psychiatry, 146,* 577-587.

Yesavage, J. A., Brink, T. L., Rose, T. L., Lum, O., Huang, V., Adey, M., & Leirer, V. O. (1993). Development and validation of a geriatric depression screening scale: A preliminary report. *Journal of Psychiatic Research, 17,* 37-49.

Chapter 7

Measuring Affect in Frail and Cognitively Impaired Elders

Valorie Shue, Cornelia Beck, and M. Powell Lawton

Psychologists and philosophers have quibbled over the precise meaning of emotion for more than a century. One of the best definitions of emotion comes from Goleman (1995). He writes:

> In its most literal sense, the *Oxford English Dictionary* defines emotion as "any agitation or disturbance of mind, feeling, passion; any vehement or excited mental state." I take emotion to refer to a feeling and its distinctive thoughts, psychological and biological states, and range of propensities to act. There are hundreds of emotions, along with their blends, variations, mutations, and nuances. Indeed, there are many more subtleties of emotion than we have words for.
>
> Researchers continue to argue over precisely which emotions can be considered primary—the blue, red, and yellow of feeling from which all blends come—or even if there are such primary emotions at all. Some theorists propose basic families, though not all agree on them.

This chapter presents a rationale for measuring affect in the frail and cognitively impaired (CI) elderly, an overview of the research on emotion, instruments for measuring affect in the frail elderly, an overview of research on affect in CI elderly, and instruments for measuring affect in the CI elderly.

MEASURING AFFECT

Rationale

Lawton (1993); Lawton, Kleban, Dean, Rajagopal, and Parmelee (1992); and Lawton, Van Haitsma, and Klapper (1996) connect emotions with well-being and use the term *emotional well-being* as an internal state serving as one component of quality of life. To them, well-being encompasses positive and negative affect and morale as well as specific emotional states, such as contentment. Lawton, Perkinson, and Van Haitsma (1996) have inferred that frequent displays of positive affect indicate increased emotional well-being, whereas frequent displays of negative affect indicate decreased emotional well-being. Further, their and others' research has shown that these constructs are neither totally independent nor totally negatively correlated with each other.

One also may conceptualize affect as an outcome measure. In this case, affect is a general indicator of the state of the organism, with positive moods suggesting a state of good function and negative moods a perturbed state (Morris, 1989 as cited in Stone, 1995).

As a practical matter, recognition of affect in the elderly may provide a means to target interventions and determine their outcomes. Positive affect is more likely to accompany interventions that meet needs (food) or bring contentment (pleasant music), whereas negative affect may signal displeasure and pending aggression. Further, elders who display positive affect may be easier to interact with or more pleasant, which may influence the amount and quality of care that caregivers provide. Conversely, elders who display negative affect may engender negative responses from caregivers.

Affect in the elderly also may signal a pathological mood disorder. For example, depression is a mood disorder characterized by pathological negative affect and lack of positive affect. Another chapter in this volume addresses depression. However, it should be noted that Starkstein et al. (1995), using the Pathological Laughter and Crying Scale (Robinson et al., 1993), found pathological affect in Alzheimer's patients without mood disorder.

Why should we study the emotions of elderly with cognitive impairment? Models of dementia posit a process of "unbecoming" or loss of self (Cotrell & Schulz, 1993; Herskovitz, 1995), such that CI elders lack subjective experience. From this perspective, it would make little sense to try to evaluate the feelings of CI elders. Researchers have tended to dismiss the possibility of gaining useful information about the experience of dementia via self-report because of the pervasive model of selfhood of CI elders, limited understanding and measurement of the concept of self-awareness, the failure to consider premorbid styles of self-expression, and methodological difficulties in assessment. Another notion suggests that CI elders lack awareness of, and, thus, emotional reactions to, their deficits as described by Danner and Friesen 1996. In general, studies fail to assess the wide variation in self-awareness and functioning among CI elders (Danner & Friesen, 1996). However, recently, a few researchers have tried to understand the feelings and preferences of CI elders (Cotrell & Schulz, 1993; Bahro, Silber, & Sunderland, 1995; Herskovitz, 1995). This approach holds great promise for informing our understanding of the emotional life of CI elders. Such understanding also may assist in the care of CI elders. Specifically, Lawton et al. (1996) suggest that emotions hold the key to their likes and dislikes. Caregivers may improve the quality of care by their ability to recognize preferences and aversions, and the quality of their relationships with CI elders from understanding the elders' inner state better.

Methods

The most common technique for studying emotion is the experiential level when people speak of their emotions or rate their feelings; whereas, the behavioral level involves observation of people's verbal behavior, such as temper tantrums, or nonverbal behavior, such as facial expressions and body movements (Lawton et al., 1996).

Global ratings, both experiential and behavioral, are based on the idea that affect states recur in the same people frequently enough to be thought of as traits. "How depressed is Mr. F. usually?" is an example of a global rating. "Usually" denotes the trait form.

The rating of affective states involves a consideration of intensity, duration, and frequency. Although intensity is of major importance as an individual experience and as a variable in research on emotion, it is difficult to measure and remains underinvestigated. Measuring occurrence of an affect state requires detection of the onset of the feeling regardless of whether frequency or duration is the metric. The duration of an affect state is also important. The person experiencing a feeling can judge how long it endures better than an observer can. However, if one accepts facial expression and affect state as totally congruent, the duration of the expression might allow an observer the opportunity to judge duration of the feeling accurately. Nonetheless, judgment of duration is at best an approximation (Lawton et al., 1996). Frequency is related to duration. Frequency is easier to judge than duration is, however, because the observer does not have to note when the state ends as required in the duration estimate. Unfortunately, if the observer only counts the number of occasions (frequency), short states are overrepresented, whereas long ones are underrepresented (Lawton et al., 1996). Thus, description of both frequency and duration will yield the clearest representation of affect. Prevalence or frequency ratings are simply global ratings given additional anchoring points of number of occasions and relatively short periods. "In the past month, how many times have you felt depressed?" (Lawton et al.).

Behavioral observations of affect states can be structured in four ways. *Real time* measures the onset of a feeling and its cessation, and the times are cumulated over occasions. *Estimated time* also produces time measures, but the observer notes and cumulates the time mentally and estimates total time (or proportion of time) at the end of the observation. *Frequency count* requires the observer to note the onset of a feeling, count that as one occasion, note its cessation without regard to duration of feeling and count a second occasion, and so on, ending with a count of the number of onsets over a specified period. The observer must decide when one occasion ends and another begins. *Incidence approaches* denote a series of judgments made at specified times when the observer notes the presence or absence of a state. Making the present or absent judgment at specified times (e.g., every 30 seconds) gives more appropriate weighting to the more enduring states than does the simple frequency count (Lawton et al., 1996).

RESEARCH ON EMOTION AND ITS MANIFESTATIONS

Emotion may be characterized on psychophysiological and neurological levels. Scientists can measure psychophysiological variates, such as heart rate, blood pressure, and muscular tension, which emotional stimulation affects (Levenson, Carstensen, Friesen, & Ekman, 1991). On the neurological level, new technologies have shown the activation of specific areas of the brain during emotional stimulation (National Advisory Mental Health Council, 1995) and that different types of smiles generate different patterns of regional brain activity (Ekman & Davidson, 1993).

Some have argued that facial expression represents the most basic form of emotion. A strong body of psychological research has shown that specific facial expressions accompany interest or excitement, enjoyment or joy, surprise or startle, distress or anguish, fear or terror, shame or humiliation, contempt, disgust, and anger or rage (Tomkins, 1984). Combinations of activity in various facial muscles produce these expressions in people across countries and cultures (Ekman et al., 1987).

The research that has linked these expressions to basic emotions has required the intensive, fine-detailed, and time-consuming analysis of the patterns of facial muscles while the person is experiencing or reacting to a stimulus depicting some presumed emotion. The best known system is the Facial Action Coding System (FACS) (Ekman & Friesen, 1978). Only the FACS manual can convey the richness of the coding system for facial expressiveness (Ekman & Friesen, 1978). This system requires long training, videotaping people's facial expressions, and coding videotaped sequences. Researchers need to develop an easier approach for families and professionals to use in everyday care.

Research as detailed and painstaking as that on facial expression has validated voice as an indicator of emotion. Emotion is revealed by the pitch, volume, and pace when the voice is used. Most people can recognize an angry, soothing, or sad voice even if the words are indistinct. Older people recognize "baby talk" even when the meaning of the words has been blotted out (Caporael, Lukaszewski, & Culbertson, 1983). In the case of CI elders, caregivers have the opportunity to judge vocalizations not framed in words for their emotional meaning. Thus, Lawton et al. (1996) suggest that observers listen for cues to the emotional meaning of vocalizations.

Body language (interpersonal communication through body movements and position) and proxemics (the rules that govern people's placement of distance between themselves and another person or object) have received considerable attention in the general population (Lawton et al., 1996). In 1970, DeLong reasoned that such communication media would become more important as cognitive impairment becomes more pervasive. Despite this insight, little empirical research has occurred since then.

This background on nonverbal body communication serves to illustrate the possibilities inherent in giving closer attention to muscular behavior. Few data exist to link body movement to affect. Nonetheless, most people probably have subliminal awareness of the behaviors' meaning and use body movement to convey messages and interpret the messages of others.

FRAIL ELDERS

Several instruments are available to measure affect in frail and CI elders. Frail elders, because of their physical weakness and limitations, need short valid instruments to mitigate fatigue. Those without cognitive impairment can use self-report scales. Schulz, O'Brien, and Tompkins (1994) reviewed several short self-report instruments. They suggested: Clyde Mood Scale (Clyde, 1963); Nowlis Mood Adjective Checklist (Nowlis, 1965); Differential Emotions Scale-IV (Kotsch, Gerbing, & Schwartz, 1982); and Semantic Differential Mood Scale (Lorr & Wunderlich, 1988).

Recent research on affect measurement has led to developing scales that assess one or two fundamental dimensions rather than the previous multidimensional instruments. The newer measures contain only 6 to 20 items. These instruments take less time to complete and may prove less fatiguing to frail elders. The primary problem with using these measures is the lack of information on their reliability and validity particularly with older respondents (Schulz et al., 1994). Schulz et al. (1994) recommended: Positive and Negative Affect Schedule (Watson, Clark, & Tellegen, 1988); Diener and Emmons Affect Scales (1985); Philadelphia Geriatric Center Positive and Negative Affect Scales (Lawton et al., 1992); Positive States of Mind Scale (Horowitz, Adler, & Kegeles, 1988); and Neutral Word Ratings (Kuykendall, Keating, & Wagaman, 1988). Please refer to Schulz et al. (1994) for descriptions of these scales.

The Affect Balance Scale (Bradburn, 1969) also has been used to measure affect in the elderly. It measures overall psychological well-being with 10 items (5 positive; 5 negative). Respondents indicate whether or not they had experienced each affect within "the past few weeks." The scale generates three scores for each respondent: positive affect, negative affect, and affect balance.

CI ELDERS

Approaches to Measuring Affect

Objective measures of affect in elderly with CI present challenges. With central nervous system damage making major inroads in both behavioral competence and cognitive function, it may not be evident that function continues in the affective realm. In a group of extremely CI elders, Asplund, Norberg, Adolfsson, and Waxman (1991) documented only gross responsiveness to environmental stimuli and failed to show differentiated responses to positive and negative emotional stimuli. Similarly, a study of exploratory eye movement reflecting curiosity (or "interest") showed diminished reactivity in Alzheimer's disease (AD) (Daffner, Scinto, Weintraub, Guinessey, & Mesulam, 1992). Albert, Cohen, and Koff (1991) demonstrated decreased ability of CI elders to recognize emotion in faces or pictured situations, label emotions correctly, or identify emotion names with verbal descriptions compared with intact elders. Allender and Kaszniak (1989) reported similar findings. Albert et al. (1991) asked whether the deficit represented a specific inability to process emotional stimuli or was secondary to the cognitive deficit. They showed that differences in affective functioning disappeared after accounting for the degree of cognitive impairment.

Evidence shows that control and communication of affect may revert to more primitive modes as cognition declines (Hurley, Volicer, Hanrahan, Houde, & Volicer, 1992; Mace, 1989; R. M. Tappen, personal communication, 1993). This often makes it difficult for untrained caregivers to identify affect in CI individuals correctly (Mace, 1990; R. M. Tappen, personal communication, 1993).

Approaches to measuring CI elders' affective state are asking the elder, questioning the family member or the professional caregiver, or observing the elder.

Asking the Elder. Cognitive impairment occurs with varying degrees of severity. When researchers have attempted to accommodate their special needs, they have found that CI elders can report some awareness of their illness, often in a highly emotional manner (Danner & Friesen, in press). For example, Parmelee, Katz, and Lawton (1989) found the validity indicators for the Geriatric Depression Scale (Yesavage, Brink, & Rose, 1983) to be as acceptable for mildly to moderately CI elders as for the nonimpaired. Stewart, Sherbourne, and Brod (1996) are trying to develop instruments for CI elders to report their inner states. Stewart et al. (1996) found mildly and moderately CI elders able to respond to a structured questionnaire on quality of life. They began by constructing items that subjects could answer in a dichotomous fashion (agree-disagree, true-false, etc.), but subjects objected to such a confining format. Therefore, they used a 5-point Likert response format. Stewart et al. (1996) selected subjects who scored 15 and higher on the Mini-Mental Status Examination (Folstein, Folstein, & McHugh, 1975).

Simmons et al. (1996, accepted for publication) suggested that exclusion of elders from satisfaction surveys based on low MMSE scores eliminated up to 80% of most nursing home populations. Instead, they developed screening criteria based on cognition, activities of daily living, and involvement items from the Minimum Data Set that allow up to 47% of residents the opportunity to respond to satisfaction surveys. These studies remind us that we often err in assuming that CI elders cannot respond in a valid manner.

Tappen and Barry (1995) administered the Dementia Mood Picture Test, (Allender, 1984) to 85 elders with moderate to severe AD (MMSE scores 1 to 11) in adult day care and nursing homes. In all but two instances, the pictures elicited a relevant response. The examiner showed the individual a picture of a face depicting a good mood and asked the individual, "Are you in a good mood?" If the answer was "yes," the examiner then asked, "Are you in a very good mood?" The examiner rated the answers as "yes," "no," or "very much," and assigned a score of 0 to 2, respectively. The examiner used the same procedure to determine whether the individual was in a bad mood or happy, sad, angry, or worried. Interrater reliability was consistently high (95% to 100%). Correlation with the Montgomery-Asberg Depression Rating Scale (1979) was $r = -.51$ and the Geriatric Depression Scale (O'Rourke, 1996) was .51. This instrument appears to stimulate reflection and enable persons with advanced AD to communicate and express their moods.

The need to translate CI elders' distorted communication constitutes one of several methodological obstacles to accurately interpreting self-report information. The ability to "read" a patient increases by studying the person's verbal, facial, postural, and contextual signals, as well as establishing rapport, which allays elders' fears and mistrust and minimizes emotional barriers to self-revelation (Cotrell & Schulz, 1993). Further, fluctuations in CI elders' level of lucidity or self-awareness require interviewing patients at their "good times" (Cotrell & Schulz, 1993).

Asking the Family Member or Caregiver. The larger area of proxy reporting has received considerable attention (Magaziner, 1991). Indeed, many major longitudinal surveys depend on substituting a family member's judgment for that of the subject if the latter is unable to respond (Longitudinal Study of Aging, National Health Interview Survey, the Assets and Health Dynamics Survey); sometimes this procedure requires that proxy responses supplant self-responses midway through a longitudinal study. Asking one person to speak for another presents a clear hazard (evidence reviewed by Magaziner, 1991). Nonetheless, Stone (1995) and Costa and McCrae (1988) have documented reasonably good validity in ratings on affect states and personality traits as rated by *spouses of adult and older-adult normal subjects.*

Several applications of the same basic line of reasoning have depended on the possibility that a close family member has expertise in recognizing and reporting inner states of a relative with dementing illness. Danner and Friesen (1996) designed the Emotional Status Interview (ESI) as a guide to the researcher in eliciting the experience of emotion in a CI elder. The ESI inquires about the occasions, conditions, and people known to have elicited emotions in the elder.

Teri and Logsdon (1991) have explored the ability of the family informant to name events that provide pleasure to the CI person. Based on the Lewinsohn and Graf (1973) Pleasant Events Schedule (PES), Teri and Lewinsohn (1982) constructed a Pleasant and Unpleasant Events Schedule for the older person, followed by the PES for Alzheimer's dementia (PES-AD, Teri & Logsdon, 1991). This schedule consists of 53 activities (active and passive; solitary and social). The caregiver rates each activity on a 3-point scale by frequency of performance and availability of the activity during the past month. The caregiver also rates enjoyment (present vs. absent) in the present (now) and the past. The scale can take less than 30 minutes to complete. Experience with the PES-AD indicates that, in mildly to moderately CI elders, having the caregiver and elder work together on the ratings is most helpful. The patient, because of memory problems, is usually unable to rate frequency or availability, but may provide valuable input on enjoyability. Activity-participated-in-now and frequency-of-enjoyed-activities scores are cumulated across items. Internal consistency is good. Both participation now and enjoyment scores were higher among the less impaired and the less depressed (as determined clinically), thus affirming the earlier findings that enjoyable events counteract depression. Logsdon and Teri (in press) also showed that a shorter 20-item version displayed similarly positive psychometric characteristics, making it the measure of choice. Lawton et al. (1996) used the PES-AD as a core and augmented the activities list with a broader array of events that could occur in nursing homes with possible positive valence.

Tappen (1995) found that both family caregivers and nursing home staff could describe displays of positive and negative affect by individuals in late AD.

No one has subjected the family proxy measures to the ultimate validity test of comparing family estimates with elders' responses. Given the availability of a group of AD subjects capable of making judgments as they did for Stewart et al. (1996), such a comparison is theoretically possible.

Behavioral Observation. The research on facial expression of emotion suggests that it may be possible to bypass CI patients' inability to introspect and report verbally on intrapsychic feeling states (Lawton et al., 1996).

In trying to give clinical care to reduce agitation, Hurley et al. (1992) developed the Discomfort Scale–Dementia of the Alzheimer Type (DS-DAT), which assesses a set of behaviors and emotion indicators, including absence of contented look and sad look. Internal consistency is $\alpha = .77$. The test-retest reliability ($r = .6$, $p < .001$) was considered appropriate for the measurement of baseline discomfort. A paired t-test yielded $t(67) = .74$, $p = .46$, indicating no significant change in repeated administration. While psychometrically sound, DS-DAT treats only one single complex affect state, discomfort.

Three reports have used the Ekman and Friesen FACS. Two studies indicate that they could use the technique with Alzheimer patients, which supports the idea that one can detect variability in emotions in this group (Clark & Bowling, 1989; Mace, 1989); however, neither provides data on measurement methods. Danner and Friesen (in press) used the system on 10 CI patients and presented case studies attesting to the CI patients' appropriate display of affective states when discussing their illness. Because of its complexity, the FACS procedure has limited clinical utility.

Lawton et al. (1996) developed the six-item Philadelphia Geriatric Center Affect Rating Scale to document behavioral displays of emotions in CI elders. The scale provides an equal number of positive affective states (pleasure, interest, and contentment) and negative affective states (anger, worry/anxiety, and sadness). Several behavioral descriptors accompany each affective state. They directly observed facial expression, body movement, and other cues that do not depend on self-report in 253 CI and 43 non-CI residents. They found each affect scale highly reliable as expressed in estimated durations over 10-minute observation periods. Further, validity estimates showed correlation between the positive states and various independent measures of social behavior and between negative states and other measures of depression, anger, anxiety, and withdrawal.

The seemingly incoherent verbalizations of CI elders probably contain a lot of information about affect. For example, Danner and Friesen (1996) describe an elder with angry affect during their semistructured interview. Careful examination of video-tapes revealed that, "although less than ten percent of her utterances were understandable and much of what could be understood was profanity" her anger actually varied with what others were doing. Jansson, Norberg, Sandman, Athlin, and Asplund (1993) found that expression of emotion in the face, voice, and body matched the overall situation: negative response to body care and positive response to food. Similarly, Hallberg, Luker, Norberg, Johnsson, and Eriksson (1993) found that Alzheimer's elders who engaged in vocally disruptive behavior reacted in comprehensible emotional ways. Cohen-Mansfield, Werner, and Marx (1990) found that patients who were alone displayed more agitated behaviors than they did when others were with them, illustrating their affective sensitivity to context.

Beck (1995) developed the Observable Displays of Affect Scale to measure facial expressions, vocalizations, and body movements as indicators of affect in CI elders. This 34-item instrument allows researchers to observe videotaped events repeatedly in actual time and slow motion (Ekman & Friesen, 1978). Such measurements are more sensitive since researchers can evaluate subtle behaviors. From videotape analysis, interrater correlation coefficients ranged from .46 to .80. Intrarater reliabilities ranged from .97 to 1.00. The interrater results indicate a need to refine the instrument. Although not as high as desired, these reliabilities are acceptable for the developmental stage of the instrument. This instrument could be shortened for use in the clinical setting.

Measuring Affect in CI Elders

Weiner et al. (1996) reviewed 14 comprehensive scales on psychiatric symptoms in AD. To review all the scales, see Weiner et al. (1996). The authors chose to describe (as published by Weiner et al., 1996) three of these scales because they are brief and measure some aspects of affect.

Behavioral and Emotional Activities Manifested in Dementia Scale (BEAM-D) (Sinha et al., 1992). This scale is a 16-item scale developed with 45 AD patients and rates 7 inferred behaviors (such as appropriateness or stability of affect). Clinicians administer the scale, which takes 15 minutes to complete, to the patient and caregiver. Each rating item is clearly defined with the descriptors 0 = no information available, behavior is not assessed or behavior cannot be assessed; 1 = consistent absence of the behavior; and 2 to 4 = severity and intensity of behavior. Interrater reliability is $\kappa = .71$, $r = .85$ for inferred behaviors; the scale has construct, content, and convergent validity. Compared with the Sandoz Clinical Assessment-Geriatric (Shader et al., 1974) and the Brief Psychiatric Rating Scale (Overall & Gorham, 1962), all items except hallucinations yielded r values significant at $p \geq .001$.

Behavioral Syndromes Scale for Dementia. (BSSD) (Devenand et al., 1992). Based on interviews of caregivers of 106 AD patients, this scale includes disinhibition (such as mood items) and apathy-indifference. The BSSD takes 20 to 30 minutes to complete. On some items, the frequency range is 1 = none to 6 = constant, whereas severity is measured from 0 = no information to 6 = extreme. Interrater, intraclass correlation coefficients range from .40 to .90. The BSSD has construct and content validity, but places disparate behavior and emotional items under single headings, does not rate most items for frequency, has no guidelines for severity, and would miss infrequent behaviors.

Neuropsychiatric Inventory. (NPI) (Cummings et al., 1994). This inventory, developed from an expert panel using the Delphi method, assesses a wide range of behaviors with potential to differentiate between dementia syndromes. The format used (screening strategy, evaluation of both frequency and severity) minimizes administration time while optimizing the capture of information. Clinicians administer the NPI, which takes 20 minutes, to caregivers of elderly dementia patients. The NPI includes measures of dysphoria, euphoria, apathy/indifference, and irritability/lability. Frequency is measured from 1 = < 1 to 4 = ≥ 1/day, and severity is measured from 1 = mild to 3 = severe. Interrater reliability is $r = .96$ to 1.0 (frequency) and .98 to 1.0 (severity). Test-retest reliability is $r = 0.79$ (frequency) and 0.86 (severity) with overall (Cronbach α) at $r = .88$. The NPI has construct and content validity and convergent validity with HAM-D (Hamilton, 1967) and BEHAVE-AD (Reisberg et al., 1987). For each item, total score equals frequency times severity.

SUMMARY

The measurement of affect in frail and CI elderly is important in evaluating their quality of life and the quality of care received. Instruments for measuring affect include self-report, reports of others, and observational instruments. The intensity, duration, and frequency of affective states deserve consideration in measurement. Although several instruments exist for measuring affect in frail and CI elderly, additional instruments with clinical utility need development. Attention to expressions of affect may allow caregivers to target their interventions to the frail and CI elders' needs more accurately. Appropriate response to displays of affect may help humanize the care of this vulnerable population.

REFERENCES

Albert, M. S., Cohen, C., & Koff, E. (1991). Perception of affect in patients with dementia of the Alzheimer type. *Archives of Neurology, 48,* 791-795.

Allender, J. R. (1984). Perception of emotional and personality change in dementia of the Alzheimer's type. Unpublished dissertation. University of New Mexico.

Allender, J., & Kaszniak, A. W. (1989). Processing of emotional cues in patients with dementia of the Alzheimer's type. *International Journal of Neuroscience, 46,* 147-155.

Asplund, K., Norberg, A., Adolfsson, R., & Waxman, H. M. (1991). Facial expressions in severely demented patients: A stimulus-response study of four patients with dementia of the Alzheimer type. *International Journal of Geriatric Psychiatry, 6,* 599-606.

Bahro, M., Silber, E., & Sunderland, T. (1995). How do patients with Alzheimer's disease cope with their illness? A clinical experience report. *Journal of the American Geriatrics Society, 43,* 41-46.

Beck, C. (1995). *Affect changes as outcomes of behavioral interventions.* NIA funded grant # 2R01 AG10321-04.

Bradburn, N. M. (1969). Two dimensions of psychological well-being: Positive and negative affect. In N. M. Bradburn & C. E. Hill (Eds.), *The structure of psychological well-being.* (pp. 53-70). Chicago: Aldine Publishing Co.

Caporael, L. R., Lukaszewski, M. P., & Culbertson, G. H. (1983). Secondary baby talk: Judgments by institutionalized elderly and their caregivers. *Journal of Personality and Social Psychology, 44,* 746-754.

Clark, P., & Bowling, A. (1989). Observational study of quality of life in nursing home and a long-stay ward for the elderly. *Ageing and Society, 9,* 123-148.

Clyde, D. (1963). *Manual for the Clyde Mood Scale.* Coral Gables, FL: University of Miami.

Cohen-Mansfield, J., Werner, P., & Marx, M. (1990). Screaming in nursing home residents. *Journal of the American Geriatrics Society, 38,* 785-792.

Costa, P. T., & McCrae, R. R. (1988). Personality in adulthood: A six-year longitudinal study of self-reports and spouse ratings on the NEO Personality Inventory. *Journal of Personality and Social Psychology, 54,* 853-863.

Cotrell, V., & Schulz, R. (1993). The perspective of the patient with Alzheimer's disease: A neglected dimension of dementia research. *The Gerontologist, 33,* 205-211.

Cummings, J. L., Mega, M., Gray, K., Rosenberg-Thompson, S., Carusi, D. A., & Gornbein, J. (1994). The Neuropsychiatric Inventory: An efficient tool for comprehensively assessing psychopathology in dementia. *Neurology, 44,* 2308-2314.

Daffner, K. R., Scinto, L. F. M., Weintraub, S., Guinessey, J. E., & Mesulam, M. M. (1992). Diminished curiosity in patients with probable Alzheimer's disease as measured by exploratory eye movements. *Neurology, 42,* 320-328.

Danner, D. D., & Friesen, W. V. (1996). Are severely impaired Alzheimer's patients aware of their environment and illness? *Journal of Clinical Gero-Psychology, 2,* 321-336.

DeLong, A. J. (1970). The microspatial structure of the older person: Some implications of planning the social and spatial environment. In L. A. Pastalan & D. H. Carson (Eds.), *Spatial behavior of older people* (pp. 68-87). Ann Arbor, MI: University of Michigan, Wayne State University Press.

Devenand, D., Brockington, C. D., Moody, B. J., Brown, R. P., Mayeux, R., Endicott, J., Sackeim, H. A. (1992). Behavioral syndromes in Alzheimer's disease. *International Psychogeriatrics, 4*(Suppl. 2), 161-184.

Diener, E., & Emmons, R. A. (1985). The independence of positive and negative affect. *Journal of Personality and Social Psychology, 47,* 1105-1117.

Ekman, P., & Davidson, R. J. (1993). Voluntary smiling changes regional brain activity. *Psychological Science, 4,* 342-345.

Ekman, P., & Friesen, W. V. (1978). *Facial action coding system.* Palo Alto, CA: Consulting Psychologists Press.

Ekman, P., Friesen, W. V., O'Sullivan, M., Diacoyanni-Tarlatzis, I., Krause, R., Pitcairn, T., Scherer, K., Chan, A., Heider, K., LeCompte, W. A., Ricci-Bitti, P. E., Tomita, M., & Tzavaras, A. (1987). Universal and cultural differences in the judgments of facial expressions of emotion. *Journal of Personality and Social Psychology, 53,* 712-717.

Folstein, M. F., Folstein, S., & McHugh, P. R. (1975). Mini-mental state: A practical method for grading the cognitive state of patients for the clinician. *Journal of Psychiatric Research, 12,* 189-198.

Goleman, D. (1995). *Emotional intelligence.* New York: Bantam Books.

Hallberg, I. R., Luker, K. A., Norberg, A., Johnsson, K., & Eriksson, S. (1990). Staff interaction with vocally disruptive demented patients compared with demented controls. *Aging, 2,* 163-171.

Hamilton, M. (1967). Development of a rating scale for primary depressive illness. *British Journal of Social and Clinical Psychology, 6,* 278-296.

Herskovitz, E. (1995). Struggling over subjectivity: Debates about the "self" and Alzheimer's disease. *Medical Anthropology Quarterly, 9,* 146-164.

Horowitz, M., Adler, N., & Kegeles, S. (1988). A scale for measuring the occurrence of positive states of mind: A preliminary report. *Psychosomatic Medicine, 50,* 477-483.

Hurley, A. C., Volicer, B. J., Hanrahan, P. A., Houde, S., & Volicer, L. (1992). Assessment of discomfort in advanced Alzheimer patients. *Research in Nursing and Health, 15,* 369-377.

Jansson, L., Norberg, A., Sandman, P., Athlin, E., & Asplund, K. (1982). Interpreting facial expressions in patients in the terminal stage of Alzheimer's disease. *Omega, 28,* 309-324.

Kotsch, W. E., Gerbing, D. W., & Schwartz, L. E. (1982). The construct validity of the Differential Emotions Scale as adapted for children and adolescents. In C. E. Izard (Ed.), *Measuring emotions in infants and children.* (pp. 251-278). Cambridge, England: Cambridge University Press.

Kuykendall, D., Keating, J. P., & Wagaman, J. (1988). Assessing affective states: A new methodology for some old problems. *Cognitive Therapy and Research, 12,* 279-294.

Lawton, M. P. (1993). Quality of life in Alzheimer's disease. *Alzheimer Disease and Associated Disorders, 8*(Suppl. 3), 138-150.

Lawton, M. P., Kleban, M. H., Dean, J., Rajagopal, D., & Parmelee, P. A. (1992). The factorial generality of brief positive and negative affect measures. *Journals of Gerontology: Psychological Sciences, 47,* 228-237.

Lawton, M. P., Perkinson, M., & Van Haitsma, K. (1996). *Rating emotion states in dementing illness.* Philadelphia: Philadelphia Geriatric Center.

Lawton, M. P., Van Haitsma, K., & Klapper, J. (1996). Observed affect in nursing home residents with Alzheimer's disease. *Journals of Gerontology, 51B,* P3-P14.

Levenson, R. W., Carstensen, L. L., Friesen, W. V., & Ekman, P. (1991). Emotion, physiology, and expression in old age. *Psychology and Aging, 6,* 28-35.

Lewinsohn, P. M., & Graff, M. (1973). Pleasant activities and depression. *Journal of Consulting and Clinical Psychology, 41,* 261-268.

Logsdon, R. G., & Teri, L. (in press). The Pleasant Events Schedule–AD: Psychometric properties and relationship to depression and cognition in Alzheimer's disease patients. *The Gerontologist.*

Lorr, M., & Wunderlich, R. A. (1988). A semantic differential mood scale. *Journal of Clinical Psychology, 44,* 33-36.

Mace, N. (1989). A new method for studying the patient's experience of care. *The American Journal of Alzheimer's Care and Related Disorders & Research, 4*, 4-6.

Mace, N. L. (1990). *The management of problem behaviors in dementia.* Baltimore, MD: Johns Hopkins University Press.

Magaziner, J. (1991). The use of proxy respondents in health surveys of the aged. In R. B. Wallace & R. F. Wodson (Eds.), *The epidemiologic study of the elderly.* New York: Oxford University Press.

Montgomery, S. A., & Asberg, M. A. (1979). A new depression scale designed to be sensitive to change. *British Journal of Psychiatry, 134*, 382-389.

Morris, W. (1989). *Mood: The frame of mind.* New York: Springer.

National Advisory Mental Health Council. (1995). Basic behavioral science research for mental health: A national investment: Emotion and motivation. *American Psychologist, 50*, 838-845.

Nowlis, V. (1965). Research with the Mood Adjective Checklist. In S. S. Tomkins & C. E. Izard (Eds.), *Affect, cognition, and personality* (pp. 352-389). New York: Springer.

O'Rourke, L. F. (1996). *Depression and cognitive impairment in person with dementia.* Unpublished master's thesis, University of Tennessee.

Overall, J. E., & Gorham, D. R. (1962). The Brief Psychiatric Rating Scale. *Psychological Reports, 10*, 799-812.

Parmelee, P. A., Katz, I. R., & Lawton, M. P. (1989). Depression among institutionalized aged: Assessment and prevalence estimation. *Journals of Gerontology: Medical Sciences, 44*, M22-M29.

Reisberg, B., Borenstein, J., Franssen, E., Salob, S., & Steinberg, G. (1987). BEHAVE-AD: A clinical rating scale for the assessment of pharmacologically remediable behavioral symptomatology in Alzheimer's disease. In A. Altman (Ed.), *Alzheimer's disease problems, prospects, and perspectives* (pp. 1-16). New York: Plenum.

Robinson, R. G., Parikh, R. M., Lipsey, J. R., Starkstein, S. E., & Price, T. R. (1993). Pathological laughing and crying following stroke: Validation of a measurement scale and a double-blind treatment study. *American Journal of Psychiatry, 150*, 286-293.

Schulz, R., O'Brien, A. T., & Tompkins, C. A. (1994). The measurement of affect in the elderly. In M.P. Lawton & J. A. Teresi (Eds.), *Annual review of gerontology and geriatrics: Focus on assessment techniques* (pp. 210-233). Pittsburgh, PA: University of Pittsburgh, Department of Psychiatry.

Shader, R. I., Harmatz, J. S., & Salzman, C. (1974). A new scale for clinical assessment in geriatric populations: Sandoz Clinical Assessment-Geriatric (SCAG). *Journal of the American Geriatrics Society, 12*, 107-113.

Simmons, S. F., Schnelle, J. F., Uman, G. C., Kulvicki, A., Lee, K. O., & Ouslander, J. G. (1996). *Selecting nursing home residents for satisfaction surveys.* Accepted for publication. Reseda, CA: Borun Center for Gerontological Research, University of California at Los Angeles School of Medicine.

Sinha, D., Zemlan, F. P., Nelson, S., Bienenfeld, D., Thienhaus, O., Ramaswamy, G., & Hamilton, S. (1992). A new scale for assessing behavioral agitation in dementia. *Psychiatry Research, 41*, 73-88.

Starkstein, S. E., Migliorelli, R., Teson, A., Petracca, G., Chemerinsky, E., Manes, F., & Leiguarda, R. (1995). Prevalence and clinical correlates of pathological affective display in Alzheimer's disease. *Journal of Neurology, Neurosurgery, and Psychology, 59*, 55-60.

Stewart, A. L., Sherbourne, C. D., & Brod, A. (1996). Measuring health-related quality of life in older and demented populations. In B. Spilker (Ed.), *Quality of life and pharmacoeconomics in clinical trials* (2nd ed.). Philadelphia: Lippincott-Raven.

Stone, A. A. (1995). Measurement of affective response. In S. Cohen, R. C. Kessler, & G. L. Underwood (Eds.), *Measuring stress: A guide for health and social scientists* (pp. 148-171). New York: Oxford University Press.

Tappen, R. M., & Barry, C. (1995). Assessment of affect in advanced Alzheimer's disease: The dementia mood picture test. *Journal of Gerontological Nursing, 21*, 44-46.

Teri, L., & Lewinsohn, P. M. (1982). Modification of Pleasant and Unpleasant Events Schedule for use with the elderly. *Journal of Consulting and Clinical Psychology, 50*, 444-445.

Teri, L., & Logsdon, R. G. (1991). Identifying pleasant activities for Alzheimer's disease patients: The Pleasant Events Schedule–AD. *The Gerontologist, 31*, 124-127.

Tomkins, S. (1984). Innate affect activators. In K. Scherer & P. Ekman (Eds.), *Approaches to emotions*. (pp. 167-168). Hillsdale, NJ: Erlbaum.

Watson, D., Clark, L. A., & Tellegen, A. (1988). Development and validation of brief measures of positive and negative affect: The PANAS Scales. *Journal of Personality and Social Psychology, 54*, 1063-1079.

Weiner, M. F., Koss, E., Wild, K. V., Folks, D. G., Tariot, P., Luszczynska, H., & Whitehouse, P. (1996). Measures of psychiatric symptoms in Alzheimer patients: A review. *Alzheimer Disease and Associated Disorders, 10*, 20-30.

Yesavage, J. A., Brink, T. L., & Rose, T. L. (1983). Development and validation of a geriatric depression scale: A preliminary report. *Journal of Psychiatric Residents, 17*, 37-49.

Chapter 8

Comorbidity in Alzheimer's Disease

Ladislav Volicer and Ann Hurley

The investigation of a clinical course or treatment interventions in Alzheimer's disease is often complicated by the presence of other diseases in the research study population. The prevalence of Alzheimer's disease increases with age, reaching up to 47% in individuals 85 years old or older (Evans et al., 1989). Since most other diseases are also more common in the elderly population, many Alzheimer patients have other comorbid conditions. Thus studies that would eliminate patients with comorbid conditions would have two methodological problems: difficulties recruiting sufficient numbers of subjects and poor applicability of results to the general Alzheimer population.

However, the existence of comorbidity should not be viewed only as a complication in study design and subject selection. Studies on comorbidity can provide valuable insights into mechanisms that lead to the development of various diseases. An example is presence of familial hypercholesterolemia in patients with coronary artery disease. It is possible that similar insights into the pathogenesis of Alzheimer's disease will be provided in the future.

This article will discuss the types of comorbidity to consider when planning dementia studies and two main approaches to the evaluation of the effects of comorbidity on the course of Alzheimer's disease. One of these approaches calculates a composite score indicating the degree of comorbidity. Four methods for calculation of this comorbidity score will be presented and their application to dementia studies will be discussed.

TYPES OF COMORBIDITY

Comorbidity can be defined as "any distinct additional clinical entity that has existed or that may occur during the clinical course of a patient who has the index disease under study" (Feinstein, 1970). In a strict sense, comorbidity applies only to coexistent diseases, not symptoms. We can distinguish two types of comorbidity: random and pathogenic.

In some cases, the coexistence of both conditions is merely due to random association. The prevalence of this random comorbidity is such as would be expected from

Acknowledgment: This work was supported by the USPHS grant 1P30 AG13846 and by the Veterans Administration.

prevalences of both conditions in the general population. Some diseases occur more frequently in patients suffering from Alzheimer's disease than in the general population. An example of this comorbidity is the incidence of aspiration pneumonia in patients with advanced Alzheimer's disease (Chandra, Bharucha, & Schoenberg, 1986). Increased incidence of aspiration pneumonia is due to the relationship between the pathogenesis of both diseases because Alzheimer's disease causes impaired swallowing and aspiration (Harkness, Bentley, & Roghmann, 1990). Therefore, this comorbidity is pathogenic (Kaplan & Feinstein, 1974).

RANDOM COMORBIDITY

Alzheimer patients suffer from a whole range of diseases at a rate similar to the rate in a general population. For instance, since Alzheimer's disease affects 10% of individuals over the age of 65 (Evans et al., 1989) and hypertension is present in 28% of this age group (Shurtleff, 1974), it would be expected that 2.8% of general population suffer from both Alzheimer's disease and hypertension. According to consequences of the coexisting disease, it is possible to distinguish three subtypes of random comorbidity (Kaplan & Feinstein, 1974).

Diagnostic Comorbidity

Diagnostic comorbidity exists when two diseases have the same symptoms. The diagnosis of Alzheimer's disease is made primarily by the exclusion of other possible causes of dementia. Gradual onset is one of the main clinical and diagnostic features of Alzheimer's disease. This makes it difficult to determine the exact time of the onset of the disease; although it is important to take the duration of Alzheimer's disease into consideration when designing therapeutic trials. This difficulty is further enhanced if the patient suffered from depression, which may cause cognitive impairment even in individuals who do not suffer from a progressive dementia (Mitchell & Dening, 1996).

Often, the families ascribe the onset of Alzheimer's disease to a specific occasion, such as hospitalization for surgery or an infection. Elderly patients sometimes develop confusion and delirium during a hospitalization, which may not completely resolve (Kolbeinsson & Jonsson, 1993). However, in many cases, detailed questioning reveals symptoms of cognitive impairment that were present before the hospitalization. On the other hand, it is possible that the development of Alzheimer's disease was induced or at least accelerated by an iatrogenic cause, such as hypoxia.

The clinical diagnosis of probable Alzheimer's disease according to the NINCDS-ADRDA (McKhann et al., 1984) and DSM-IV criteria is primarily a diagnosis of exclusion, although measurement of A-beta and tau proteins in the cerebrospinal fluid, together with determination of apolipoprotein E status, may lead to a definitive diagnosis in a small fraction of patients (Munroe et al., 1995; Southwick et al., 1996). The presence of a cerebrovascular disease, manifested by transient ischemic attacks or strokes, does not exclude the possibility of coexisting Alzheimer's disease, because combined Alzheimer and multi-infarct changes are found in 1.9% -27.5% of autopsies (Jellinger, Danielczyk, Fischer, & Gabriel, 1990).

Prognostic Comorbidity

Prognostic comorbidity exists when the presence of another disorder affects the prognosis of a patient. This may involve effectiveness of a therapeutic intervention or the length of survival.

Therapeutic Intervention. At present, the options for treatment of cognitive impairment are quite limited. The only drugs approved for treatment of Alzheimer's disease are cholinesterase inhibitors, which act by inhibiting breakdown of acetylcholine (Knapp et al., 1994). The first drug approved was tacrine which causes liver damage in a significant number of patients (Watkins, Zimmerman, Knapp, Gracon, & Lewis, 1994); preexisting liver damage might prevent administration of an effective tacrine dose.

Length of Survival. Several comorbid conditions were reported to decrease the 2-year survival rate in patients with dementia (Van Dijk, Van de Sande, Dippel, & Habbema, 1992): myocardial infarction, heart failure, atrial fibrillation, Parkinson's disease, respiratory tract infection, anemia, pressure sores and malignancies. In that study, hypertension and stroke were not associated with increased mortality rate. However, in a follow-up study by the same authors (Van Dijk, Dippel, Van der Meulen, & Habbema, 1996), stroke significantly increased the effect of pulmonary infection and the mortality rate was also increased by urinary incontinence, diabetes mellitus and visual problems. The authors conclude that comorbidity and severity of dementia independently influence mortality.

Burns, Lewis, Jacoby and Levy (1991) found a higher mortality rate in patients with the diagnosis of *possible* Alzheimer's disease than in patients with diagnosis of *probable* Alzheimer's disease. They postulated that this difference occurred because the diagnosis of possible Alzheimer's disease was used whenever there was a coexisting other physical disease such as hypertension or cerebrovascular disease. In contrast, Walsh, Welch, and Larson (1990) found no effect of comorbid conditions on survival of Alzheimer patients. The authors stated that this was probably due to the relatively small sample which was further divided into subgroups.

Incidental Comorbidity

Incidental comorbidity is that which has no influence on either disease detection or course. Examples of incidental comorbidity are gout, or other chronic nonlife threatening conditions.

EPIDEMIOLOGICAL COMORBIDITY

Other conditions exist in Alzheimer patients more commonly than would be expected on the basis of their prevalence in the general population. In this case we may speak of epidemiological or pathogenic comorbidity. Such a relationship between two conditions may indicate that the conditions have a common cause, or that one predisposes an individual for development of the other. At the current level of knowledge, it is sometimes difficult to distinguish between these two possibilities. For instance, a history of depression is known to increase the probability of developing Alzheimer's disease (Speck et al., 1995). It is not clear, however, if depression in these individuals is due to the early preclinical stage of Alzheimer's disease, or if depression affects the biochemical processes of the brain in such a way that the individual is more likely to develop Alzheimer's disease.

Epidemiological comorbidity may be extended to a situation when two or more conditions coexist in a family unit. The increased incidence of Down syndrome in families of Alzheimer patients (Heyman et al., 1984; Huff, Auerbach, Charkravarti, & Boller, 1988) is an example of familial comorbidity. Epidemiological comorbidity may provide clues to the pathogenesis of Alzheimer's disease. Thus, the increased incidence of Alzheimer's disease in individuals who suffered a brain injury (Mayeux et al., 1993; Mortimer et al., 1991) points to the possible role of tissue repair processes in the development of Alzheimer's disease. One possible scenario is that injury induces an increased production of growth factors, which include the amyloid precursor protein (Mucke et al., 1994). The increased production of amyloid precursor protein may overwhelm its processing mechanisms, resulting in the formation of toxic fragments which cause further cell damage (Mattson & Goodman, 1995).

Several diseases are more common in Alzheimer's disease because they are a consequence of the dementing process. These diseases include new onset seizures (Volicer, Smith, & Volicer, 1995), respiratory and urinary infections (Carson, 1988; Marrie, Durant, & Kwan, 1986), and pressure sores (Chandra et al., 1986). Seizures occur in about 20% of patients with advanced Alzheimer's disease. They may be due to compensatory changes which occur in the brains of Alzheimer patients, such as increased kainic acid binding sites or axon sprouting (Geddes, Ulas, Brunner, Choe, & Cotman, 1992; Geddes et al., 1985). The increased incidence of infections in patients with advanced Alzheimer's disease is due to changes of the immune system, incontinence, decreased mobility, and aspiration. Pressure sores are a secondary consequence due to decreased mobility and the presence of a nutritional deficit (Berlowitz & Wilking, 1989).

It is also possible that some diseases are less common in patients with Alzheimer's disease. Adolfsson and his coworkers (1980) reported that diabetes mellitus was less common in hospitalized Alzheimer patients. Patients with Alzheimer's disease had lower fasting blood glucose and higher insulin levels during oral glucose tolerance tests than did hospitalized cognitively intact patients (Adolfsson, Bucht, Lithner, & Winblad, 1980; Bucht, Adolfsson, Lithner, & Winblad, 1983). Although this finding was not supported by other investigators (De Leon et al., 1988; Winograd et al., 1991), Nielson et al. (1996) recently reported that diabetes is much rarer in Alzheimer's disease than in other dementias. They proposed that the protective effect could be mediated by the insulin-degrading enzyme which degrades also beta-amyloid peptide. Other possible explanations of this relationship is that chronic hyperglycemia may improve brain metabolism and decrease beta-amyloid peptide production, and that weight loss observed in some Alzheimer patients may prevent development of diabetes (Halter, 1996).

Incidence of diabetes was also compared in dementia and control patients using both autopsy and clinical samples (Thorpe, Widman, Wallin, Beiswanger, & Blumenthal, 1994). These investigators found significantly lower prevalence of diabetes only in a female clinical sample. However, they combined all dementia types and the prevalence of diabetes was lower in nonvascular than in vascular dementias. In this study, there was also lower prevalence of cardiomegaly/hypertension and myocardial infarction in dementia patients than in control individuals.

MEASUREMENT OF COMORBIDITY

There are two main approaches to the evaluation of the effects of comorbidity on the course of Alzheimer's disease or outcomes of treatment strategies. The first approach involves the investigation of the effect of each individual disease and the second combines all comorbid conditions into a single comorbidity score. The evaluation of individual diseases results in a large number of variables, which makes the analyses difficult and would require large sample sizes to detect differences in research variables. Also, the impact of rare diseases may be difficult to determine because the number of patients with these conditions may be too small. A single comorbidity score simplifies the analyses and permits the inclusion of all conditions. However, currently there is no consensus about the optimal way of combining comorbid conditions.

A computerized literature search did not reveal any approach to the measurement of comorbidity which was specifically developed for individuals with dementia, but there are four major recognized methods for classifying comorbidity that have been used with other populations. In the remainder of this article, we will describe these methods and discuss their empirical support.

Kaplan and Feinstein (1974) developed one of the first systems for classifying comorbidity. They studied the effect of comorbidity on vascular complications and survival in patients with diabetes. The comorbid index was developed in two steps. First, comorbid conditions were divided: into cogent conditions which are those ailments that are expected to impair a patient's long-term survival, and noncogent conditions are those ailments that have no known long-term effects on vital organs. The noncogent conditions could be either chronic conditions which are well controlled with or without medication (varicose veins, hemorrhoids, controlled hypothyroidism, etc.), or a single period of morbidity that completely resolved (passed ureteral stones, removed pheochromocytoma, diverse infections, fractures, etc.).

The cogent conditions included hypertension, cardiac, cerebral or psychic, respiratory, renal, hepatic, gastrointestinal, peripheral vascular, malignancy, locomotor impairment, alcoholism, and miscellaneous. For each of these cogent conditions, three grades of severity were defined. Grade 1 was used for a slight decompensation of a vital system and for episodes of chronic conditions that were not life threatening. Grade 2 was used for an impaired but not full decompensation of a vital system, and for episodes and chronic conditions that were potentially life threatening. Grade 3 was used for a recent full decompensation of a vital system, and for recent life-threatening events and chronic conditions.

For instance, hypertension Grade 1 was defined as diastolic pressure 90-114 mm Hg without secondary effects of symptoms, Grade 2 as diastolic pressure 115-129 mm Hg or at any level below 130 with secondary cardiovascular or symptomatic effects such as headaches, vertigo, and epistaxis, and Grade 3 as severe or malignant hypertension with papilledema, encephalopathy or diastolic pressure 130 mm of Hg or higher. Each patient was then assigned a comorbidity index according to the highest severity of any cogent comorbid condition, except in the case where two or more Grade 2 ailments occurred in different organ systems. In this case, the patient's comorbid index was designated Grade 3.

The survival analysis of 188 patients followed for 5 years indicated that the comorbid index was significantly related to the mortality rate. The mortality rate of Grade 0 (no cogent comorbidity) was 7%, Grade 1, 28%, Grade 2, 42%, and Grade 3, 69%. The differences between Grades 0 and 1 and Grades 2 and 3 were significant, while the difference between Grades 1 and 2 was not. The authors, therefore, combined Grades 1 and 2 into one category labeled Moderate. Grade 0 was labeled None, and Grade 3 was labeled Severe. Using these three degrees of severity, the investigators divided patients further into groups of those whose comorbidity was due to vascular conditions, those whose comorbidity was due to nonvascular conditions, and into a younger and older group. There was a significant relationship between comorbidity and mortality rate in both vascular and nonvascular subgroups, and in both age groups.

Weighted Index of Comorbidity (WIC; Charlson, Pompei, Ales, & MacKenzie, 1987). In contrast to Kaplan and Feinstein (1974), who developed their classification scheme on the basis of clinical experience without using specific data about prognosis, Charlson, Pompei, Ales, and MacKenzie (1987) developed their classification scheme on the basis of the actual impact of various diseases on mortality during acute hospitalization and 1 year later. They analyzed records from 607 patients admitted to a medical service for the number and severity of comorbid diseases at the time of admission and recorded 1 year survival status. From these data, they then calculated adjusted relative risk for 1 year mortality for each comorbid disease using a proportional hazard model (Cox, 1972). Conditions with relative risks of 1.19 or less were dropped from consideration. Conditions with a relative risk of >1.2<1.5 were assigned a weight of 1, conditions with a risk of >1.49<2.5 a weight of 2; conditions with a weight of >2.49<3.5 a weight of 3; and conditions with weights of 3.5 or more were assigned a weight of 6.

Conditions with weight of 1 included myocardial infarct, congestive heart failure, peripheral vascular disease, cerebrovascular disease, dementia, chronic pulmonary disease, connective tissue disease, ulcer disease, mild liver disease, and diabetes. Conditions with weight 2 included hemiplegia, moderate or severe renal disease, diabetes with end-organ damage, any tumor, leukemia, and lymphoma. The condition with weight 3 was moderate or severe liver disease; weight 6 was assigned to metastatic solid tumor and AIDS. The detailed description of each individual condition was provided in the Appendix to Charlson et al. (1987). The WIC was computed for each patient by adding weights for all coexisting conditions. The WIC was a significant predictor of 1 year survival and explained a higher proportion of variance than a model based on the number of comorbid diseases (Charlson et al., 1987).

The WIC was further validated in a cohort of 685 breast cancer patients who had received their first treatment at least 10 years previously. Their records were analyzed and the death was attributed to either breast cancer or to a comorbid disease. The method of Hutchinson, Thomas, and MacGibbon (1982) was used to create a scoring system which combined both age and comorbidity. The data analysis showed that the relative risk for each increasing level of comorbidity index was 2.3 and the relative risk for each decade of age was 2.4. Therefore, the age-comorbidity index was constructed by adding 1 point to the WIC for each decade of age over the fourth decade (age >49<59 1 point, age >59<69 2 points, etc.). Thus a 62-year old patient with a comorbidity score of 1 would have an age-comorbidity index of 3. A composite age-comorbidity score was calculated for each patient and the actual 10-year survival was evaluated. The observed survival was 93% for an age-comorbidity index of 0, 73% for an index of 1, 52% for an index of 2, and 45% for an index of 3, which was very close to a predicted 10-year survival calculated for a theoretical low-risk population (Charlson et al., 1987).

Charlson et al. (1987) also compared their method with the method of Kaplan and Feinstein (1974) in predicting a 10-year survival rate in the cohort of breast cancer patients. They found that both methods did equally well in demarcating patients at a very low risk of comorbid deaths and that the amount of variance explained was virtually identical with both methods.

Index of Coexistent Disease (ICED; Greenfield, Apolone, McNeil, & Cleary, 1993). This index was developed to study the effect of comorbidity on postoperative complications and recovery in patients undergoing total hip replacement. It is based on previous work of the same authors in which they documented that coexisting conditions were related to physicians' choice and intensity of treatment in cancer patients (Bennett et al., 1991; Greenfield et al., 1987). The authors defined comorbidity as "overall severity of illness due to diseases other than hip disease that could affect recovery from surgery" and identified two dimensions of comorbidity: individual disease severity and functional status.

According to an unpublished manual (Apolone & Greenfield, 1991), individual disease severity (IDS) represented the physiological severity of 12 categories of specific conditions: organic heart disease, ischemic heart disease, primary arrhythmias and conduction problems, congestive heart failure, hypertension, cerebrovascular accident, peripheral vascular disease, diabetes mellitus, respiratory problems, malignancies, hepatobiliary disease, and renal disease. For each condition, five mutually exclusive severity stages were described using symptoms, signs and laboratory tests, based on an approach derived from the Gonella (1985) staging system.

IDS of 0 indicated absence of a coexistent decease; IDS of 1 indicated a comorbid condition which is asymptomatic or mildly symptomatic (e.g., controlled hypertension with no medications, chemical diabetes, sporadic urinary tract infections); IDS of 2 indicated a mild to moderate condition that is generally symptomatic and requires medical intervention or a past condition, presently benign, that presents a moderate risk of morbidity (e.g., hypertension or asthma controlled with medications, history of myocardial infarction with no residual effects); IDS of 3 indicated an uncontrolled condition which causes moderate to severe disease manifestations (e.g., chronic renal or hepatic failure, symptomatic coronary heart disease); and IDS of 4 indicated an uncontrolled condition which causes severe manifestations, requiring immediate intervention and carrying an extremely high risk of mortality (e.g., respiratory failure, coma, diabetic ketoacidosis).

Functional status (FS) was included to measure the global impact of all conditions, diagnosed or not, on patients' functional ability. Ten functional areas were identified: circulation, respiration, neurological, mental, urinary, fecal, feeding, vision, hearing, and speech. Each of these areas was classified into one of three ranks with increasing level of impairment. FS 0 indicated no significant impairment or normal function, FS 1 indicated mild or moderate impairment (e.g., walking with assistance, chronic cough), and FS 2 indicated serious/severe impairment (e.g., bedridden, requiring oxygen) (Apolone & Greenfield, 1991).

Patients were given the highest IDS and FS scores achieved in any of the categories. The investigators stated that "earlier analysis showed that having additional coexistent conditions at the same or lower level added no additional risk." The final ICED index was assigned according to the combination of both IDS and FS scores. Patients with IDS 0 and FS 0 or 1 were assigned ICED 0, patients with IDS 1 or 2 and FS 0 were assigned ICED 1. Patients with IDS 1 or 2 and FS 1 were assigned ICED 2, and patients with either IDS 3 or FS 2 were assigned ICED 3.

Analysis of data from 356 patients showed that IDS and FS were only weakly associated ($r = 0.27$) indicating that they measured different domains. The incidence of complications during the hospitalization for total hip replacement increased with increasing ICED scores, from 3% in patients with ICED 0, to 41% in patients with ICED 3. Similarly the functional outcomes, determined 1 year after the surgery, were strongly related to ICED scores (Greenfield et al., 1993).

Chronic Disease Score (CDS; Von Korff, Wagner, & Saunders, 1992). Use of computerized data bases for the estimation of comorbidity was first investigated by Mossey and Roos (1987). They used automated insurance claims data to measure health care status. However, this approach is limited by differences in perceived need for visits by different health care professionals and by nonhealth-related influences, such as supply of hospital beds and supply of physicians. Therefore, Von Korff and coworkers (1992) investigated the use of another data base-automated pharmacy data.

A multidisciplinary group of physicians, pharmacists, epidemiologists and health services researchers developed scoring rules for prescriptions used by HMO enrollees. They started with the assumptions that the score should increase with the number of chronic diseases treated and with complexity of treatment, potentially life-threatening or progressive diseases should receive higher scores, and treatment used for CDS score should target diseases not symptoms. Therefore, they excluded prescriptions for symptomatic conditions, such as analgesics, anti-inflammatory drugs, antidepressants, and sedatives/hypnotics. The group assigned weights to drugs used in the treatment of 17 diseases or classes of diseases. Treatments for heart disease, respiratory illness and hypertension, which may simultaneously use several drug classes for the same illness, were weighted according to the number of drug classes used for an individual patient. The CDS score was calculated by adding weights assigned to all relevant prescriptions that the patient was receiving (Von Korff et al., 1992).

Using data from 122,911 HMO enrollees, the CDS was correlated with total ambulatory visits and age, but not with gender. In contrast, ambulatory visits correlated less with age, but had a significant correlation with gender due to more frequent visits by females. The CDS was relatively stable, with little change from year to year, and in a subgroup of 941 patients correlated with ratings of the severity of physical disease made by primary care physicians. The CDS also correlated with self-rated health status and with graded chronic pain. The CDS was not correlated with depression and anxiety scores, while the numbers of visits were. Both CDS and visits were correlated with a measure of severity of diffuse physical symptomatology (somatization). The CDS was also associated with functional disability and with subsequent probability of death and being hospitalized. In patients with a CDS score of 7 or higher, the odds ratio for hospitalization was 5 times higher, and the odds ratio for death 10 times higher than in patients with a CDS score of 0 (Von Korff et al., 1992).

The use of CDS was replicated in another study, using more than 375,000 enrollees of another HMO (Johnson, Hornbrook, & Nichols, 1994). This study found that CDS scores increased during one year, but there was very good correlation between CDS scores in two subsequent years. The CDS correlated with the number of chronic conditions diagnosed by a physician (based on patient recall) and with following-year health care visits and hospitalizations. The correlation between CDS scores and episodes of hospitalization persisted after adjustment for age, gender, same year health care visits (or hospitalization), and perception of general health (Johnson et al., 1994).

In conclusion, there are four acceptable methods for calculating comorbidity. Each of the methods has positive and negative features when considering their direct applicability to dementia studies.

IMPLICATIONS FOR DEMENTIA STUDIES

None of the four methods described above is clearly superior to another. The Kaplan and Feinstein and ICED methods base the comorbidity score on the severity of the most severe comorbid conditions, while WIC and CDS use a weighted score of all comorbid conditions. The similarity of information obtained by the Kaplan and Feinstein and WIC methods indicates that both approaches are acceptable and better than a simple count of comorbid conditions. In a recent study, the Kaplan and Feinstein, WIC and ICED methods were calculated in the same patient population (Albertsen, Fryback, Storer, Kolon, & Fine, 1995). Detailed results were not presented, but the authors stated that the three indexes were highly correlated and ICED accounted for "somewhat more variation in survival than did the other two indexes."

A method used for controlling comorbidity in dementia studies should not be confounded by severity of dementia itself. This problem is most significant with the ICED method, which combines a score indicating disease severity with a score indicating functional impairment. Many of the 10 items in the functional impairment part are affected by the progression of dementia. Those which are not affected, such as circulation and respiration, are reflected by the IDS score. Therefore, it is possible to eliminate the functional impairment part and use the IDS score as the comorbidity index instead of the full ICED score. The Kaplan and Feinstein method includes as one of the cogent co-morbid ailments "locomotor impairment" which may be also a consequence of advanced dementia. The WIC method includes "dementia" as one of the conditions without specifying the stage or severity.

Another problem in using these methods for measuring comorbidity in patients with dementia is that the list of coexistent medical conditions does not include some comorbid conditions that are cogent for dementia patients, such as pressure ulcers. However, it would be possible to consider pressure ulcers a consequence of dementia because of decreased mobility, incontinence and eating difficulties instead as unrelated comorbid condition.

The CDS method is promising for studies where an automated pharmacy database is available. However, it may be biased by different levels of insurance drug benefit which would influence how many patients will not fill their prescriptions, and by differences in patients' adherence to their treatment regime. People treated with the same medications may also have differences in their health status. Furthermore, the prescribing may be influenced by prescriber characteristics. The CDS scoring may also not correctly represent the importance of different conditions because it was derived by a group consensus rather than from empirical hard data. However, this method seems to be preferable to the estimation of a chronic disease status from insurance claims.

We hope that this article will help to clarify the concept of comorbidity and help in planning studies involving demented individuals. None of the methods for comorbidity determination was designed specifically for this subject population. The final decision about which method to use to control for comorbid conditions depends on the nature and objectives of an individual study.

Operational explicitness in the definitions and precise measurement of comorbid conditions are required to identify correctly those causal or associative relationships that may affect the course of Alzheimer's disease. The inclusion of rigorously constructed comorbidity factors in the study of Alzheimer's disease is essential and may provide new insights into this disease.

REFERENCES

Adolfsson, R., Bucht, G., Lithner, F., & Winblad, B. (1980). Hypoglycemia in Alzheimer's disease. *Acta Medica Scandinavica, 208*, 387-388.

Albertsen, P. C., Fryback, D. G., Storer, B. E., Kolon, T. F., & Fine, J. (1995). Long-term survival among men with conservatively treated localized prostate cancer. *Journal of the American Medical Association, 274*, 626-631.

Apolone, G., & Greenfield, S. (1991). *Co-morbidity manual: How to score the revised approach to ICED*. Boston, MA: Institute for the Improvement of Medical Care and Health, New England Medical Center.

Bennett, C. L., Greenfield, S., Aronow, H., Ganz, P., Vogelzang, N. J., & Elashoff, R. M. (1991). Patterns of care related to age of men with prostate cancer. *Cancer, 67*, 2633-2641.

Berlowitz, D. R., & Wilking, S. V. B. (1989). Risk factors for pressure sores: A comparison of cross-sectional and cohort derived data. *Journal of the American Geriatrics Society, 37*, 1043-1050.

Bucht, G., Adolfsson, R., Lithner, F., & Winblad, B. (1983). Changes in blood glucose and insulin secretion in patients with senile dementia of Alzheimer type. *Acta Medica Scandinavica, 213*, 387-392.

Burns, A., Lewis, G., Jacoby, R., & Levy, R. (1991). Factors affecting survival in Alzheimer's disease. *Psychological Medicine, 21*, 363-370.

Carson, C. C., III. (1988). Nosocomial urinary tract infection. *Surgical Clinics of North America, 68*, 1147-1155.

Chandra, V., Bharucha, N. E., & Schoenberg, B. S. (1986). Conditions associated with Alzheimer's disease at death: Case-control study. *Neurology, 36*, 209-211.

Charlson, M. E., Pompei, P., Ales, K. L., & MacKenzie, C. R. (1987). A new method of classifying prognostic comorbidity in longitudinal studies: development and validation. *Journal of Chronic Diseases, 40*, 373-383.

Cox, D. R. (1972). Regression models and life tables. *Journal of the Royal Statistical Society, 34*, 187-220.

De Leon, M. J., McRae, T., Tsai, J. R., George, A. E., Marcus, D. L., Freedman, M., Wolf, A. P., & McEwen, B. (1988). Abnormal cortisol response in Alzheimer's disease linked to hippocampal atrophy. *Lancet, 2*, 391-392.

Evans, D. A., Funkenstein, H. H., Albert, M. S., Scherr, P. A., Cook, N. R., Chown, M. J., Hebert, L. E., Hennekens, C. H., & Taylor, J. O. (1989). Prevalence of Alzheimer's disease in a community population of older persons. Higher than previously reported. *Journal of the American Medical Association, 262*, 2551-2556.

Feinstein, A. R. (1970). The pre-therapeutic classification of co-morbidity in chronic disease. *Journal of Chronic Diseases, 23*, 455-468.

Geddes, J. W., Monaghan, D. T., Cotman, C. W., Lott, I. T., Kim, R. C., & Chui, H. C. (1985). Plasticity of hippocampal circuitry in Alzheimer's disease. *Science, 230*, 1179-1181.

Geddes, J. W., Ulas, J., Brunner, L. C., Choe, W., & Cotman, C. W. (1992). Hippocampal excitatory amino acid receptors in elderly, normal individuals and those with Alzheimer's disease: Non-N-methyl-D-aspartate receptors. *Neuroscience, 50*, 23-34.

Gonella, J. S., (Ed.) (1985). *Clinical criteria for disease staging: Version 6.0*. Santa Barbara, CA: Systemetrics/McGraw Hill.

Greenfield, S., Blanco, D. M., Elashoff, R. M., & Ganz, P. A. (1987). Patterns of care related to age of breast cancer patients. *Journal of the American Medical Association, 257*, 2766-2770.

Greenfield, S., Apolone, G., McNeil, B. J., & Cleary, P. D. (1993). The importance of co-existent disease in the occurrence of postoperative complications and one-year recovery in patients undergoing total hip replacement. *Medical Care, 31*, 141-154.

Halter, J. B. (1996). Alzheimer's disease and non-insulindependent diabetes mellitus: Common features do not make common bedfellows. *Journal of the American Geriatrics Society, 44*, 992-993.

Harkness, G. A., Bentley, D. W., & Roghmann, K. J. (1990). Risk factors for nosocomial pneumonia in the elderly. *American Journal of Medicine, 89*, 457-463.

Heyman, A., Wilkinson, W. E., Stafford, J. A., Helms, M. J., Sigman, A. H., & Weinberg, T. (1984). Alzheimer's disease: A study of epidemiological aspects. *Annals of Neurology, 15*, 335-341.

Huff, F. J., Auerbach, J., Chakravarti, A., & Boller, F. (1988). Risk of dementia in relatives of patients with Alzheimer's disease. *Neurology, 38*, 786-790.

Hutchinson, T. A., Thomas, D. C., & MacGibbon, B. (1982). Predicting survival in adults with end-stage renal disease—an age equivalence index. *Annals of Internal Medicine, 96*, 417-423.

Jellinger, K., Danielczyk, W., Fischer, P., & Gabriel, E. (1990). Clinicopathological analysis of dementia disorders in the elderly. *Journal of the Neurological Sciences, 95*, 239-258.

Johnson, R. E., Hornbrook, M. C., & Nichols, G. A. (1994). Replicating the chronic disease score (CDS) from automated pharmacy data. *Journal of Clinical Epidemiology, 47*, 1191-1199.

Kaplan, M. H., & Feinstein, A. R. (1974). The importance of classifying initial comorbidity in evaluating the outcome of diabetes mellitus. *Journal of Chronic Diseases, 27*, 387-404.

Knapp, M. J., Knopman, D. S., Solomon, P. R., Pendlebury, W. W., Davis, C. S., & Gracon, S. I. (1994). A 30-week randomized controlled trial of high-dose tacrine in patients with Alzheimer's disease. *Journal of the American Medical Association, 271*, 985-991.

Kolbeinsson, H., & Jonsson, A. (1993). Delirium and dementia in acute medical admissions of elderly patients in Iceland. *Acta Psychiatrica Scandinavica, 87*, 123-127.

Marrie, T. J., Durant, H., & Kwan, C. (1986). Nursing home-acquired pneumonia: A case-control study. *Journal of the American Geriatrics Society, 34*, 697-702.

Mattson, M. P., & Goodman, Y. (1995). Different amyloidogenic peptides share a similar mechanism of neurotoxicity involving reactive oxygen species and calcium. *Brain Research, 676,* 219-224.

Mayeux, R., Ottman, R., Tang, M.-X., Noboa-Bauza, L., Marder, K., Gurland, B., & Stern, Y. (1993). Genetic susceptibility and head injury as risk factors for Alzheimer's disease among community-dwelling elderly persons and their first-degree relatives. *Annals of Neurology, 33,* 494-501.

McKhann, G., Drachman, D., Folstein, M., Katzman, R., Price, D., & Stadlan, E. M. (1984). Clinical diagnosis of Alzheimer's disease: Report of the NINCDS-ADRDA Work Group under the auspices of Department of Health and Human Services Task Force on Alzheimer's Disease. *Neurology, 34,* 939-944.

Mitchell, A. J., & Dening, T. R. (1996). Depression-related cognitive impairment: Possibilities for its pharmacological treatment. *Journal of Affective Disorders, 36,* 79-87.

Mortimer, J. A., Van Duijn, C. M., Chandra, V., Fratiglioni, L., Graves, A. B., Heyman, A., Jorm, A. F., Kokmen, E., Kondo, K., Rocca, W. A., Shalat, S. L., Soininen, H., & Hofman, A. (1991). Head trauma as a risk factor for Alzheimer's disease: A collaborative re-analysis of case-control studies. *International Journal of Epidemiology, 20* (Suppl. 2), S28-S35.

Mossey, J. M., & Roos, L. L. (1987). Using insurance claims data to measure health status: the Illness Scale. *Journal of Chronic Diseases, 40* (Suppl. 1), 41S-50S.

Mucke, L., Masliah, E., Johnson, W.B., Ruppe, M. D., Alford, M., Rockenstein, E. M., Forss-Petter, S., Pietropaolo, M., Mallory, M., & Abraham, C. R. (1994). Synaptotrophic effects of human amyloid ß protein precursors in the cortex of transgenic mice. *Brain Research, 666,* 151-167.

Munroe, W. A., Southwick, P. C., Chang, L., Scharre, D. W., Echols, C. L., Jr., Fu, P. C., Whaley, J. M., & Wolfert, R. L. (1995). Tau protein in cerebrospinal fluid as an aid in the diagnosis of Alzheimer's disease. *Annals of Clinical and Laboratory Science, 25,* 207-217.

Nielson, K. A., Nolan, J. H., Berchtold, N. C., Sandman, C. A., Mulnard, R. A., & Cotman, C. W. (1996). Apolipoprotein-E genotyping of diabetic dementia patients: Is diabetes rare in Alzheimer's disease. *Journal of the American Geriatrics Society, 44,* 897-904.

Shurtleff, D. (1974). Some characteristics related to the incidence of cardiovascular disease and death. Section 30. In W.B. Kannel & T. Gordon (Eds.), *Framingham Study, 18 Year Follow-up* (DHEW publication no. NIH 74-599). Washington, DC: U.S. Government Printing Office.

Southwick, P. C., Yamagata, S. K., Echols, C. L.,Jr., Higson, G. J., Neynaber, S. A., Parson, R. E., & Munroe, W. A. (1996). Assessment of amyloid ß protein in cerebrospinal fluid as an aid in the diagnosis of Alzheimer's disease. *Journal of Neurochemistry, 66,* 259-265.

Speck, C. E., Kukull, W. A., Brenner, D. E., Bowen, J. D., McCormick, W. C., Teri, L., Pfanschmidt, M. L., Thompson, J. D., & Larson, E. B. (1995). History of depression as a risk factor for Alzheimer's disease. *Epidemiology, 6,* 366-369.

Thorpe, J., Widman, L. P., Wallin, A., Beiswanger, J., & Blumenthal, H. T. (1994). Comorbidity of other chronic age dependent diseases in dementia. *Aging Clinical and Experimental Research, 6,* 159-166.

Van Dijk, P. T. M., Dippel, D. W. J., Van der Meulen, J. H. P., & Habbema, J. D. F. (1996). Comorbidity and its effect on mortality in nursing home patients with dementia. *Journal of Nervous and Mental Diseases, 184*, 180-187.

Van Dijk, P. T. M., Van de Sande, H. J., Dippel, D. W. J., & Habbema, J. D. F. (1992). The nature of excess mortality in nursing home patients with dementia. *Journals of Gerontology, Medical Sciences 47*, M28-M34.

Volicer, L., Brandeis, G., & Hurley, A. C. (1997). Infections in advanced dementia. In: Volicery & Hurley (Eds.). *Hospice care for patients with advanced progressive dementia*. New York: Springer Publishing Co. (in press).

Volicer, L., Smith, S., & Volicer, B. J. (1995). Effect of seizures on progression of dementia of the Alzheimer type. *Dementia, 6*, 258-263.

Von Korff, M., Wagner, E. H., & Saunders, K. (1992). A chronic disease score from automated pharmacy data. *Journal of Clinical Epidemiology, 45*, 197-203.

Walsh, J. S., Welch, H. G., & Larson, E. B. (1990). Survival of outpatients with Alzheimer-type dementia. *Annals of Internal Medicine, 113*, 429-434.

Watkins, P. B., Zimmerman, H. J., Knapp, M. J., Gracon, S. I., & Lewis, K. W. (1994). Hepatotoxic effects of tacrine administration in patients with Alzheimer's disease. *Journal of the American Medical Association, 271*, 992-998.

Winograd, C. H., Jacobson, D. H., Minkoff, J. R., Peabody, C. A., Taylor, B. S., Widrow, L., & Yesavage, J. A. (1991). Blood glucose and insulin response in patients with senile dementia of the Alzheimer's type. *Biological Psychiatry, 30*, 507-511.

Chapter 9

ADL Assessment Measures for Use With Frail Elders

John N. Morris and Shirley A. Morris

This chapter addresses issues relevant to the assessment of ADL status among frail and cognitively impaired residents of nursing facilities, focusing on a discussion of the areas of functional performance that have been found to comprise the ADL "palette." Information is presented on which ADL elements to assess, how they can be measured, and how performance levels on these measures are distributed within the nursing home population—with a presentation of both cross-sectional and rate of change estimates.

ADL status indicators have a long, established tradition of use within the rehabilitative and long-term-care arenas. Although ADL has at times been used as a synonym for physical function or performance, ADL item batteries actually assess the pattern of subject involvement in the performance of the basic personal activities of daily life. As such, they represent a relatively narrow range of performance. Typically, ADL performance activities have been arranged hierarchically, from the most basic of human functions (i.e., eating and moving the body while in bed, which are often referred to as "late-loss" ADLs) to somewhat higher types of functioning (e.g., dressing, personal hygiene, and bathing activities, which are often referred to as "early-loss" ADLs).

For less impaired elders, instrumental activities of daily living (IADL) have been used to assess higher self-performance levels, including the performance of household chores, use of a telephone, medications administration, and shopping. The advantage of standard ADL and more specialized IADL scales is that when combined, they assess the full range of basic activities that are critical for the person to remain in a community setting. Once having entered a nursing home, it is the more focused activities of the ADL palette that take center stage.

For each ADL measure there is an initial need to determine the basic nature of the functional concept to be assessed. This involves focusing on what the person does, either during a specific test or over a specified observation period—e.g., performance patterns over a day, a week, or longer. By adopting a performance-based approach to measurement, one excludes as basic measurement elements the more abstract indicators of subject capacity to perform functional activities or the structural parameters that focus on deficiencies in different bodily systems—e.g., difficulty using limbs,

Acknowledgments. This chapter acknowledges support by the National Institute on Aging, grant #U01 AG10305, Evaluating a Family Partnership Program in SCUs, and National Institute on Aging grant #P50 AG11719, HRCA Center of Research on Applied Gerontology.

contractures, or missing limbs. To be useful for tracking subject status, a variety of ADL activities will have to be monitored. At program intake, the functional status of the typical client is likely to be quite volatile; changes in many different ADL areas are possible, and one cannot limit measurement to only two or three key areas. Many clients will have experienced a recent acute or catastrophic problem, and any number of ADLs may be impaired.

ADL change trajectories tend to be hierarchical in character. The first area of loss is usually bathing, followed by dressing and personal hygiene. At this stage, the subject will likely retain some capabilities in locomotion, bed mobility and eating, and it is not surprising to find that an elder who is totally dependent in dressing and personal hygiene may still have retained ability to participate in bringing food to his or her mouth or turning or sitting up in bed, or even moving in the environment without having to be fully supported by others. Eventually, within the typical hierarchical paradigm of ADL loss, as frailty becomes more pervasive, eating and bed mobility will be the last areas of retained ability in which the typical elder will have at least a minimal involvement.

Not withstanding these hierarchical tendencies, there are significant variations among nursing home residents in their ADL disability profiles and rates of change. Some will exhibit early-loss ADL problems, while others will exhibit problems in middle- or late-loss areas. Interestingly, if one compares subjects at different points along the loss spectrum, no matter where they started, the underlying risk of decline over any 3-month period is strikingly similar—about 10% to 15% will experience decline, and about half as many will improve. For those who are newly admitted to a nursing home, since they are more likely to have experienced a recent acute event, their improvement rates will be somewhat higher. Over a longer period of time, decline rates continue to become more pervasive, with the ratio of decline to improvement in a population becoming increasingly one-sided.

In tracking ADL status and change trajectories over time, four measurement issues should be considered:

1. The spectrum of functional activities to be assessed, including the mix of early-, middle-, and late-loss ADL indicators.
2. The time period over which ADL performance is assessed—a session, a day, a week.
3. The number of categories used to describe subject performance for each ADL, ensuring that they are sufficient to capture both variability and change, while at the same time ensuring that assessors can arrive at a reliable estimate of subject disability status. The many extant ADL measures vary widely in the number of response choices offered— ranging from simple dichotomous (yes-no) scales, such as the self-care dependency factor of the Physical and Mental Evaluation Scale (PAMIE) (Gurel, Linn, & Linn, 1972), to the 11-point Sickness Impact Profile (SIP) scale (Bergner, Babbitt, Carter, & Gibson, 1981). There are also many intermediate measurement systems, such as the 7-category FIM system (Hamilton, Laughlin, Fiedler, & Granger, 1994; Research Foundation, 1987) and the 5-category MDS system (Morris, Nonamaker, Murphy, Hawes, Fries, Mor, & Phillips, in press). The advantage of a yes-no response system is that untrained persons or those with very little formal training can reliably rate the answers. The disadvantage is that less variance in behavior can be described, and thus the measures are not sensitive to treatment changes or to discrimination between levels of functioning.

4. Each ADL, as well as each of the categorical responses for each ADL, must have explicit definitions. Definitions and examples must make clinical sense, and the process for gathering the necessary assessment data from subjects, family, and caregivers must be consistently described and followed. Lack of specificity in item definitions and the assessment process can lead to unreliability.

ADL MEASUREMENT BARRIERS

The methods for classifying subjects with respect to functional status during the course of illness were initially developed by Katz and colleagues at the Benjamin Rose Hospital, a geriatric hospital in Cleveland, Ohio (Staff of Benjamin Rose Hospital, 1958), where observations were made of a large number of activities performed by a group of patients with hip fracture. These activities were described more systematically in 1963 in a seminal article on activities of daily living (Katz, Ford, Moskowitz, Jackson, & Jaffee, 1963), with a series of follow-up descriptive articles (Katz & Akpom, 1976; Katz, Downs, Cash, & Grotz, 1970) further extending this important body of work. For Katz, six ADL measures are presumed to be lost in disabled older persons in roughly the opposite order to their initial acquisition in childhood, progressing from bathing, dressing, going to the toilet, transferring, continence, and ultimately feeding. The presumption is that, generally, a frail older person will be least likely to bathe without the support of others; while conversely, a person who cannot feed herself will likely be unable to perform any of the other ADL tasks. The scores from these individual functional performance items are used either in a simple count of the number of dependent areas or are ordered in a hierarchical topology.

Virtually every developer of functional assessment instruments since the publication of Katz and his colleagues' early work has acknowledged an intellectual debt to this pioneering effort. The Katz measure in its various adaptations has been shown to be useful in predicting death, hospitalization, and the increased use of institutional long-term care (Spector, Katz, Murphy, & Fulton, 1987; Siu, Hays, Ouslander, Osterwell, Valdez, Krynski & Gross, 1993).

However, an interesting question posed by this body of work is whether individual ADLs can be combined to form a single hierarchical structure or Guttman scale. In addressing this issue, Lazaridis, Rudberg, Furner, and Cassel (1994) used data from the baseline year of the Longitudinal Study of Aging. For each of the 360 permutations of the ADLs within the original Katz hierarchy, they calculated the standard measures of fit of ordered data to a Guttman scale: the coefficient of reproducibility, the minimum marginal reproducibility, the percentage improvement, and the coefficient of scalability. Their finding was that although the Katz hierarchy does satisfy the traditional requirements for scalability, many other ADL hierarchies also satisfy these criteria. Specifically, the analysis shows that there are four hierarchies at least as good as the Katz hierarchy, and 103 hierarchies that satisfy the minimum standard for scalability. Their conclusion: "The typical scalogram methodology may not be sufficient to summarize data, and a multiplicity of disability profiles may exist."

Historically, many organizations (typically, rehabilitation hospitals and long-term-care facilities) have preferred to construct measures to fit their particular situation— "the present state of the trade seems to be one in which each investigator feels an inner compulsion to make his own scale and to cry that other existent scales cannot possibly fit his own setting," wrote M.P. Lawton and Brody (1969)—and since many of these instruments have not been particularly well developed, they continue to have uncertain validity for clinical, research, or program evaluation purposes.

As of 1989, Law and Letts (1989) report that five widely used measures had no published reliability data—ADL Test (Lawton, 1980); Burke Stroke Time-Oriented Profile (Feigenson, Polkow, Meikle, & Ferguson, 1979); Donaldson ADL Evaluation Form (Donaldson, Wagner, & Gresham, 1973); Kenny Self-Care Evaluation (Schoening, Anderegg, Bergstrom, Fonda, Steinke & Ulrich, 1965); and Time Care Profile (Halstead & Hartley, 1975). Reliability data for five others were found to be limited—ADL Rating Scale (Dinnerstein, Lowenthal, & Dexter, 1965); Index of ADL (Katz et al., 1963); LORS-II (Carey & Posavac, 1982); Physical Self-Maintenance Scale (M.P. Lawton & Brody, 1969); and Simulated ADL Examination (Potvin, Tourtellotte, Dailey, Albers, Walker, Pew, Henderson & Snyder, 1972). Measures that had demonstrated adequate observer and test-retest reliability are the Barthel Index (Granger, Albrecht, & Hamilton, 1979); the Klein-Bell ADL Scale (Law & Usher, 1988); the PULSES Profile (Granger et al., 1979); FIM (Dodds, Martin, Stolov, & Deyo, 1993); and the MDS-ADL (Hawes, Morris, Phillips, Mor, Fries & Nonamaker, 1995; Morris et al., in press).

Beyond the issues of reliability, an assessment instrument should also be sensitive to clinically important changes in the subject's status. Many ADL batteries address a very limited range of human performance with a too limited scoring range. In such cases, subjects who function outside this narrow range can have clinically meaningful changes that go undetected. One main reason why an index may not detect important changes is that the items are rated using coarse categorical assignment systems (Merbitz, Morris, & Grip, 1989; Wright & Linacre, 1989). For instance, the OARS multidimensional functional assessment questionnaire asks whether the subject can ambulate without assistance, with assistance, or not at all (Fillenbaum, 1988); the degree of difference between the categories cannot be inferred.

In most indexes of disability, the individual subscale ratings are aggregated into a single "output" rating. The aggregation can be formed with a simple addition of rating scores, as in the Barthel Index (Mahoney & Barthel, 1965), or with an ordinal clustering of categories, which may then be given either numerical ratings or lettered values, as in the A-B-C-D and so on arrangement of the Katz index (Katz et al., 1963). Instruments that are summaries of scores of individual variables may be useful for describing overall function, but can conceal as much information as they reveal. Sometimes, a change in one or two key variables may be critical in terms of outcome or patient preferences or degree of social support received, but changes in these individual variables may have little effect on the overall score of multiple-item indexes. Thus, in this article we are focusing our discussion on the self-performance elements themselves, rather than on the extensive literature related to the summing of these items into aggregated indicators of subject status.

SELECTED ADL AREAS

The following presents a brief exposition of ADL batteries that have followed in the tracks of the original Katz articles. We show ADL batteries that have been used by persons other than the originator of the scales, as well as a few batteries of more recent

TABLE 9.1 ADL Inventories

Name of instrument	Purpose	Major citation
Katz Index of Independence in Activities of Daily Living	To distinguish between independent and dependent status, establishing the ordered relationship among ADLs.	Katz et al., 1963
Seven Levels of Subsistence	To differentiate various levels for each ADL in a way that is universally applicable and requires no special training or equipment.	Gauger, Brownell, Russell, & Retter, 1964
Barthel Index	To measure functional levels of self-care and mobility in the physically impaired.	Mahoney and Barthel, 1965
Kenny Self-Care Evaluation	To develop an ADL form that is simple, short, and self-explanatory.	Schoening et al., 1965
Abilities in Activities of Daily Living Scale	To obtain a numerical rating in a hospital rehab unit of a patient's ability in 66 behaviors within 11 areas of functioning.	Dinnerstein et al., 1965
Stockton Geriatric Rating Scale (SGRS)	To develop a scale based on observation of day-to-day behavior of geriatric psychiatric patients in a hospital setting, and to include behavior relevant to leaving hospital as improved.	Meer and Baker, 1966
Adaptive Behavior Measurement Scale	To develop a descriptive system for measuring adaptive behavior in mental retardates.	Nihira, Foster & Spenser, 1968
Physical Self-Maintenance Scale (PSMS)	To "tap representative behavior" at each level of functionality and within range of competence appropriate to the individual.	Lawton and Brody, 1969
Simulated Activities of Daily Living Examination (SADLE)	To provide measures of a patient's capability to carry out functional activities by focusing on performance testing of simple motor skills	Potvin el al., 1972
Physical and Mental Impairment -of-function Evaluation in the Aged (PAMIE)	To create a multifactorial assessment instrument for the chronically ill elderly.	Gurel et al., 1972
Performance Test of Activities of Daily Living (PADL)	To measure the self-care capacity of geriatric psychiatric patients.	Kuriansky and Gurland, 1976

(Continued)

TABLE 9.1 *(Continued)*

Name of instrument	Purpose	Major citation
Burke Stroke Time-Oriented Profile (BUSTOP)	To create a functional profile for the quantitative assessment of stroke patients' progress during rehabilitation.	Feigenson et al., 1979
Functional Capacity Evaluation	To assess functional capacity of noninstitutional clients with polyarticular disability.	Jette, 1980
Sickness Impact Profile (SIP)	To provide a measure of perceived health status sensitive enough to detect changes that occur over time or between groups	Bergner et al., 1981
Klein-Bell ADL Scale	To identify critical or easily observable components of ADL behavior and to express these in generic terms.	Klein and Bell, 1982
Level of Rehabilitation Scale (LORS-II)	To gather and summarize functional ratings of patients in hospital-based rehabilitation programs.	Carey and Posavac, 1982
Rapid Disability Rating Scale (RDRS-2)	To discern degrees of disability and rates of deterioration in older chronically ill patients.	Linn and Linn, 1982
Functional Independence Measure (FIM)	To assess disabilities in everyday life, measuring a minimum number of activities intended to be valid indicators of level or cost of disability.	Research Foundation, 1987
OARS Multidimensional Functional Assessment Questionnaire—ADL	To assess overall personal functional status and service use of adults, and in particular the elderly, indicating which areas of functioning are impaired	Fillenbaum, 1988
ADL Situational Test	To devise four experimental tasks that provide a direct measure of ADL	Skurla, Rogers, & Sunderland, 1988

(Continued)

TABLE 9.1 *(Continued)*

Name of instrument	Purpose	Major citation
Direct Assessment of Functional Status (DAFS)	To examine areas of functional competence that may become impaired in Alzheimer's disease patients or other dementia patients.	Loewenstein, Amigo, Duara, Guterman, Hurwitz, Berkowitz, Wilkie, Weinberg, Black, Gittelman, & Eisdorfer, 1989
Physical Performance Test (PPT)	To assess physical function using observed performance of tasks that simulate ADLs of various degrees of difficulty.	Reuben and Siu, 1990
Minimum Data Set—ADL (MDS-ADL)	To provide a reliable measure for assessing resident self-performance and associated support levels in nursing homes.	Morris, Fries, Phillips, Mor, Hawes, & Morris, 1995
Structured Assessment of Independent Living (SAILS)	To develop a set of standardized behavioral tools that measure the functional abilities of patients with dementia.	Mahurin, DeBettignies, & Pirozzolo, 1991
ADL Scale	To determine to what extent six ADL items can describe the functional status of elders living at home.	Fredericks, teWierik, Visser & Sturmans, 1991
IADL Functional Status Measures	To compile a 50-item IADL questionnaire that is suitable for patient self-completion.	Myers, 1992
Physical Disability Index (PDI)	To detect differences in function among functionally impaired elderly and to identify differential change over time.	Gerety, Mulrows, Tuley, Hazuda, Lichtenstein, Bohannon, Kanten, O'Neil, & Gordon, 1993
Physical Performance and Mobility Examination (PPME)	To develop a performance-based instrument that assesses 6 domains of physical functioning and mobility for hospitalized and frail elderly.	Winograd, Lemsky, Nevitt, Nordstrom, Stewart, & Miller, 1994

While there is general agreement on the types of areas to be covered, ADL batteries vary in their specific item content and level of coding specificity. The following discussion focuses on the major categories of ADL that have been included in measurement instruments; a subsequent section focuses on how a subset of ADL batteries addresses the more complex task of segmenting or monitoring many of the small subactivities that comprise the more global ADL activities.

TABLE 9.2 ADL Areas Assessed

	Katz	OARS	PAMIE	Kenny	PSMS	Barthel	FIM	MDS
Bathing	X	X	X		X	X		X
Dressing	X	X	X	X	X	X	X	X
Upper body				X	X	X	X	X
Lower body				X		X	X	
Brace/prosthesis						X		
Grooming/Personal Hygiene		X	X	X	X	X	X	X
Transfer	X	X		X		X	X	X
Chair						X		
Tub/shower						X	X	
Locomotion				X	X	X	X	X
Walking		X				X		X
Stairs						X	X	
Wheelchair						X		(a)
Continence								
Bladder		X	X		X	X	X	(a)
Bowel						X	X	(a)
Toileting	X	X	X	X		X	X	X
Bed mobility				X				X
Eating/Feeding	X	X	X	X	X	X	X	X

(a) Measured in MDS, not part of ADLs

vintage. As you look at Table 9.1 it is obvious that there are many options available within the ADL measurement area. The following sections of this article detail a selected array of these batteries.

While there is general agreement on the types of areas to be covered, ADL batteries vary in their specific item content and level of coding specificity. The following discussion focuses on the major categories of ADL that have been included in measurement instruments; a subsequent section focuses on how a subset of ADL batteries addresses the more complex task of segmenting or monitoring many of the small subactivities that comprise the more global ADL activities. Table 9.2 lists nine activities that have been found in standard ADL batteries: bathing; dressing; personal hygiene (grooming); transfer; locomotion; continence; toileting; bed mobility; and eating (feeding).

The seminal work by Katz referenced five of these areas, all of which have been widely adopted in other ADL batteries. These include bathing, dressing, transfer, toileting, and eating. Other measures which have come into use in multiple batteries include personal hygiene and locomotion. Bed mobility has been identified as a crucial element in several ADL batteries. Finally, continence, although it has been identified

TABLE 9.3 Level of ADL Item Specificity

ADL activity and components of functional performance item definition	Katz	PSMS	FIM	MDS
BATHING				
• Bathing one or more parts of body	X	X	X	X
• Transfer in/out of tub	X			X
• Face/hands				(c)
• Exclusions:				
Back			•	•
Hair				•
DRESSING				
• Gets clothes	X	X	X	(a)
• Puts on street clothes	X	X	X	X
• Takes off street clothes				X
• Distinction between upper and lower body			X	
• Donning prosthesis	X		X	X
• Fastening tasks (bra, zippers)	X		X	X
• Exclusion:				
Tying shoes	•			
GROOMING/PERSONAL HYGIENE	(b)			
• Hair		X	X	X
• Nails		X		
• Hands and face		X	X	X
• Neatness		X		
• Shaving		X		X
• Make-up			X	X
• Oral care			X	X
• Perineum care				X
• Exclusion:				
Baths and showers				•
TRANSFER		(b)		
• Bed	X		X	X
• Chair	X		X	X
• Wheelchair	X		X(d)	X
• Standing position			X	X
• Exclusions				
Bath/toilet				
TOILETING				
• Go to toilet room	X		X	X
• Transfer on/off toilet				X
• Arrange clothing	X		X	X
• Cleansing self	X	X	X	X
• Bed pan, urinal, commode, etc.	X			X
• Change pads			X	X
• Manage ostomy, catheters				X
EATING/FEEDING				
• Moves food to mouth	X	X	X	X
• Parenteral feeding, tubes, IV	X		X	X
• Food set-up		X		
• Drinks from cup, etc.			X	X
• Exclusion				
Set-up	•		•	•

(a) Set up help scored in separate item in the MDS
(b) Not assessed in this ADL battery
(c) Under grooming in MDS
(d) Subtasks described in some detail

TABLE 9.4 ADL Scale Response Alternatives

	Kats	OARS	PAMIE	Kenny	PSMS	Barthel	FIM	MDS
Number of Response Alternatives for Each Item	3	3	2	5	5	4	7	5(a)
Measures Actual Performance of ADLs	X	X	X	X	X	X	X	X

(a) A special sixth category is used when the activity did not occur during the measurement period.

in many systems, is not really a functional support item in its own right; the functional component of continence is captured under toileting.

The operational definitions and associated scoring criteria for these ADL items can vary considerably. Disparities can occur in: (1) item definition; (2) response code specificity; and (3) the time period to which the assessment applies. To a large extent, these differences are a function of when the instrument was created: the more recent the instrument, the more specific and detailed the operational criteria. Table 9.3 shows these differences for six widely used ADL items (bathing, dressing, grooming, transfer, toileting, and eating) as operationalized within four commonly used ADL systems: Katz, PSMS, FIM, and MDS-ADL.

Table 9.3 indicates which aspects of ADL function are specially referenced in the item definition, as well as instances in which specific subsets of activities are explicitly excluded from consideration. As indicated, certain types of subtasks are mentioned in one ADL battery but not another. For example, Katz and MDS include transfer in and out of the tub (or shower), but PSMS and FIM do not. Similarly under toileting, only Katz references going to the toilet room, while only the MDS references transfer on and off the toilet, and management of ostomies and catheters. The inescapable conclusion is that in using an ADL battery or interpreting data derived from a battery, one must be acutely aware of how the items have been defined.

A second, basic difference existing across ADL batteries relates to the character of the available response alternatives for the items. Table 9.4 describes the response alternative structure for the eight ADL batteries referenced in Table 9.2.

The definition of response alternatives is as crucial as the specification of the functional parameters of a specific ADL element. If the response alternatives are unclear, assessors will predictably misclassify significant numbers of persons. Thus, average reliabilities (of all types) will decline and the clinical utility of the battery will be compromised. Because of the importance of this issue, the following design parameters should be considered in reviewing any ADL coding system:

1. Over what time period are ADL functions assessed?
2. How are the subject's retained patterns of self-involvement in an ADL area distinguished from what others do for the subject in that area?
3. Does the instrument consider help from all sources, or only from formal sources (e.g., nursing aide)?
4. How is set-up help weighed (e.g., bringing a brace for the subject to put on)?

5. How are nonphysical and supervisory activities weighed?
6. How does the instrument differentiate between weight-bearing and nonweight-bearing supports?
7. How does the instrument deal with exceptions to normal patterns (e.g., in the last week the subject dressed and undressed independently on all but one occasion—when a daughter helped her mother get ready to go to the doctor)?
8. How does the instrument deal with the extent of involvement of the client and others in the activities?
9. How does the instrument deal with situations when the activity did not occur during the assessment period (e.g., the subject was bed-bound for the entire period and did not transfer or dress in normal street clothes)?
10. How does the instrument score an ADL with multiple subtasks—i.e., where the subject does some tasks independently and receives help with others?
11. Do the coding categories for each ADL have the same meaning—e.g., does a code of 2" for dressing indicate the same general mix of self-involvement and help by others as does a "2" for personal hygiene?
12. Does each ADL have the same number of response alternatives?

In the discussion below we look at how a selected subset of ADL batteries—Katz, PSMS, FIM and MDS—addresses these fundamental issues.

The Katz Index of ADL uses a three-category scoring model. For each function on the Evaluation Form, the observer checks one of three given descriptions that is most appropriate to the subject. According to Katz et al. (1963): "Two descriptions would permit distinguishing between independent and dependent states; however, introduction of an intermediate description increases observer awareness of subtle distinctions, and thereby increases reliability. The form includes all the terms needed in the evaluation and has the advantage of needing no extensive guides." From this perspective, the system is a significant improvement over a dichotomous model, and client assessments more closely approximate the daily functioning of the person. Yet, when we scrutinize the scoring schema on the basis of the set of questions on design parameters given above, several conceptual problems become apparent:

- The most dependent of the three scoring options does not always represent total dependency. For transfer it represents the activity not occurring (bed bound), while the middle category includes all levels of assistance—from limited nonweight-bearing physical help to total performance by others on all occasions of transfer. Contrast this with either dressing or feeding, where the most dependent score encompasses a wide diversity of support activities, starting with receiving assistance in getting clothes for dressing, and receiving assistance in feeding or eating.
- In some ADLs, set-up help is mentioned (e.g., feeding and dressing); in others, it is not mentioned (e.g., bathing, toileting, transfer).
- No mention is made of cueing or supervisory activities.
- No mention is made of the frequency with which support activities are provided.

In evaluating the Katz ADL Index, there is a limited body of work that addresses the psychometric property of the items. For example, Spector et al. (1987) say that when using ADL to measure dysfunction for a community's elderly population, only between 2% and 8% were found to be dysfunctional, depending on the definitions used. "Scales of ADL underestimate the number of elders who need assistance with the full range of activities of daily living because ADL does not measure adaptation to the environment," they write. Accordingly, they devised a three-level hierarchical scale comprised of both ADL (bathing, dressing, transferring, and feeding) and IADL (shopping and transportation) items that would "likely be a more sensitive measure of functional decline than ADL alone."

Validation included discriminant validity and predictive validity. With respect to discriminant validity, the negative association between functional ability (as measured by the scale) and age was observed. With respect to predictive validity, the negative relationship between functional ability (as measured by the scale) and risk of decline to ADL, death, and hospitalization in a year was observed.

In a second study relative to the psychometric properties of the Katz ADL Index, Siu et al. (1993) studied 155 new residents of a long-term-care institution to assess the validity of various brief, multidimensional measures of health. Among the interviewer-assisted self-reported instruments they administered was the Katz ADL. They found that compared to other measures, the correlation of self-reported lower extremity mobility was highest with performance-based gait and balance. Self-reported ADLs correlated "about equally strongly" with timed manual performance and with gait and balance.

The Physical Self-Maintenance Scale (PSMS) was built by Lawton and Brody (1969) on the Langely-Porter Scale (Lowenthal, 1964). The Langley-Porter scale asks an observer to rate the client for competence in behaviors of toileting, feeding, dressing, grooming, locomotion, and bathing. Lawton and Brody felt it would be more useful to "treatment personnel" if each scale had the same number of points and if content was broadened in some instances so as to be applicable to either community residents or residential care patients. The six types of behavior assessed by the Langley-Porter scale and many of the points from their scale were retained. Within the five-category PSMS scoring schema, a score of "one" (1) always indicates that the person is independent, performing the activity without the help of others. However, the meaning of the code responses for the remaining four categories is not consistent across ADLs. Once again, looking at the set of questions given above, what conceptual difficulties exist in the design of the PSMS?

- For toileting, supervision or cueing is referenced, but this concept is not referenced for other ADLs.
- The meaning of the intermediate code responses is not consistently defined. In some instances there is a time and frequency distinction (toileting codes 3 and 4), though this concept is not referenced in other ADLs.
- Undefined terms, such as moderate assistance, major assistance, and extensive assistance, are used. In feeding, code 4 is defined as "Requires extensive assistance for all meals," while for dressing Code 4 is defined as "Needs major assistance in dressing, but cooperates with efforts of others to help." What is the difference between "extensive" and "major," how is the assessor to operationalize these terms?

Regarding the scale properties of the PSMS, Lawton and Brody state that Guttman scaling criteria are "adequately met," as demonstrated by (1) the major range of item difficulty being represented, without extreme splits; (2) the percentage of errors on each item being substantially less than percentage of nonerror; and (3) the high reproducibility coefficient of .96. In testing, pairs of licensed practical nurses were asked to rate independently 36 patients with varied self-care deficits. The Pearsonian *r* between the pairs of ratings was .87. Two research assistants independently rated 14 other impaired and nonimpaired patients, with a correlation of .91 between their ratings. Finally, they report data on the correlations of the PSMS with other measures, including .38 with the Mental Status Questionnaire (MSQ) and .62 with a 6-point scale of functional health rated by physicians (the Physical Classification).

The Functional Independence Measure (FIM) battery is a significant extension of the Barthel Index Measurement System (Research Foundation, 1987). Granger et al. (1979) first introduced the 4-level adaptation of the Barthel Index, moving from independent to nonphysical help to physical help to total dependence. With FIM, however, an even more useful extension of the coding metric has been attempted. Under FIM, each area of ADL performance is scored from 1 (Total Assistance) to 7 (Complete Independence).

Within the FIM system, Code 1 is for clients who expend less than 25% of the effort to perform an ADL. Code 2 records instances where the client expends less than 50% but at least 25% of the effort. Codes 3, 4, and 5 fit into what FIM refers to as a Modified Dependence range. For these codes, another person is required for supervision or physical assistance, but the client expends half (50%) or more of the effort. Code 5 includes both the concepts of supervision and equipment setup. Codes 6 and 7 are differentiated on the basis of whether help goes beyond tracking the client, and the percentage of the ADL activity done by the client or others. Code 6 retains the Barthel concept of adaptive equipment. For example, for feeding, code 6 (Modified Independent) is defined as "uses an adaptive or assistive device such as a straw, spork, rocking knife or requires more than a reasonable time to eat."

The FIM system, with its relatively complex 7-category system, was designed for use in rehabilitative hospitals, and has been the basis for extensive research, tracking rates of improvement of clients cared for in these environments. When used in such controlled settings and accompanied by detailed manuals, extensive case examples, and mandatory assessor training, FIM has been an unqualified success. But if it is to be adapted to other environments, several design considerations must be addressed:

- The FIM has terms that are not operationally defined—e.g., "safety (risk) considerations," or carrying out an activity within "reasonable" time limits.
- There are no operational rules given for knowing exactly what is meant by the percentage of effort expended by the subject (e.g., 25%, 50%, 75%).
- Code 1 (Total Dependence) includes subjects who are still highly involved in their own care; it is not a true "total dependence on others" category.
- Set-up help is equated with supervisory help. But one is a single time activity, the other can be a continuous activity.

Reports on the psychometric properties of the FIM have been reported since its introduction. Hamilton, Laughlin, Fiedler, and Granger (1991) reported on interrater agreement. Two or more pairs of clinicians assessed each of 263 patients undergoing inpatient medical rehabilitation at 21 U.S. hospitals subscribing to the uniform data system (UDS) for medical rehabilitation. Only facilities meeting standard UDS criteria for acceptable I-RA on their first evaluation were reported. Criteria were intraclass correlation coefficient (ICC) (ANOVA) for total FIM and FIM subscores greater than or equal to 0.90 (five of six subscores must be .90 or more; no ICC could be 0.75 or less) and Kappa (unweighted) for individual FIM items greater than or equal to 0.45 for at least 15 of the 18 items. Results were: total FIM intraclass correlation coefficient—0.97; self-care—0.96; sphincter control—0.94; mobility (transfers)—0.96; locomotion—0.93; communication —0.95; social cognition—0.94. FIM item Kappa mean was 0.71 (range 0.61 to 0.76). In another study of FIM's interrater reliability published several years later by Hamilton et al. (1994), they concluded that the FIM "is reliable when used by trained/tested inpatient medical rehabilitation clinicians."

Using a sample of 27,669 patients (mean age, 62.1 years) undergoing rehabilitation in UDS hospitals, Heinemann, Linacre, Wright, Hamilton, and Granger (1993) scaled the FIM with Rasch analysis to determine the similarity of scaled measures across 13 UDS-defined impairment groups. Stroke was further subdivided into left hemiparesis, right hemiparesis, and bilateral.

The results showed that:

- the FIM contains two fundamental subsets of items: one measures motor, and the second measures cognitive function. Motor and cognitive aspects of function were important to be distinguished, and were treated separately.
- the FIM could be scaled as an interval measure for each of the 13 impairment groups. Item difficulty varied slightly across impairment groups, reflecting the unique impact of various kinds of impairments. The validity of the FIM is supported by this pattern of item difficulties and by the factor analysis performed. "The results make clear the fact that raw scores are not linear and should not be used in parametric statistical analysis," say the researchers.
- Discharge expectancies could be established based on these scaling results, and programs could evaluate their outcomes in terms of attainment of discharge performance. Demonstration of patient function as consisting of two distinct aspects of behavior suggests that both domains are important in helping patients live independently and in estimating caregiver requirements.

The Minimum Data Set (MDS) ADL battery is used in the assessment of almost all nursing home residents in the United States (Hawes et al., 1995; Morris et al., in press), and it has now been shown to be equally applicable in community care settings (Morris, Fries, Ikegami, Bernabei, Carpenter, Gilgen, Hirdes, & Topinkovia, in press). On an annual basis, approximately 3 million different residents in U.S. nursing homes are assessed with this battery of items, with approximately 5 million total assessments completed per year. Table 9.5 gives the detailed definitions for the coding used with all MDS ADL items—except for bathing which uses the same number of code responses but has different wording, since the average nursing home resident has only two baths per week.

In nursing homes, to be able to promote the highest level of functioning among residents, clinical staff must first identify what the resident actually does for himself or herself, noting when assistance is received and clarifying the types of assistance provided—verbal cueing, physical support, etc. A resident's ADL self-performance may vary from day to day, shift to shift, or within shifts. The MDS scoring system recognizes this reality by requiring a review performance over the prior 7-day period (Morris, Hawes, Murphy, Nonamaker, Phillips, Fries & Mor, 1991; Morris et al., 1995). There are many possible reasons for functional performance variations, including

TABLE 9.5 Coding Schema for MDS ADL Items

ADL SELF-PERFORMANCE—(**Code** for resident's **PERFORMANCE OVER ALL SHIFTS during last 7 days**—Not including setup—which is coded separately).

---

0. INDEPENDENT—No help or oversight—OR—Help/oversight provided only 1 or 2 times during last 7 days
1. SUPERVISION—Oversight, encouragement or cueing provided 3 or more times during last 7 days—OR—Supervision (3 or more times) plus physical assistance provided only 1 or 2 times during last 7 days
2. LIMITED ASSISTANCE—Resident highly involved in activity; received physical help in guided maneuvering of limbs or other nonweight bearing assistance 3 or more times—OR—More help provided only 1 or 2 times during last 7 days
3. EXTENSIVE ASSISTANCE—While resident performed part of activity, over last 7-day period, help of following type(s) provided 3 or more times: —Weight-bearing support —Full staff performance during part (but not all) of last 7 days
4. TOTAL DEPENDENCE—Full staff performance of activity during entire 7 days
8. ACTIVITY DID NOT OCCUR during entire 7 days

---

fatigue, mood, medical condition, relationship issues (e.g., willing to perform for a nurse assistant he or she likes), client motivation, and medications. The responsibility of the person completing the assessment, therefore, is to capture the total picture of the resident's ADL self-performance over the 7-day period, 24 hours a day—i.e., not only how the evaluating clinician sees the resident, but how the resident performs on other shifts as well.

In order to accomplish this, it is necessary to gather information from multiple sources—i.e., interviews/discussion with the resident and direct care staff on all three shifts, including weekends, and review of documentation used to communicate with staff across shifts. This involves asking questions pertaining to all aspects of the ADL activity definitions. For example, when discussing Bed Mobility with a nurse assistant, staff are to inquire specifically how the resident moves to and from a lying position, how the resident turns from side to side, and how the resident positions himself or herself while in bed. A resident can be independent in one aspect of Bed Mobility yet require extensive assistance in another aspect.

The wording used in each coding option is intended to reflect real-world situations in nursing homes, where slight variations in performance capability are common. Where variations occur, the coding ensures that the resident is not assigned to an excessively independent or dependent category. For example, by definition, codes 0, 1, 2, and 3 (Independent, Supervision, Limited Assistance, and Extensive Assistance) permit one or two exceptions for the provision of heavier care. Thus, if a resident carried out an activity every day, every shift without the help of others, but received nonweight bearing support on two days because of scheduling issues, the relevant ADL can still be scored as independent. In our experience, having such exceptions increased the average interassessor weighted Kappa reliabilities by some 10% to 15%.

Figure 9.1 depicts how the ADL scoring system for the MDS is actually applied by the assessor in assigning a score to the subject for a given ADL.

How does the MDS ADL scoring system rate against the design criteria given earlier? Each code response has a distinct definition; the same response structure is used for each ADL (with the exception of bathing); intensity and frequency of help is built

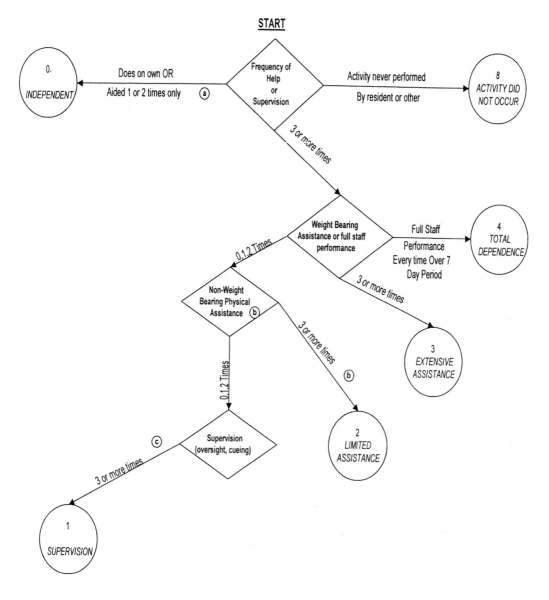

a. Can include one or two events where received supervision, non-weight bearing help, or weight bearing help.

b. Can include one or two episodes of weight bearing help--e.g., two events with non-weight bearing plus two of weight bearing would be coded as a "2".

c. Can include one or two episodes where physical help received--e.g., two episodes of supervision, one of weight bearing, and one of non-weight bearing would be coded as a "1".

Figure 9.1 Scoring ADL self performance.

into the scoring system, and the same time period (7 days) is used for each ADL. Yet, there are conceptual issues with the MDS that should be recognized.

- While there is a volume distinction on the extent of help provided, there can be significant variations in performance patterns across a single day or 7-day period.
- Set-up help is not explicitly included in the MDS; it is measured as a separate item.
- For multiple task ADLs (e.g., personal hygiene), there is no way to differentiate subtask activities performed independently from those that involved the help of others. The MDS scores such ADL items based on the subtask that involved the most help from others.

As a final indication of the utility of the MDS ADL items, Table 9.6 presents information on interassessor weighted Kappa reliability values (Morris, Nonamaker, in press; Morris, Fries et al. in press). These reliability values are based on 187 dual assessments by trained nurse assessors for a random sample of residents in 21 nursing facilities and 241 dual assessments in home care agencies in five countries. In completing these independent assessments, the two nurse assessors at each facility did not discuss the residents or their findings. In evaluating the reliability values in Table 9.6, note that Kappa values lower than 0.4 indicate poor reliability; .40-.75 is considered adequate, and .75 or above is considered evidence of excellent reliability (Fleiss, 1981).

NURSING HOME RESIDENTS' ADL PROBLEM DISTRIBUTIONS

The following figures describe the functional performance of nursing home residents (as identified by staff in the MDS assessment instrument), both for the total cohort of residents and for the subgroup of residents with Alzheimer's disease. These estimates are based on the MDS ADL Self-Performance items and are derived from a 10-state cluster sample of some 2,089 residents generated for use in a HCFA-funded study of the

TABLE 9.6 Weighted Kappa Reliabilities for MDS ADL Self-performance Items

ADL item	Weighted Kappa inter-rater reliability	
	In nursing homes	In home care
Bed mobility	.91	.92
Transfer	.91	.90
Locomotion on unit (in home)	.99	.90
Locomotion off unit	.89	—
Walk in room	.92	—
Walk in corridor	.89	—
Dressing	.90	.94
Eating	.94	.84
Toilet use	.93	.94
Personal Hygiene	.87	.92
Bathing	.86	.91

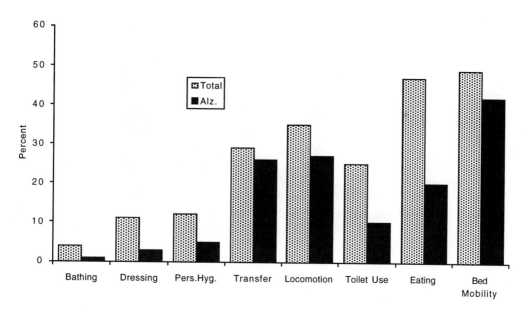

Figure 9.2 ADL independence levels.

MDS (Hawes, Phillips, Morris, Mor, Fries, Steele-Friedlob & Greene, in press). Figure 9.2 presents information on the percent who are independent in ADLs. As expected, based on the extensive research on the hierarchy of loss of ADLs, almost no residents are fully independent in bathing. (Note: While the vast majority of residents entering nursing homes are not independent in bathing, it is also true that staff support is almost always mandated once the elder enters the nursing home.) If one enters a nursing home, one's performance in this area is likely to be impaired. According to the concepts of early- and late-loss ADLs, dressing and personal hygiene are predictably the next areas where there is little remaining independence of functioning, while locomotion, eating, and bed mobility represent the highest levels of retained functioning. These distributions make clear that there is a distinct pattern of loss for elders in nursing homes, although there can be considerable variation in the pattern of loss at the individual level.

Figure 9.3 presents a full picture of ADL self-performance for three selected ADLs: dressing, locomotion, and eating. Several key features of ADLs in nursing home populations can be seen in this figure. ADL distributions tend to be either slightly skewed, with a single high prevalence point (as for dressing), or have a bipolar distribution (as for locomotion and eating); and the number of residents who are totally dependent is usually equal to or greater than the number receiving limited or extensive physical assistance.

Using these same three ADLs, Figure 9.4 depicts how residents of nursing homes change over a 6-month period (either becoming more or less dependent on the scoring categories for the MDS ADL items—see Figure 9.1). The estimates are based on data derived from the 10-state HCFA sample. The rates of decline are about the same for each ADL, both in total and for those with Alzheimer's disease: a little over 20% decline over a 6-month period. Improvement rates are also about the same for the three ADLs—about

Dressing

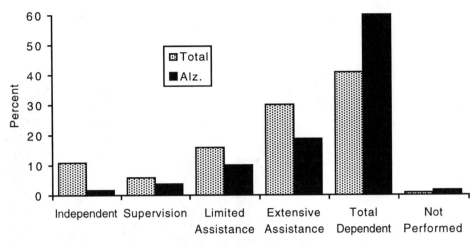

Locomotion

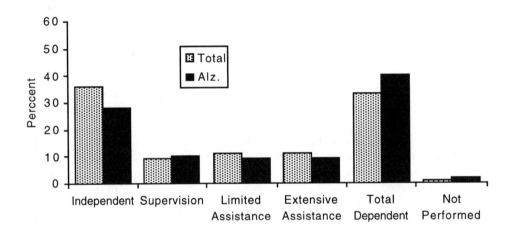

Eating

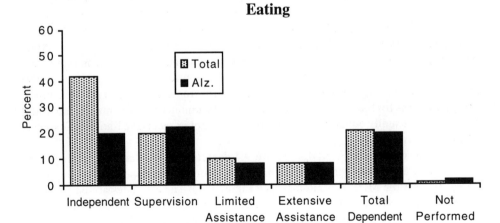

Figure 9.3 ADL Self Performance profile for 3 selected ADLs.

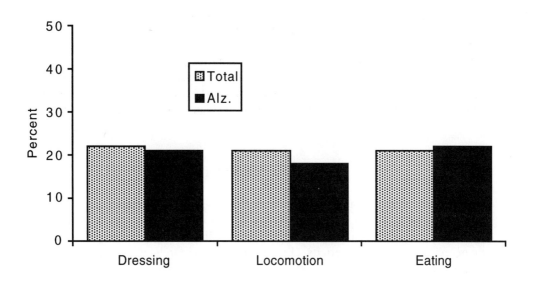

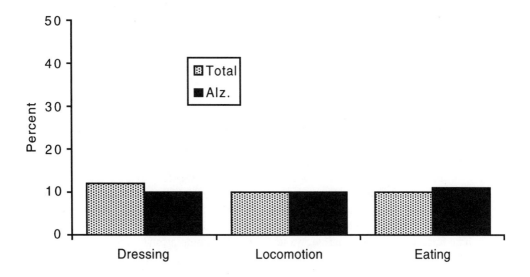

Figure 9.4 Proportion of residents who improve & decline in ADL over a 12 month period.

11% improve in status over a 6-month period. As one would expect, the decline rate is about twice the improvement rate.

These rates increase somewhat if we first exclude residents from the decline estimate who could not further decline (i.e., they were already totally dependent in the ADL at the baseline measurement point). When estimated in this way, over a 6-month period about 35% of residents decline: 32% in locomotion, 36.6% in dressing, and 26.4% in eating. The comparable rates for the Alzheimer's subgroup are 38.3%, 38.4%, and 36.0%.

For our improvement estimates, if we exclude residents who could not improve further (i.e., they were independent at baseline), the rates are still considerably below the decline rates: 20.1% improved in locomotion, 12.0% in dressing, and 19.5% in eating. The comparable improvement rates for residents with Alzheimer's disease are 14.2%, 11.2%, and 15.2%.

TASK SEGMENTATION

Task segmentation, although closely related to physical performance, is a relatively unique approach to ADL measurement, so we are describing it separately from the main-line approaches discussed above. In some applications, particularly those involving people with cognitive deficits, clinical and some research approaches, the concept of task segmentation has driven specification of ADL elements. For example, in the Barthel Index, dressing ability is measured separately for upper and lower body, while transfer is disaggregated into transfer to/from chair and transfer to/from bed.

For clinical purposes, however, one has the option of going much further. What are some of the driving forces, and what do these measures look like? Clinicians have distinguished between disability directly related to physical or cognitive impairment, and "excess disability," which often results from external factors. Caregivers who fail to allow or encourage elders with cognitive impairment to perform ADLs "to the full extent of their abilities" may, in fact, be contributing to premature functional decline. It is through a review of subtasks that the need for effective programs to maintain or improve function may be indicated (Beck, Heacock, Mercer, Walton, & Shook, 1991).

Task segmentation involves breaking down an ADL activity into smaller steps. Dressing, for instance, involves a complex set of physical and cognitive skills. The single task of putting on one's sock, for example, involves much more than slipping the sock onto the foot. Rather, its successful completion requires that the resident identify the sock, understand what the sock is used for, manipulate the sock so that the toe is pointed upward, reach down to the foot or bring the foot closer to the lap, pull the sock onto the foot, roll the sock up the lower leg, and repeat this set of activities for the second foot.

Once staff are aware of how a task can be broken down into its component parts, caregivers may provide set-up help, and use verbal and/or physical cues to encourage the individual to complete each step of an ADL activity.

The following discussion reviews several task segmentation batteries that have been created. Their use tends to be more clinical in nature; they take time to complete. The more general measures described earlier are excellent tools for assessing changing subject status and program effects, and these task segmentation batteries have a more limited but important role in clinical care practice. Katz, Drugovitch, Morris, Cornelius, Granger, Sloan, Murphy & Seltzer, 1991, in working on the MDS system, designed a task segmentation inventory for dressing, bathing, toileting, locomotion, transfer, and eating. Using toileting as an example, seven subtasks are described: going to the toilet room; removing/opening clothes; transfer/positioning self; eliminating into toilet; tears/using paper to clean self; flush; and adjust clothes/wash hands. This example indicates the level of detail at which subtasks for a given ADL can be described. In designing these lists one needs to stand back and treat the ADL from an engineering point of view. What does the task involve? How are arms, legs, and the trunk used? What external devices, clothing, or equipment are used? How does the nature of the environment impact on the activity—does it require a special location or can it be done anywhere? How does the subject's decision-making ability impact on recognition of the need to complete the activity?

To indicate how these issues have been addressed, we will describe how a series of investigators have developed operational task segmentation instruments. In 1968, Nihira and colleagues included a checklist for eating in their Adaptive Behavior Measurement Scale. Their "Use of Utensil for Eating" included five items: eats with spoon; eats with fork; uses table knife for cutting; uses table knife for spreading; and uses knife and fork correctly without difficulty. Contrast this list to the level of detail in the eating list of Katz et al. (1990), and one can begin to see the true complexity in assessing each of the basic ADLs. Katz added the concepts of opening, pouring, unwrapping, grasping, chewing/drinking/swallowing, repetitions until food is consumed, and cleansing after meal.

The only informant-based instrument included in this review, the Functional Capacity Evaluation, was developed to assess the functional capacity of individuals with polyarticular disability (Jette, 1980). Forty-five IADL and ADL items were selected based on a review of earlier work by Katz (Katz, et al., 1963; Katz, et al., 1970). Personal care activities included combing hair and turning on bathroom faucets, as well as six separate components of dressing ability: putting on/tying shoes; putting on hose/pants; putting on underclothes; putting on a shirt/blouse; putting on buttons/zippers; and putting on a sweater coat.

The Burke Stroke Time-Oriented Profile (BUSTOP) was created to provide a functional profile for assessment of stroke patients (Feigenson et al., 1979). However, the authors note the importance of evaluating the degree of behavioral abnormality, communication deficit, visual/perceptual difficulty, and sensory function, and relating them to a patient's actual function. Several ADL or self-care activities were separated into two or more components: functional performance at mealtime was coded separately for bimanual tasks and one-handed tasks; bathing was scored separately for upper body and lower body; and dressing included upper dressing, lower dressing, and shoes/socks.

The Klein-Bell ADL Scale was an attempt to identify critical and observable components of ADL behavior that could be expressed in generic terms (Klein & Bell, 1982). Each ADL was broken down into a number of subtasks, resulting in 170 items scored either as "achieved" (behavior performed without verbal or physical assistance from another person) or "failed" (assistance is needed). For example, dressing tasks were defined for each type of clothing (i.e., shorts/pants, pullover shirt/button shirt and sweater/coat/jacket), with the items ordered as follows: reach shirt to top of head; pull head through neck hole; put R hand through R armhole; put R elbow into sleeve; put L hand through one armhole; put L elbow into sleeve; pull L hand through L armhole; put L elbow into sleeve; and pull shirt down over trunk. Total points within each ADL category are added and can be combined to yield an overall independence score.

Loewenstein and colleagues (1989) developed the Direct Assessment of Functional Status (DAFS) as an operational procedure for examining areas of functional competence that would identify subtle changes in specific subskills during the progression of Alzheimer's disease. Among the domains in DAFS were subscales for grooming and eating. For grooming, the subject is asked to perform a number of subtasks including: take cap off toothpaste; put toothpaste on brush; turn on water; and brush teeth. Other grooming items include subtasks for washing and dressing. As in the Klein-Bell ADL Scale, only independent performance was evaluated, and level of assistance by others that might allow the subject to complete the task was not considered. Interestingly, on a sample of 30 cognitively impaired and 18 normal controls, the scale failed to detect a significant difference in dressing/grooming skills.

The Structured Assessment of Independent Living Skills (SAILS) (Mahurin, DeBettignies, & Pirozzolo, 1991) included individual items selected from a review of existing behavioral assessment techniques, rating scales and informant report measures. Inclusion of items in the SAILS was based on three criteria: (a) theoretical relevance to specific constructs of functional competence (e.g., dressing, language abilities); (b) practicality of implementing the task in a laboratory setting, and (c) graduation of task difficulty within each area of functioning. Two ADL items, dressing and eating, are among 11 categories measured. Five subtasks under dressing are coded and summed to create a subscore for the dressing category. These tasks represent basic dressing skills: puts on shirt; buttons cuffs of shirt; puts on jacket; ties shoelaces; and puts on gloves.

Whereas earlier scales had separated some ADLs into several components in order to more accurately assess the individual's functional ability, the Beck Dressing Performance Scale (Beck, 1988) is a task segmentation scale for assessing the performance level of cognitively impaired individuals when different behavioral strategies are employed. Dressing performance is measured for the following items: underwear, bra or undershirt, slip, blouse or dress, pants, socks, and shoes. For each of these items, smaller tasks are scored according to type of assistance received to complete the task. Scores range from (0) No assistance, verbal, nonverbal or physical by a caregiver to (7) Subject performs no actions that would help in completing component. Intermediate scores of 1 through 6 represent a hierarchical ranking of type of assistance required by subject in order to complete the task: stimulus control, initial verbal prompt, repeated verbal prompts, gestures or modeling, occasional physical guidance, and complete physical guidance.

FINAL COMMENTS

Chronic care deficits, including Alzheimer's and other neurological diseases, cancer, arthritis, and circulatory problems, all carry an associated risk of lessened self-sufficiency. With each increment in disease status there is a stepped increase in subject dependency status (Kiely et al., submitted). For a nursing home population, as well as for high-risk elders in the community, ADLs are the key functional parameters of interest (Morris, Sherwood, & Gutkin, 1988). Nursing home residents are at risk of physical decline, and the vast majority have some level of deficit upon admission. Almost all have comorbid illnesses, including neurological impairments, that can negatively impact on self-sufficiency during their stay. As a consequence of the many adverse influences, the typical resident will experience accelerated decline during the stay. At the same time some residents improve and rates of decline can be slowed. Thus, one's ADL measures must be broad enough to capture the relevant areas of change, using a coding metric that can maximally capture subject variation while ensuring that high levels of reliability are maintained.

REFERENCES

Beck C. (1988). Measurement of dressing performance in persons with dementia. *American Journal of Alzheimer's Care and Related Disorders & Research, May/ June,* 21-25.

Beck, C., Heacock, P., Mercer, S., Walton, C. G., & Shook, J. (1991). Dressing for success: Promoting independence among cognitively impaired elderly. *Journal of Psychosocial Nursing, 29,* 30-35.

Bergner, M., Babbitt, R. A., Carter, W. B., & Gilson, B. S. (1981). The Sickness Impact Profile: development and final revision of a health status measure. *Medical Care, 19,* 787-805.

Carey, R. G., & Posavac, E. J. (1982). Rehabilitation program evaluation using a revised Level of Rehabilitation Scale (LOS-II). *Archives of Physical Medicine and Rehabilitation, 63,* 367-370.

Dinnerstein, A. J., Lowenthal, M., & Dexter, M. (1965). Evaluation of a rating scale of ability in activities of daily living. *Archives of Physical Medicine and Rehabilitation, 46,* 579-584.

Dodds, T. A., Martin, D. P., Stolov, W. C., & Deyo, R. A. (1993). A validation of functional independence measurement and its performance among rehabilitation inpatients. *Archives of Physical Medicine and Rehabilitation, 74,* 531-536.

Donaldson, S. W., Wagner, S. W., & Gresham, G. E. (1973). A unified ADL evaluation form. *Archives of Physical Medicine and Rehabilitation, 54,* 175-179, 185.

Feigenson, J., Polkow, L., Meikle, R., & Ferguson, W. (1979). Burke Stroke Time-Oriented Profile (BUSTOP): An overview of patient function. *Archives of Physical Medicine and Rehabilitation, 60,* 508-511.

Fillenbaum, G. G. (1988). *Multidimensional functional assessment of older adults: the Duke older Americans resources and services procedures.* Hillsdale, NJ: Lawrence Erlbaum Associates.

Fleiss, J. L. (1981). *Statistical methods for rates and proportions, 2nd Ed.* New York: Wiley.

Frederiks, C. M. A., teWierik, M. J. M., Visser, A. P., & Sturmans, F. (1991). A scale for the functional status of the elderly living at home. *Journal of Advanced Nursing, 16,* 287-292.

Gauger, A. B., Brownell, W. M., Russell, W. W., & Retter, R. W. (1964). Evaluation of levels of subsistence. *Archives of Physical Medicine and Rehabilitation, 45,* 286-292.

Gerety, M. B., Mulrow, C. D., Tuley, M. R., Hazuda, H. P., Lichtenstein, M. J., Bohannon, R., Kanten, D. N., O'Neil, M. B., & Gorton, A. (1993). Development and validation of a physical performance instrument for the functionally impaired elderly: The Physical Disability Index (PDI). *Journals of Gerontology: Medical Sciences, 48,* M33-M38.

Granger, C. V., Albrecht, G. L., & Hamilton, B. B. (1979). Outcome of comprehensive medical rehabilitation: measurement by PULSES Profile and the Barthel Index. *Archives of Physical Medicine and Rehabilitation, 60,* 145-154.

Gurel, L., Linn, M. W., & Linn, B. S. (1972). Physical and mental impairment-of-function evaluation in the aged: the PAMIE scale. *Journal of Gerontology, 27,* 83-90.

Halstead, L., & Hartley, R. B. (1975). Time Care Profile: An evaluation of a new method of assessing ADL dependence. *Archives of Physical Medicine and Rehabilitation, 56,* 110-115.

Hamilton, B. B., Laughlin, J. A., Granger, C. V., & Krayton, R. M. (1991). Interrater reliability of the 7-level Functional Independence Measure (FIM). *Archives of Physical Medicine and Rehabilitation, 72,* 790 (abstract).

Hamilton, B. B., Laughlin, J. A., Fiedler, R. C., & Granger, C. V. (1994). Interrater reliability of the 7-level Functional Independence Measure (FIM). *Scandinavian Journal of Rehabilitative Medicine, 26,* 115-119.

Hawes, C., Morris, J. N., Phillips, C. D., Mor, V., Fries, B. E., & Nonemaker, S. (1995). Reliability estimates for the minimum data set for nursing home residents and care screening (MDS). *The Gerontologist, 35,* 172-178.

Hawes, C., Phillips, C., Morris, J., Mor, V., Fries, B., Steele-Freidlob, E., Greene, A. The impact of the RAI on indicators of process quality in nursing homes, (In press). *Journal of the American Geriatrics Society.*

Heinemann, A. W., Linacre, J. M., Wright, B. D., Hamilton, B. B., & Granger, C. (1993). Relationship between impairment and physical disability as measured by the Functional Independence Measure. *Archives of Physical Medicine and Rehabilitation, 74,* 566-573.

Jette, A. M. (1980). Functional capacity evaluation: An empirical approach. *Archives of Physical Medicine and Rehabilitation, 61,* 85-89.

Katz, S., & Akpom, C. A. (1976). A measure of primary sociobiological functions. *International Journal of Health Services, 6,* 493-507.

Katz, S., Downs, T. D., Cash, H. R., & Grotz, R. C. (1970). Progress in development of the index of ADL. *The Gerontologist, 10,* 20-30.

Katz, S., Ford, A. B., Moskowitz, R. W., Jackson, B. A., & Jaffee, M. W. (1963). Studies of illness in the aged: the index of ADL: A standardized measure of biological and psychosocial function. *Journal of the American Medical Association, 185,* 914-919.

Katz, S., Drugovich, M., Morris, J. N., Cornelius, E., Granger, C., Sloan, P., Murphy, K., & Seltzer, G. (1991). ADL/Functional Rehabilitation Potential. A Resident Assessment Protocol (RAP). In J.N. Morris et al. (Eds.), *Resident assessment instrument training manual and resource guide.* Natick, MA: Eliot Press.

Kiely, D. K., Morris, J. N., Cupples, L. A., Ooi, W. L., Morris, S. A., & Sherwood, S. (Submitted). The effect of specific medical conditions on functional decline.

Klein, R. M., & Bell, B. B. (1982). Self-care skills: Behavioral measurement with Klein-Bell ADL scale. *Archives of Physical Medicine and Rehabilitation, 63,* 335-338.

Kuriansky, J., Gurland, B. (1976). The performance test of activities of daily living. *International Journal of Aging and Human Development, 7,* 343-352.

Law, M., & Letts, L. (1989). A critical review of scales of activities of daily living. *American Journal of Occupational Therapy, 43,* 522-528.

Law, M., & Usher, P. (1988). Validation of the Klein-Bell ADL Scale for pediatric and occupational therapy. *Canadian Journal of Occupational Therapy, 55,* 63-68.

Lawton, E. B. (1980). Activities of daily living test: Geriatric consideration. *Physical and Occupational Therapy in Geriatrics, 1,* 11-20.

Lawton, M. P., & Brody, E. M. (1969). Assessment of older people: Self-maintaining and instrumental activities of daily living. *The Gerontologist, 9,* 179-186.

Lazaridis, E. N., Rudberg, M. A., Furner, S. E., & Cassel, C. K. (1994). Do activities of daily living have a hierarchical structure? An analysis using the longitudinal study of aging. *Journal of Gerontology: Medical Sciences, 49,* M47-M51.

Linn, M. W., & Linn, B. S. (1982). The rapid disability rating scale—2. *Journal of the American Geriatrics Society, 30,* 378-382.

Loewenstein, D. A., Amigo, E., Duara, R., Guterman, A., Hurwitz, D., Berkowitz, N., Wilkie, F., Weinberg, G., Black, B., Gittelman, B., & Eisdorfer, C. (1989). A new scale for the assessment of functional status in Alzheimer's disease and related disorders. *Journals of Gerontology: Psychological Sciences, 44,* P114-P121.

Lowenthal M. F. (1964). *Lives in distress: The paths of the elderly to the psychiatric ward.* New York: Basic Books.

Mahoney, F. I., & Barthel, D. W. (1965). Functional evaluation: The Barthel Index. *Maryland State Medical Journal, 14,* 61-65.

Mahurin, R. K., DeBettignies, & Pirozzolo, F. J. (1991). Structured assessment of independent living skills: Preliminary report of a performance measure of functional abilities in dementia. *Journals of Gerontology: Psychological Sciences, 46,* P58-P66.

Meer, B., & Baker, J. A. (1966). The Stockton geriatric rating scale. *Journal of Gerontology, 21,* 392-403.

Merbitz, C., Morris, J., & Grip, J. C. (1989). Ordinal scales and foundations of misinference. *Archives of Physical Medicine and Rehabilitation, 70,* 308-312.

Morris, J. N., Fries, E., Steel, K., Ikegami N., Bernabei, R., Carpenter, G. I., Gilgen, R., Hirdes, J. P., Topinková, E. Comprehensive clinical assessment in com-munity setting—applicability of the MDS-HC. (In press). *Journal of Geriatrics Society.*

Morris, J. N., Fries, B. E., Phillips, C., Mor, V., Hawes, C., & Morris, S. (1995). MDS—ADL self-performance index (MDS-ADL). Presented at the Gerontological Society of America Annual Meeting.

Morris, J. N., Hawes, C, Murphy, K., Nonemaker, S., Phillips, C., Fries, B. E., & Mor, V. (1991). *Resident assessment instrument training manual and resource guide.* Natick, MA: Eliot Press.

Morris, J. N., Sherwood, S., & Gutkin, C. E. (1988). Inst-Risk II: An approach to forecasting relative risk of future institutional placement. *HSR: Health Services Research, 23*(4), 511-536.

Morris, J. N., Nonemaker, S., Murphy, K., Hawes, C., Fries, B. E., Mor, V., & Phillips, C. (In press). A commitment to change: Revision of HCFA's RAI. *Journal of the American Geriatrics Society.*

Myers, A. M. (1992). The clinical Swiss army knife: Empirical evidence on the validity of IADL functional status measures. *Medical Care, 30,* MS96-MS111.

Nihira, K., Foster, R., & Spenser, L. (1968). Measurement of adaptive behavior: A descriptive system for mental retardates. *American Journal of Orthopsychiatry, 38,* 622-634.

Potvin, A. R., Tourtellotte, W. W., Dailey, J. S., Albers, J. W., Walker, J. E., Pew, R. W., Henderson, W. G., & Snyder, D. N. (1972). Simulated activities of daily living examination. *Archives of Physical Medicine and Rehabilitation, 53,* 476-487.

Research Foundation of the State University of New York, Buffalo (1987). *Guide for use of the uniform data set for medical rehabilitation.*

Reuben, D. B., & Siu, A. L. (1990). An objective measure of physical function of elderly outpatients: The Physical Performance Test. *Journal of the American Geriatrics Society, 38,* 1105-1112.

Schoening, H. A., Anderegg, L., Bergstrom, D., Fonda, M., Steinke, N., & Ulrich, P. (1965). Numerical scoring of self-care status of patients. *Archives of Physical Medicine and Rehabilitation, 46,* 689-697.

Siu, A. L., Hays, R. D., Ouslander, J. G., Osterwell, D., Valdez, R. B., Krynski, M., & Gross, A. (1993). Measuring functioning and health in the very old. *Journals of Gerontology: Medical Sciences, 48,* M10-M14.

Skurla, E., Rogers, J. C., & Sunderland, T. (1988). Direct assessment of activities of daily living in Alzheimer's disease: A controlled study. *Journal of the American Geriatrics Society, 36,* 97-103.

Spector, W. D., Katz, S., Murphy, J. B., & Fulton, J. P. (1987). The hierarchical relationship between activities of daily living and instrumental activities of daily living. *Journal of Chronic Diseases, 40,* 481-489.

Staff of Benjamin Rose Hospital (1958). Multidisciplinary study of illness in aged persons, I. Methods and preliminary results. *Journal of Chronic Diseases, 7,* 332-345.

Winograd, C. H., Lemsky, C. M., Nevitt, M. C., Nordstrom, T. M., Stewart, A. L., & Miller, C. J., (1994). Development of a physical performance and mobility examination. *Journal of the American Geriatrics Society, 42,* 743-749.

Wright, B. D., & Linacre, J. M. (1989). Observations are always ordinal; measurements, however, must be interval. *Archives of Physical Medicine and Rehabilitation, 70,* 857-860.

Chapter 10

Social Support Measurement in Group Residences for Older Adults

Jason T. Newsom, Jamila Bookwala, and Richard Schulz

Social support is one of the most widely studied psychosocial risk factors of physical and mental health. Social support has been found to be associated with lower incidence of heart disease (Eriksen, 1994; Smith & Gallo, 1994), higher cancer survival (Ell, Nishimoto, Mediansky, & Mantell, 1992), less hypertension (Henry, 1988), and lower mortality rates (Berkman, 1995; House, Landis, & Umberson, 1988). Associations with mental health also are well documented, showing that a lack of social support resources is associated with greater depression (Barnett, & Gotlib, 1988; George, 1989; Newsom & Schulz, 1996), lower psychological well-being (Finch, Okun, Barrera, Zautra, & Reich, 1989), and suicide (Rudd, 1993).

Although social support research has frequently focused on older adults, there has been a surprising lack of attention to social support and its importance for health and well-being among institutionalized individuals. Researchers working in the institutional setting have examined issues related to social support, such as dependence, visitation, and conflict with staff, but, by comparison to the more elaborate theoretical constructs developed by social support researchers interested in community settings (see Barrera, 1981; Heitzman & Kaplan, 1988; Sarason, Sarason, & Pierce, 1990; Turner, 1992, for reviews), they represent only a small set of the possible support-related dimensions that can be investigated. The well documented importance of social support for mental and physical health suggests a great need to improve our understanding of the role of support systems among institutionalized elders. An important first step toward this understanding is a thorough consideration of social support measurement issues relevant to these populations and settings. The purpose of this paper is to review measures related to social support that have been used with residents of nursing homes and congregate housing for older adults.

Institutional settings have a number of unique features that have implications for how we think about and measure social support. Those who live in these settings are more likely to have physical and cognitive functioning difficulties than are those residing in the community, and these limitations present difficult challenges for measuring support. Assistance with at least some daily living activities such as meal preparation or housekeeping is both more needed and more readily available in

Acknowledgment. Preparation of this manuscript was supported by grants from the National Institute on Aging (AG09291) and the National Institute of Mental Health (MH42247, MH46015).

institutional settings than in the community. The regular provision of this type of support means that residents interact more frequently with professional care providers and health care workers, and that such interactions provide potential sources of both companionship and conflict. In addition, residents interact more frequently with and live in closer proximity to a greater number of nonrelatives of a similar age group which may influence the size, structure, and functions of support networks for these individuals (Friedman, 1966).

In this review, we consider three types of residences (Moos & Lemke, 1994)—nursing homes, residential care facilities, and congregate apartments. Nursing homes can be characterized by the regular availability of health care services, meals, housekeeping, and personal care assistance. Residential care facilities provide meals, housekeeping services, supervision and assistance with daily living but do not have health services regularly available. Congregate apartments typically provide meal services but no personal care or health care services. Although these types of residences vary in the amount of personal and health care that is regularly available, there are similarities in their social environments. Our review includes research conducted in all three of these types of facilities, which we will refer to collectively as "group residences."

The description of measures and their psychometric properties is preceded by a brief overview of social support measurement concepts and the special considerations that are needed when measuring these constructs in group residences. This is followed by a description of the psychometric standards by which we evaluate the measures reviewed and the methodological approaches available for assessing social support among cognitively impaired individuals. Finally, individual measures will be discussed, organized around the basic concepts of social support. First described are perceived support measures, followed by social network measures, and then observational measures of social interactions. This review does not include any measures used with community-residing older adults because such measures have been more comprehensively reviewed elsewhere (Oxman & Berkman, 1990; Rook, 1994).

DEFINING AND DESCRIBING SOCIAL SUPPORT

There have been many approaches to the definition and measurement of social relationships. Because there have been a number of thorough treatments that classify and define the types, functions, and sources of social support elsewhere (Barrera, 1986; Berkman, Oxman, & Seeman, 1992; Cohen & Wills, 1985; Heitzman & Kaplan, 1988; Rook & Pietromonaco, 1987; Winemiller, Mitchell, Sutliff, & Cline, 1993), we present only an abbreviated description of the relevant concepts here.

Perhaps the broadest classification that can be made in measuring social relationships is the distinction between perceived support and social networks. *Perceived support* involves an individual's subjective assessment of support received within a particular time frame, support available if needed, or satisfaction with or perceived adequacy of support. The measurement of *social networks*, on the other hand, usually involves counting the number of family and friends, the frequency of contact with network members, proximity to network members, and occasionally the amount of contact that members of the network have with one another (i.e., *network density*). Contrary to what might be expected, perceived support and social network measures are not always strongly associated with one another (e.g., Cutrona, 1986; Newsom & Schulz, 1996). Some have also argued that, in terms of consequences for mental health, the perception of support is of greater importance than network size or the frequency of contact with network members (e.g., Barrera, 1981; Schaefer, Coyne, & Lazarus, 1981).

Researchers most often identify two basic functions of social support: *emotional* support, which involves affection from others, sharing feelings, or a general sense of belonging; and *instrumental* support, which involves the tangible or material assistance from others and can include anything from financial assistance to help with daily chores. A less frequently studied function of support, *informational* or appraisal support, is advice or knowledge provided by others. Emotional, tangible, and informational support are often included as separate factors in perceived support measures but are not typically features of network measures.

One of the unique characteristics of institutional settings is the high level of instrumental support available. Assistance provided by both formal and informal caregivers, such as housekeeping, transportation, meal preparation, finances, or personal care, can be classified as instrumental support (Litwin & Auslander, 1990; Pearlman & Crown, 1992). For individuals living in group residences, instrumental support is more likely to be provided by professional staff than by family and friends. Although such assistance is more likely to be available when needed, residents are more dependent on it for daily functioning. Thus, individuals in group residences may be more sensitive to discrepancies between the amount of instrumental support received and the amount perceived to be needed.

Who provides support, or the *source* of support, is an important aspect of social relationships. It is common to identify whether support is provided by relatives or friends. Some researchers also attempt to identify confidants—friends or family members with whom individuals share their most personal feelings (e.g., Connidis & Davies, 1990; Schulz, Tompkins, & Rau, 1988). For older adults in nursing homes or those who receive in-home assistance, professional staff are a potential source of support. Professional staff are not typically included as an independent source of support in most measures, yet for physically and cognitively impaired individuals, they are likely to provide a substantial amount of tangible support and will often be an important source of emotional support as well (Pearlman & Crown, 1992).

Relationships with paid staff differ from relationships with friends and family in several important ways. First, unlike friends and family, residents are not able to choose the staff members they must regularly interact with, and they may have little control over when interactions take place. Second, receiving assistance with personal activities, such as bathing or toileting, from individuals that residents do not know well may be awkward and uncomfortable. In general, older adults prefer to receive assistance from family members rather than professionals or friends (Chappell, 1991), and this preference may be stronger if the assistance is of a more personal nature. Third, paid care providers are a potential source of companionship and emotional support, but the nature of the relationship between care provider and recipient may be merely professional for many. Fourth, while most support relationships are reciprocal (Ingersoll-Dayton & Antonucci, 1988), formal care relationships are decidedly more one-sided.

The positive aspects of social relations are the most often studied and are the focus of most social support-related measures, but a growing body of research suggests that negative aspects of social interaction may have the greatest impact on mental health (Fiore, Becker, & Coppel, 1983; Pagel, Erdley, & Becker, 1987; Rook, 1984; Finch et al., 1989; Ruehlman & Wolchik, 1988). Negative social relations may be a result of actions intended to be supportive or from interactions that create interpersonal conflict (Rook & Pietromonaco, 1987). In some instances, social support from network members is intended to be positive but is perceived negatively because network members are overly helpful or do not help appropriately. Interpersonal conflict may arise from interactions initiated by either the respondent or network members in the form of criticism, invasion of privacy, or unequal exchange.

MEASUREMENT METHODOLOGY ISSUES

In order to evaluate the adequacy of existing social support measures, we briefly note some methodological considerations when examining the reliability of measures of social support in group residences.

Reliability

Cronbach's alphas are the most commonly used metric of internal reliability and are generally considered to be acceptable if over .80. Because alpha is not only a reflection of interitem correlations, but is also influenced by the number of items in a scale, we also present an adjusted alpha, based on the Spearman-Brown Prophecy formula (Ferguson, 1971; Nunnally, 1978), to facilitate comparisons of the reliability of scales of different lengths. The adjusted alpha we use is computed assuming a scale length of 10 items. In some instances reliability estimates based on interitem associations may not be appropriate. For example, there may be no theoretical basis to expect a strong association between frequency of contact with network members and network size. This does not mean that reliability of such measures should not be examined, but in such cases other methods of testing reliability, such as test-retest reliability, may be more appropriate. Psychometricians also frequently recommend that multiple items be used to assess a single construct in order to increase reliability and assure that the theoretical domain is fully assessed (e.g., Nunnally, 1978), so individual items that have low correlations with other items should be supplemented with additional items if possible.

Approaches to Measurement Among Cognitively Impaired

In general, an important consideration in measuring social support in group residences, particularly nursing homes, is the large number of residents that suffer from substantial cognitive impairment. Although exact figures differ across studies, between 60% and 80% of nursing home residents are cognitively impaired (e.g., Class et al., 1996; Rovner, Kafonek, Filipp, Lucas, & Folstein, 1986). Other group residences such as residential care facilities or congregate apartments have lower rates of cognitive impairment and residents are likely to be less severely impaired on average. Cognitive impairment makes it difficult for researchers to measure certain aspects of social support. Because perceived support measures involve an individual's subjective assessment of support, these measures are by nature self-report. Therefore residents with severe cognitive impairment levels that interfere with the ability to comprehend or accurately respond to interview questions cannot complete perceived support measures.

Researchers desiring to measure social support in these settings have three general approaches available for dealing with measurement problems caused by cognitive impairment of respondents. One option is to eliminate participants who have a certain level of impairment. For researchers wishing to study the subjective aspects of support, such as perceived availability or satisfaction with support, there may be no alternative to excluding individuals who are severely cognitively impaired. The primary drawback to eliminating participants is that the generalizability of the results may be limited. If the study involves a comparison group (e.g., an intervention or a clinical trial), however, the number of potential respondents who are eliminated because of cognitive impairment should not differ between comparison groups, because such differences are potential confounds.

Researchers have debated whether cognitive impairment affects the accuracy of self-report and if it does, what level of impairment is problematic. Studies investigating the effect of cognitive impairment on self-reported depression and physical functioning accuracy have had mixed results. Some authors have concluded that mild or moderate impairment has no effect on self-report accuracy (Little, Hemsley, Volans, & Bergmann, 1986; Parmelee, Lawton, & Katz, 1989; Rogers, Holm, Goldstein, & McCue, 1994; Teri & Wagner, 1991), and others have concluded that impairment does have important effects (McGivney, Mulvihill, & Taylor, 1994; Sager et al., 1992; Weinberger et al., 1992). The discrepancies in these findings may stem from a number of variables, including different cognitive tests, different "gold standards" of comparison, varying exclusionary criteria for the most severely impaired, and differences in cutoffs.

The contradictory findings in the area leave researchers in a quandary about how to deal with cognitively impaired participants. Even if one chooses to eliminate those with cognitive impairments from the sample, there seems to be no consensus on which cutoff is most appropriate. For example, McGivney and colleagues (1994) used a cutoff of 15 on the Mini-Mental State Examination whereas Sager and colleagues (1992) used a cutoff of 24. Until more is known about the potential problems with cognitively impaired respondents, researchers are advised to formally measure cognitive functioning and set a predetermined cutoff for inclusion in the study. Subjective judgments by interviewers should be avoided, because they may not be reliable assessments, may impose variable selection criteria, and may often be difficult decisions for interviewers to make.

A second approach to the measurement problems posed by cognitive impairment is to use observational methods. Most aspects of social networks, for example, can be measured successfully with cognitively impaired individuals through observation. Frequency of contact with friends and family, proximity, conflict and network size can all be assessed using these approaches. Researchers should check reliability of observers by using a second observer of the same behaviors for at least 20% of their sample and reporting total interrater agreement or correlations. Information about perceived support, such as satisfaction with support or perceived availability of support cannot be adequately measured with these approaches, however.

A third option is for researchers to obtain data from proxy informants who are familiar with the impaired individual. Research on the comparability of proxy and self-report data, however, suggests that systematic biases in proxy-rated information often occurs (Zimmerman & Magaziner, 1994). In general, proxies tend to overestimate disability and negative affect. Proxy reports more accurately reflect self-reports when the measure assesses more concrete and observable phenomena. The accuracy of proxy reports of social support has not been widely studied. In one study of AIDS patients and their primary caretakers, Berk (1995) found that caregiver proxies consistently indicated a greater need for care, less personal support, and a more impoverished social network for the patient than did the patient, although the differences did not reach statistical significance. More research on the accuracy of proxy reports of social support is needed, but based on research with other types of measures, it would be expected that proxy reports of observable social behaviors such as contact with friends and relatives will be more accurate, whereas proxy reports of more subjective aspects of support will be the less accurate. One suggestion is to estimate the amount of bias by examining the agreement between proxy and self-report for a portion of the sample that does not suffer from cognitive impairment (Magaziner, 1988).

REVIEW OF MEASURES

Next, we review social support measures that have been used with group residence populations. We first examine measures of perceived support, followed by social network measures, and then observational measures. A list of all support and network measures reviewed, subscales, length of measure, Cronbach's alphas, and adjusted alphas can be found in Table 10.1. Observational measures are described in the text.

Perceived Support Measures

This category includes measures that assess perceptions of support availability, support received, and adequacy or satisfaction with support. In most cases, it will not make sense for spouses, family members, or friends to provide proxy reports for perceived support measures, since a key component to the measure is the subjective appraisal of support. Thus, these measures require the participant to have an acceptable level of cognitive functioning.

The Sheltered Care Environment Scale (SCES; Lemke & Moos, 1987) is a general measure designed to assess the quality of nursing home environments on seven dimensions (cohesion, conflict, independence, self-disclosure, organization, resident influence, physical comfort). The measure consists of 63 yes/no items, with nine items for each subscale. Only the Cohesion and Conflict subscales are related to social support. The cohesion subscale examines how involved residents are with each other and how supportive they are of one another. Conflict items concern how much residents express anger and are critical of each other. Cronbach's alpha for the Conflict subscale is good (.78, adjusted alpha = .80) but the alpha for the Cohesion could be improved (.69, adjusted alpha = .71; Timko & Moos, 1991). The scale has been used with nursing homes, residential care facilities, and congregate apartments and can be completed by residents or staff. Although information is obtained from individual residents and can be used at this level, the intention of the scale is to assess the quality of the social environment of the institution rather than to examine aspects of perceived support or social networks. Ratings by individuals are typically aggregated into a summary measure, and analyses are based on each facility's average rating. Moos and Lemke

(1994) report a correlation of .41 between residents and staff total scale scores of the SCES (the resident-staff correlations for the subscales were not reported), suggesting that staff may not serve as very suitable proxies for residents.

The Iowa Self-Assessment Inventory (ISAI; Morris & Buckwalter, 1988; Morris et al., 1990) is a 56-item multidimensional scale that includes social support items. Items for the 8-item support subscale were taken from the larger Social Provisions Scale (Cutrona, Russell, & Rose, 1986) and involve statements such as "there is no one I can turn to in times of stress" and "there is someone I can talk to about important decisions." Items from the 24-item Social Provisions Scale were selected using an exploratory factor analysis with orthogonal rotation on all subscales with a sample of older adults from housing projects, congregate meal sites, and community residents. Neither loadings nor percentage of variance accounted for by the factors were reported. Gilmer and colleagues (Gilmer et al., 1991) conducted both exploratory (maximum likelihood with oblique rotation) and confirmatory factor analyses with the ISAI. Half of their sample consisted of retirement community residents, with the remainder drawn from congregate meal sites and housing projects. Although the exploratory factor analyses with the scale indicated loadings of sufficient magnitude, the fit of the confirmatory factor model was not optimal, suggesting that additional items may need to be deleted or modifications are needed in the factor structure. Individual loadings from the confirmatory analysis were not reported. Alphas for the subscale obtained from two different samples approached the .80 cutoff (.75 by Morris et al., 1990 and .79 by Gilmer et al., 1991).

Armer (1993) administered a modified version of the Perceived Social Support scale (PSS; Procidano & Heller, 1983) to participants in two congregate residential facilities who had no cognitive impairment and no debilitating health problems. The measure consists of dichotomous response items that ask if the respondent's support, information, and feedback needs are met by family and friends in the network. Armer revised the friends scale to create an additional scale to measure support received from neighbors in the facility. Cronbach's alphas for the total scale and subscales were low (.24-.64), especially given the relatively large number of items (adjusted alphas between .14 and .47). Interestingly, Procidano and Heller reported substantially higher alphas (.88 for friends and .90 for family) and a high test-retest over a 1-month period ($r = .83$), raising concerns that the internal reliability of the scale may not be consistent across age groups. Although Armer reports moderate correlations with the Philadelphia Geriatric Center Morale scale (Lawton, 1975) and the Index of Relocation Adjustment (Prager, 1986), more information about the reliability of this scale when used with institutionalized elders is needed before it can be considered to be a valid instrument for this population.

Social Network Measures

Self-report and Interview Network Measures. The Norbeck Social Support Questionnaire (NSSQ; Norbeck, Lindsey, & Carrieri, 1981) was originally developed for the general population but has been used successfully with nursing home residents. The NSSQ represents a combination of network and perceived-support measures. Respondents are asked to list up to 20 network members and are then asked eleven follow-up questions hypothesized to cover six domains of support: affect, affirmation,

TABLE 10.1 Social Support and Social Network Measures

Measure	Reference	Type of Measure	Response Format	Subscales	# Items	Alpha	Adjusted alpha[b]	Factor Analysis
Norbeck Social Support Questionnaire (NSSQ)	Norbeck et al. (1981) Nelson (1989)	SN, R, AV	size, 5-pt	Total Functioning	6	.97	.99	NA
				Affect	2	.99		
				Affirmation	2	.91		
				Aid	2	.94		
				Total Network	3	.72	.81	
				Size	1	NA		
				Duration	1	NA		
				Frequency	1	NA		
				Total Loss	3	NA		
Sheltered Care Environment Scale (SCES)	Lemke & Moos (1987)	NI, R	Y/N	Cohesion	9	.69	.71	NA
				Conflict	9	.78	.80	
Iowa Self-Assessment Inventory (ISAI)	Morris & Buckwalter (1988) Morris et al. (1990)	AV	4-pt.	NA	8	.75-.79	.79-.82	EFA[a]
Perceived Social Support	Armer (1993)	SA	Y/N	Total	60	.63	.22	NA
				Friends	20	.52	.35	
				Family	20	.64	.47	
				Neighbors (in facility)	20	.24	.14	
Social Contact Scale	Kane et al. (1983)	SN, C	NA	Social Contact	5	NA	NA	EFA
Social network measure	Cohen et al. (1985)	SN	size	Network variables (number transactions, number linkages, reciprocity, number interlinking subgroups, number multitransaction links, number large subgroups)	7	.76	.82	EFA

(Continued)

TABLE 10.1 (*Continued*)

Measure	Reference	Type of Measure	Response Format	Subscales	# Items	Alpha	Adjusted alpha[b]	Factor Analysis
Social network measure	Wells & Macdonald (1981)	SN	size	number close relationships residents staff family friends	4	NA	NA	NA
Network composition	Pearlman & Crown (1992)	SN, NE, R	Y/N, 5-pt.	network composition spouse children paid helpers received tangible aid ADL IADL frequency of help duration of caregiving relationship	3 1 1 1 15 6 8 1 1	NA NA NA NA NA NA NA NA	NA	NA
Social network measure	Cohen-Mansfield & Marx (1992)	SN, I	size, 7-pt.	frequency of contact with staff, visitors, others, intimacy with staff, visitors, and number of visits	NA	NA	NA	EFA
Friendships	Retsinas & Garrity (1985)	SN	size, Y/N, 4-pt.	social isolation, number of friends, visits	NA	NA	NA	NA

[a] factor analysis used orthogonal rotator. [b] Adjusted Cronbach's alpha using the Spearman-Brown prophecy formula estimates the alpha value if the scale length is ten items. NA = not available or not applicable. EFA = exploratory factor analysis, PCA = principal components analysis, CFA = confirmatory factor analysis. SN = social network measures (e.g., size, frequency), R = received support, AV = available, SA = satisfaction or adequacy, NI = negative interactions, C = confidant, NE = need for support, I = perceived intimacy/closeness.

165

short- and long-term aid, duration of relationship, frequency of contact, and loss of relationship. Norbeck and colleagues derived three scores from the 11 follow-up questions, Total Functioning (affect, affirmation, and aid items), Total Network (size, duration, and frequency), and Total Loss (number of categories and amount of support lost). They report high interitem correlations and test-retest correlations with a student population. Nelson (1989), using the scale with nursing home residents, also reported high internal reliability for the scale (affect, $\alpha = .99$; affirmation, $\alpha = .91$; aid, $\alpha = .94$; Total Functioning, $\alpha = .97$; and Total Network, $\alpha = .72$). In this study, however, the Total Loss subscale was not significantly correlated with Total Function or Total Network subscales, but the correlation between Total Network and Total Function scales was quite high ($r = .92$), suggesting that these two subscales may not measure separate constructs. All three subscales correlated significantly with depression, indicating some convergent validity.

Kane, Bell, Riegler, Wilson, and Kane (1983) used a 5-item self-report "social contact" subscale as part of a multiassessment instrument for nursing home residents. The entire instrument assesses physiological health, activities of daily living, affect, cognition, and satisfaction with the nursing home in addition to social contact. The social contact items include self-reported frequency of contacts with friends inside and outside the nursing home, family, other residents, and the perceived closeness of the contacts. The authors do not report a Cronbach's alpha for the subscale but report that the interitem correlations are approximately .20. Test-retest reliability using different interviewers over 2 to 5 days was low for the short period of time ($r = .59$). An exploratory factor analysis (unspecified method) of the 6-factor multiple assessment scale indicated that social contact items formed a separate factor. One of the 5 factor loadings was low (visitation from friends, .36), but the remaining 4 were of acceptable magnitude (ranging from .57 to .69).

Cohen, Teresi, and Holmes (1985) used a self-reported interview to assess 19 aspects of social networks. Results of a factor analysis (method unspecified) of the 19 variables suggested 7 overall factors, representing the number of transactions, number of linkages deemed to be "very important," the amount of reciprocity, the number of subgroups with 100% interlinking, the total number of linkages, the number of links with more than one type of transaction, and the number of subgroups with five or more members. The factors appear to be moderately to highly correlated as indicated by an alpha of .76 for the seven subscale scores. No information on alphas or correlations among variables within each factor were provided.

Wells and Macdonald (1981) collected network information on 56 residents (47 female and 7 male) who chose to be relocated within the Toronto Homes for the Aged system. They collected self-report data on the number of close relationships with residents, staff, family, and friends before and after the move between nursing homes. Residents were asked to list the number of people with whom they felt close. No psychometric information or detailed description of the measure was reported, but information relevant to the validity of the scale was presented. Significant pre- vs. postrelocation differences in the number of close ties were found for resident relationships and staff relationships, but no differences were found in family and friend relationships. The number of close resident ties prior to the move was not related to changes in life satisfaction, physical health, cognitive impairment, or agitation, but prior ties to staff members were related to physical health and cognitive impairment.

Family and friend relationships were related to life satisfaction, physical health, and agitation. These findings suggest some evidence for the validity of the measure, but reliability data is needed.

Pearlman and Crown (1992) used a measure of network composition, frequency of assistance, type of assistance received (whether helped with ADLs or IADLs), and the adequacy of tangible assistance specifically adapted for use with institutionalized individuals. Composition was measured by grouping individuals into three groups based on marital status (married vs. not married), whether the respondent had living children, and whether there were any paid helpers. Adequacy of tangible support was based on the number of tasks for which respondents received help relative to the number of tasks for which they required help. The authors do not report any reliability information, but do report that those with ADL/IADL impairments who had higher support and network scores had fewer nursing home stays. The measure of adequacy of tangible support provides a possible future direction for assessing whether instrumental assistance meets the respondent's needs. Although this approach to measuring adequacy more objectively quantifies the amount of care provided relative to that needed, it does not measure either the perceived or actual *quality* of the assistance, nor does it capture the *frequency* with which help is received. More reliability information on these measures is needed.

Bear (1988) interviewed residents of congregate living facilities (board care home that included housing, food, and personal care, but not full-time nursing care) and their closest network member. Based on these interviews, she computed measures of network density (percentage of links among network members out of the total possible), degree (number of network members who associate with other members of the network), intensity (which combines frequency of contacts and emotional intimacy), and reciprocity. Reciprocity was based on whether material assistance with personal needs, assistance with financial matters, and giving of gifts were equally exchanged for each member of the network. Friend and family networks were examined separately. No information on reliability was reported, but *t*-tests indicated that there were no mean differences between resident and closest other reports for any of the network categories. Although the *t*-test results suggest no directional bias in the closest network member's reports, they do not provide any information on the degree of agreement between self-report and network member reports. The network measures were found to be associated with health and timing of entry into the facility. Additional validity and reliability information on the scale is needed.

Proxy Measures of Social Networks. A limited number of studies have compared responses of target individuals and their proxies on measures of social support and social networks. In a sample of university retirees with physical functioning difficulties, Epstein and colleagues (Epstein, Hall, Tognetti, Son, & Conant, 1989) compared care recipients and the proxy reports of their primary caregivers on a 6-item measure adapted from Wan (1982). The measure assesses contact with children, siblings, other relatives, neighbors, non-neighbor friends, and people in the context of organized social activities. Internal reliability of the measure was examined separately for recipients and proxies using a principal components analysis with both indicating a single underlying factor. Study participants and their proxies had similar mean responses for contact during the previous month, but proxies who reported spending more time assisting the recipient were more likely to underestimate social activity compared to recipient reports. Correspondence between proxy and respondent reports was moderate ($r = .64$).

Nursing home staff (e.g., nurses, social workers) can serve as a useful source of information about residents' social networks and friendships. Cohen-Mansfield and Marx (1992) developed a measure of social networks specifically designed for nursing home residents. Their measure taps six different dimensions: frequency of contact with staff, frequency of visitors, frequency of other contacts (i.e., letters or phone calls from family members and friends), intimacy with staff, intimacy with visitors, and number of visitors. All items except number of visitors were rated on a 7-point scale by day charge nurses, evening charge nurses, and social workers over a period of 2 weeks. There was an acceptable level of overall interrater agreement (82%), and all correlation coefficients computed to compare ratings by the day nurses, evening nurses, and social workers were statistically significant (range = .17 to .73, $p \le .05$). A factor analysis (generalized least squares with oblique rotation) of all items as rated by the three groups yielded two underlying factors—intimacy and size/density of network—that accounted for 29% of the variance.

As part of a study examining predictors of nursing home friendships, Retsinas and Garrity (1985) used staff reports of social contacts and friendships, but staff reports were not compared to resident self-reports. Each resident was given a "friendship score" signifying the number of friends the staff identified for the resident, which was then used to yield two measures—social isolation (dichotomously scored, in which residents with at least one friend were considered separate from loners) and the number of friends (ranging from 0 to 6). With the help of the floor staff, a social worker diagrammed social patterns within the nursing home. Staff were then asked to identify groups and couples on the basis of mealtime seating arrangements, visits throughout the day, and conversations at recreational or leisure periods. External contacts of the resident (i.e., whether the resident had a living spouse, living children, or a living sibling) and the frequency of visits (regular—once a week or more, occasional—between once a month and once a week, and rarely/never) was also examined. There were no psychometric characteristics reported.

Observational Measures. A number of observational methods have been used with nursing home residents or cognitively impaired individuals. These methods focus on a variety of types of social interaction and do not always use the traditional frameworks developed by social support researchers. Nevertheless, these methods can be informative about social interactions between residents in group living arrangements and may be useful to researchers wishing to adopt these methods to assess more traditional social support constructs.

Baltes and colleagues (Baltes, Kinderman, Reisenzein, & Schmid, 1987; Baltes & Reisenzein, 1986; Baltes & Wahl, 1992) have developed an extensive observation technique to record naturally occurring interaction patterns between the institutionalized elderly and their social partners in the context of dependent and independent self-care behaviors. This coding system addresses several aspects of the interaction behavior including the source of the behavior (i.e., who performed the behavior and, if the target resident was the source, was he or she alone or in the presence of others), actor identification (i.e., the type of social partner: staff, fellow-resident, visitor, volunteer, etc.), the type of behavior of the target resident (i.e., sleeping, constructively engaged, destructively engaged, nonengaged, independent self-care, and dependent self-care), the type of behavior of the social partner (i.e., the social partner's supportiveness of the resident's behaviors, departure) and the dyadic form of the behavior. Codes for the dyadic form of behavior included five types of interaction patterns: a suggestion, command, or request; an expressed intention; an act of compliance or cooperation; an act of refusal/resistance; and a conversation. If a behavior fit none of these categories or if the target resident's behavior was performed in the absence of a social partner, it was coded as "miscellaneous other." Baltes et al. (1987) obtained high interobserver agreement when this carefully structured, detailed coding system was used on two samples of institutionalized elderly (a nursing home and a home for the chronically ill, $\kappa = .87$ and .88, respectively). The narrow definition of the categories for the dyadic form of the behavior, however, can be problematic, because, as reported by Baltes and her colleagues (1987), it may encourage greater use of the "miscellaneous other" category.

A much simpler observational technique was used by Moos and colleagues (Moos, David, Lemke, & Postle, 1984) in their study of the changes in resident and staff behavior patterns following an intra-institutional relocation. Using a behavioral map- ping technique grounded in environmental psychology, resident behavior patterns were coded using a 5-category coding scheme: resident-resident interaction; assistance from staff; staff-resident interaction; interaction between residents and volunteers; relatives, or other visitors; and participation in organized facility activities. Resident-oriented behavior patterns of the staff were also coded, including staff-resident assistance, staff- resident conversation, other informal interaction (e.g., playing cards), and participation with residents in organized facility activities. Observations were made by trained observers who walked through the nursing home premises following a prearranged route. Although the purpose of this observational scheme was to assess changes in resident and staff behavior patterns, such a measure may represent a useful means to assess nursing home residents' social contacts. The simplicity of the observa- tional scheme, however, limits the richness and amount of data that can be obtained.

Observation of supportive behaviors through the use of video recordings of interac- tions could also prove to be useful in a nursing home setting. Kihlgren and colleagues (1993) analyzed video recorded interactions between nursing home staff and residents during morning care sessions in their study on nurse-patient interaction before and after training in integrity-promoting care. Most of the residents in their sample had moderate to severe dementia and were severely disabled in their self-care functions. The coding scheme contained 93 items; most items were coded in terms of whether a behavior occurred or not, whereas a few items assessed quantitative aspects of support or care provided. The items concerned eye, verbal, and body contact between patient and care provider (e.g., patient/caregiver avoided eye contact, patient/caregiver strived for verbal contact), caregiver's attempt to orient the patient (e.g., to the morning care situation, time, etc.), the patient's opportunities to participate in decisions, actions, and to take initiatives during the morning care, the patient's reactions (e.g., aggression), behaviors aimed at strengthening the patient's experience of identity (e.g., caregiver's praise or criticism of the patient, asking the patient's wishes and opinions), caregivers' behavior in relation to the patient's human territory, and struggles for power. The morning care session was divided into five phases comprising greeting or initiation, undressing, washing, dressing, and other (e.g., shaving, combing), and each phase was rated separately on all relevant questions in the coding scheme. Exact interobserver agreement obtained by Kihlgren et al. using this coding scheme was 83%, and the disagreements that existed were nonsystematic. This level of agreement, however, did not take into account the base rate of occurence of the behaviors. Data obtained through this observational technique were useful in assessing changes in nurses' behavior toward patients during morning care sessions after an intervention designed to promote the patient's experience of integrity and the quality of the nurse's communication with the patient, and to make the ward environment calmer and more homelike for the patient.

An observational system that measures a wider variety of social support behaviors was developed by Liotta, Jason, Robinson, and La Vigne (1985). Although the measure was developed explicitly to record supportive interaction behaviors between parents in the home setting, its use may be easily extended to other populations, such as nursing home residents. Building on Gottlieb's (1978) categorization of helping behaviors, Liotta and colleagues constructed a coding scheme for six different supportive behavioral categories, providing a list of behaviors that qualified for each category and a simple scoring strategy. The categories in their coding system include cognitive guidance (e.g., provision of information, advice, clarification of a problem), tangible assistance (e.g., offer of assistance after a request has been made), social reinforcement (e.g., praise, appreciation), emotional support (e.g., reassurance, encouragement), socializing and directionality of support (who was helping whom). Using trained observers to record the categories (as occurring or not occurring) and the direction of the supportive behavior at 30-second intervals, Liotta et al. obtained high interrater reliability estimates ranging from .89 to 1.0. This level of agreement, however, did not take into account the base rate of occurrence of the behaviors. Caution is also advised in the interpretation of these reliability estimates, because computations were based on the observation of a single spousal pair.

DISCUSSION

Our review of measures indicates that there are a number of network and observational measures but relatively few measures of perceived support, support satisfaction, or negative interactions that have been used in group residences for older adults. This is surprising given the growing body of research that suggests perceived support is an important predictor of physical and psychological health outcomes (e.g., Berkman, 1995; George, 1989). Perhaps one reason for the greater number of network and observational measures is the fairly high proportion of residents of nursing homes that have cognitive impairments. Research on perceived support in these settings, however, is much needed and is feasible with a large percentage of residents. Studies on the accuracy of self-report data among mildly and moderately cognitively impaired participants have often found high reliability of self-reports of physical functioning and depression (e.g., Parmelee et al., 1989; Rogers et al., 1994). Moreover, a significant proportion of nursing home residents and a larger proportion of those in group residences and congregate apartments may have sufficient cognitive functioning levels to provide accurate self-report data.

Researchers in this area have rarely measured the separate functions of support typically assessed in other populations. Relatively few network or perceived support measures we reviewed examined instrumental, emotional, and informational support separately. These factors are usually found to be empirically distinct from one another (e.g., Cohen, Mermelstein, Kamarck, & Hoberman, 1985; Krause & Markides, 1990; Newsom & Schulz, 1996). Examining instrumental or tangible aid seems particularly important in these populations, because residents are more likely to suffer from medical illness and physical impairment and require a greater amount of assistance with daily activities.

The special characteristics of group residences require more careful measurement of those who provide support. Researchers working with other populations have often found evidence that family and friend network members serve different support functions and play different roles in predicting mental health outcomes (e.g., Dean, Kolody, & Wood, 1990). Based on these findings, one might expect that residents and staff also may have distinct support functions. Staff members are an important source of instrumental and informational support but may provide significant emotional support as well. Emotional, informational, or instrumental support may also come from other residents. With only a few exceptions, however, most of the measures examined here were not developed to assess support from other residents or staff. Much more work is needed on the types of support that are provided by staff and other residents and the importance of these individuals for the physical health and psychological functioning of residents.

Measures of negative interactions and conflict are becoming increasingly important for research in other populations (Rook, 1994), yet we could find few examples of measures that were designed or adapted for use with nursing home residents or residents of other congregate living environments. Evidence suggests that negative support may be of equal or greater importance in predicting mental health than positive support (e.g., Finch et al., 1989). The number of network members who are sources of conflict, frequency of negative interactions, perceived conflicts, and negatively interpreted support all deserve greater attention. There are a number of measures available that assess negative interactions and have been used with community samples (Rook, 1984; Finch et al., 1989; Krause, 1995; Malone-Beach & Zarit, 1995), many of which may be easily adapted for use with group residence populations.

Psychometric data on measures used in these populations has also been severely lacking. Because of age differences, health differences, and differences in living environments, the reliability of measures originally used with older adults in the community should be reevaluated when used in group residences for older adults. Researchers in this area should at least routinely report internal reliability statistics with interview measures and interrater reliability statistics with observational measures or proxy reports. Many of the measures we reviewed do not meet acceptable levels of reliability. In many instances, the reliability of measures can be improved by eliminating items using factor analytic techniques or by examining item-total correlations. Given the wide variety of reliable support measures available elsewhere, there may be no need to develop completely new measures in many cases. A good strategy may be for researchers to select reliable measures used with older adults in the community and supplement them with additional scales, subscales, or items that are specific to formal instrumental support and support from residents and staff. These adapted measures then should be reevaluated for their psychometric characteristics in institutionalized populations.

When measuring social support in group residences, it is important to measure factors that are expected to be related to support in these settings. It is critical that information on the time since entry into the residence is collected because it may take time for residents to adjust socially after relocation (Kahana, Kahana, & Young, 1985). Cognitive functioning of participants may be another variable that has an important association with social support. Cognitive functioning may influence social support, it may be affected by social support, or it may be an important covariate that will increase measurement precision when controlled. Because social environments may differ fairly dramatically between the types of facilities available, researchers should be specific in their description of the residence. The type and amount of daily assistance available, the number of others in the home, the social activities available, staff/resident ratio, and characteristics of the residents are all factors that should be routinely reported, because they may have important effects on social support. Many samples may be drawn from only one or two facilities, and the variability of the residence characteristics may be a source of variation between studies, possibly accounting for inconsistent findings. Time since entry into the residence, cognitive functioning and residence characteristics should be routinely measured and reported, not only because they may be sources of variation in support within and between studies, but because they may have important theoretical relations with support as well.

Both physical and mental health problems are common in older adults living in group residences, and these problems will become more serious as the population ages. Research on social support among these individuals is overdue and will be critical for facing the health, mental health, and policy challenges that lie ahead. Advancing research on social support among this population will be important for developing interventions, establishing facility guidelines, and altering institutional norms that can reduce physical impairment and improve mental health for those who reside in these facilities. An important first step in this endeavor will be to develop instruments that can reliably and validly measure social support and interactions in this population.

REFERENCES

Armer, J. M. (1993). Elderly relocation to a congregate setting: Factors influencing adjustment. *Issues in Mental Health Nursing, 14*, 157-172.

Baltes, M. M., Kinderman, T., Reisenzein, R., & Schmid, U. (1987). Further observational data on the behavioral and social world of institutions for the aged. *Psychology and Aging, 2*, 390-403.

Baltes, M. M., & Reisenzein, R. (1986). The social world in long-term care institutions: Psychosocial control toward dependency? *The psychology of control and aging* (pp. 315-343). Hillsdale, NJ: Lawrence Erlbaum Associates.

Baltes, M. M., & Wahl, H. W. (1992). The dependency-support script in institutions: Generalization to community settings. *Psychology and Aging, 7*, 409-418.

Barnett, P. A., & Gotlib, I. H. (1988). Psychosocial functioning and depression: Distinguishing among antecedents, concomitants, and consequences. *Psychological Bulletin, 104*, 97-126.

Barrera, M. (1981). Social support in the adjustment of adolescents: Assessment issues. In B. H. Gottlieb (Ed.), *Social networks and social support* (pp. 69-96). Beverly Hills, CA: Sage.

Barrera, M., Jr. (1986). Distinctions between social support concepts, measures, and models. *American Journal of Community Psychology, 14,* 413-445.

Bear, M. (1988). Use of adult congregate living facilities: Impact of network characteristics on health severity at the time of entry. *Adult Foster Care Journal, 2,* 158-175.

Berk, R. A. (1995). Use of primary caretakers as proxies to measure the health care needs of patients with AIDS. *Public Health Nursing, 12,* 109-116.

Berkman, L. F. (1995). The role of social relations in health promotion. *Psychosomatic Medicine, 57,* 245-254.

Berkman, L. F., Oxman, T. E., & Seeman, T. E. (1992). Social networks and social support amount the elderly: Assessment issues. In R.B. Wallace & R.F. Woolson (Eds.), *The epidemiologic study of the elderly* (pp. 196-212). Oxford, England: Oxford University Press.

Chappell, N. L. (1991). Living arrangements and sources of caregiving. *Journal of Gerontology: Social Sciences, 46,* 1-8.

Class, C. A., Unverzagt, F. W., Gao, S., Hall, K. S., Baiyewu, O., & Hendrie, H. C. (1996). Psychiatric disorders in African-American nursing home residents. *American Journal of Psychiatry, 153,* 677-681.

Cohen, C. I., Teresi, J., & Holmes, D. (1985). Social networks and adaptation. *The Gerontologist, 25,* 297-304.

Cohen, S., Mermelstein, R., Kamarck, T., & Hoberman, H.M. (1985). Measuring the functional components of social support. In I.G. Sarason & B.R. Sarason (Eds.), *Social support: Theory, research, and applications* (pp. 73-94). The Hague: Martinus Nijhoff.

Cohen, S., & Wills, T.A. (1985). Stress, social support, and the buffering hypothesis. *Psychological Bulletin, 98,* 310-357.

Cohen-Mansfield, J., & Marx, M. S. (1992). The social network of the agitated nursing home resident. *Research on Aging, 14,* 110-123.

Connidis, I. A., & Davies, L. (1990). Confidants and companions in later life: The place of family or friends. *Journal of Gerontology: Social Sciences, 45,* 141-149.

Connidis, I. A., & Davies, L. (1992). Confidants and companions: Choices in later life. *Journal of Gerontology: Social Sciences, 47,* 115-122.

Cutrona, C. (1986). Objective determinants of perceived social support. *Journal of Personality and Social Psychology, 50,* 349-355.

Cutrona, C. E., Russell, D. W., & Rose, J. (1986). Social support and adaptation to stress by the elderly. *Psychology and Aging, 1,* 47-54.

Dean, A., Kolody, & Wood, P. (1990). Effects of social support from various sources on depression in elderly persons. *Journal of Health and Social Behavior, 31,* 148-161.

Ell, K., Nishimoto, R., Mediansky, L., & Mantell, J. (1992). *Journal of Psychosomatic Research, 36,* 531-541.

Epstein, A. M., Hall, J. A., Tognetti, J., Son, L. H., & Conant, L. (1989). Using proxies to evaluate quality of life: Can they provide valid information about patients health status and satisfaction with medical care? *Medical Care, 27* (Supplement), S91-S98.

Eriksen, W. (1994). The role of social support in the pathogenesis of coronary heart disease: A literature review. *Family Practice, 11*, 201-209.

Ferguson, G. A. (1971). *Statistical analysis in psychology and education.* New York: McGraw-Hill.

Finch, J. F., Okun, M. A., Barrera, M., Zautra, A. J., & Reich, J. (1989). Positive and negative social ties among older adults: Measurement models and the prediction of psychological stress and well-being. *American Journal of Community Psychology, 17*, 585-605.

Fiore, J., Becker, J., & Coppel, D. B. (1983). Social network interactions: A buffer or a stress? *American Journal of Community Psychology, 11*, 423-439.

Friedman, E. P. (1966). Spatial proximity and social interaction in a home for the aged. *Journal of Gerontology, 21*, 566-570.

George, L. K. (1989). Stress, social support, and depression over the life-course. In K. S. Markides, & C. L. Cooper (Eds.), *Aging, stress and health* (pp. 241-267). New York: Wiley.

Gilmer, J. S., Cleary, T. A., Lu, D.F., Morris, W. W., Buckwalter, K. C., Andrews, P., Boutelle, S., & Hatz, D.L. (1991). The factor structure of the Iowa Self-assessment Inventory. *Educational and Psychological Measurement, 51*, 365-375.

Gottlieb, B. H. (1978). The development and application of a classification scheme of informal helping behaviors. *Canadian Journal of Behavioral Science, 10*, 110-115.

Heitzman, C. A., & Kaplan, R. M. (1988). Assessment methods for measuring social support. *Health Psychology, 7*, 75-109.

Henry, J. P. (1988). Stress, salt, and hypertension. Special issue: Stress and coping in relation to health and disease. *Social Science and Medicine, 26*, 293-302.

House, J. S., Landis, K. R., & Umberson, D. (1988, July 29). Social relationships and health. *Science, 241*, 540-545.

Ingersoll-Dayton, B., & Antonucci, T. C. (1988). Reciprocal and nonreciprocal social support: Contrasting sides of intimate relationships. *Journal of Gerontology: Social Sciences, 43*, 65-73.

Kahana, E., Kahana, B., & Young, R. F. (1985). Social factors in institutional living. In W. A. Peterson & J. Quadagno (Eds.), *Social bonds in later life: Aging and interdependence* (pp. 389-418). Beverly Hills, CA: Sage.

Kane, R. L., Bell, R., Riegler, S., Willson, A., & Kane, R. A. (1983). Assessing the outcomes of nursing home patients. *Journal of Gerontology, 38*, 385-393.

Kihlgren, M., Kuremyer, D., Norberg, A., Brane, G., Karlson, I., Engstrom, B., & Melin, E. (1993). Nurse-patient interaction after training in integrity promoting care at a long-term ward: Analysis of video-recorded morning care sessions. *International Journal of Nursing Studies, 30*, 1-13.

Krause, N. (1995). Negative interaction and satisfaction with social support among older adults. *Journal of Gerontology: Psychological Sciences, 50B*, 59-73.

Krause, N., & Markides, K. (1990). Measuring social support among older adults. *International Journal of Aging and Human Development, 30*, 37-53.

Lawton, M. P. (1975). The Philadelphia Geriatric Center morale scale: A revision. *Journal of Gerontology, 30*, 85-89.

Lemke, S., & Moos, R. H. (1987). Measuring the social climate of congregate residences for older people: Sheltered Care Environment Scale. *Psychology and Aging, 2*, 20-29.

Little, A. G., Hemsley, D. R., Volans, P. J., & Bergmann, K. (1986). The relationship between alternative assessments of self-care ability in the elderly. *British Journal of Clinical Psychology, 25*, 51-59.

Liotta, R. F., Jason, L. A., Robinson, L., & LaVigne, V. (1985). A behavioral approach for measuring social support. *Family Therapy, 12*, 285-295.

Litwin, H., & Auslander, G. K. (1990). Evaluating informal support. *Evaluation Review, 14*, 42-56.

Magaziner, J. Simonsick, E. M., Kashner, M., & Hebel, J. R. (1988). Patient-proxy response comparability on measures of patient health and functional status. *Journal of Clinical Epidemiology, 41*, 1065-1074.

Malone-Beach, E. E., & Zarit, S. H. (1995). Dimensions of social support and social conflict as predictors of caregiver depression. *International Psychogeriatrics, 7*, 25-38.

McGivney, S. A., Mulvihill, J., & Taylor, B. (1994). Validating the GDS depression screen in the nursing home. *Journal of the American Geriatrics Society, 42*, 490-492.

Moos, R. H., David, T. G., Lemke, S., & Postle, E. (1984). Coping with an intra-institutional relocation: Changes in resident and staff behavior patterns. *The Gerontologist, 24*, 495-502.

Moos, R. H., & Lemke, S. (1994). *Group residences for older adults: Physical features, policies, and social climate.* New York: Oxford University Press.

Morris, R. H., & Buckwalter, K. C. (1988). Functional assessment of the elderly: The Iowa Self-Assessment Inventory. In C. F. Waltz and O. L. Strickland (Eds.), *Measurement of nursing outcomes, volume 1, measuring client outcomes*, (pp. 328-351). New York: Springer Publishing Co.

Morris, W. W, Buckwalter, K. C., Cleary, T. A., Gilmer, J. S., Hatz, D. L., & Studer, M. (1990). Refinement of the Iowa Self-Assessment Inventory. *The Gerontologist, 30*, 243-248.

Nelson, P. B. (1989). Social support, self-esteem, and depression in the institutionalized elderly. *Issues in Mental Health Nursing, 10*, 55-68.

Newsom, J. T., & Schulz, R. (1996). Social support as a mediator in the relation between functional status and quality of life in older adults. *Psychology and Aging, 11*, 34-44.

Norbeck, J. S., Lindsey, A., & Carrieri, V. L. (1981). The development of an instrument to measure social support. *Nursing Research, 30*, 264-269.

Nunnally, J. C. (1978). *Psychometric theory* (2nd edition). New York: McGraw-Hill.

Oxman, T. E., & Berkman, L. F. (1990). Assessment of social relationships in elderly patients. *International Journal of Psychiatry in Medicine, 20*, 65-84.

Pagel, M. D., Erdly, W. W., & Becker, J. (1987). Social networks: We get by with (and in spite of) a little help from our friends. *Journal of Personality and Social Psychology, 53*, 793-804.

Parmelee, P. A., Lawton, M. P., & Katz, I. R. (1989). Psychometric properties of the Geriatric Depression Scale among the institutionalized aged. *Psychological Assessment, 1*, 331-338.

Pearlman, D. N., & Crown, W. H. (1992). Alternative sources of social support and their impacts on institutional risk. *The Gerontologist, 32*, 527-535.

Prager, E. (1986). Components of personal adjustment of long distance elderly movers. *The Gerontologist, 26*, 676-680.

Procidano, M. E., & Heller, K. (1983). Measures of perceived social support from friends and from family: Three validation studies. *American Journal of Community Psychology, 11*, 1-24.

Retsinas, J., & Garrity, P. (1985). Nursing home friendships. *The Gerontologist, 25*, 376-381.

Rogers, J. C., Holm, M. B., Goldstein, G., & McCue, M. (1994). Stability and change in functional assessment of patients with geropsychiatric disorders. *American Journal of Occupational Therapy, 48*, 914-918.

Rook, K. S. (1984). The negative side of social interactions: Impact on psychological well-being. *Journal of Personality and Social Psychology, 46*, 1097-1108.

Rook, K. S. (1994). Assessing the health-related dimensions of older adults' social relationships. In M. P. Lawton, & J. A. Teresi (Eds.), *Annual review of gerontology and geriatrics: Focus on assessment techniques, Vol. 14* (pp. 142-181). New York: Springer Publishing Co.

Rook, K. S., & Pietromonaco, P. (1987). Close relationships: Ties that heal or ties that bind? In W. H. Jones & D. Perlman (Eds.), *Advances in personal relationships, Vol. 1* (pp. 1-35). Greenwich, CT: Jai Press.

Rovner, B. W., Kafonek, S., Fillipp, L., Lucas, M. J., & Folstein, M. F. (1986). Prevalence of mental illness in a community nursing home. *American Journal of Psychiatry, 143*, 1446-1449.

Rudd, D. M. (1993). Social support and suicide. *Psychological Reports, 72*, 201-202.

Ruehlman, L. S., & Wolchik, S. A. (1988). Personal goals and interpersonal support and hindrance as factors in psychological distress and well-being. *Journal of Personality and Social Psychology, 55*, 293-301.

Sager, M. A., Dunham, N. C., Schwantes, A., Mecum, L., Halverson, K, & Harlowe, D. (1992). Measurement of activities of daily living in hospitalized elderly: A comparison of self-report and performance based methods. *Journal of the American Geriatrics Society, 40*, 457-462.

Sarason, B. R., Sarason, I. G., & Pierce, G. R. (1990). Traditional views of social support and their impact on assessment. In B. R. Sarason, I. G. Sarason, & G. R. Pierce (Eds.), *Social support: An interactional view* (pp. 9-25). New York: Wiley.

Schaefer, C., Coyne, J., & Lazarus, R. (1981). The health-related functions of social support. *Journal of Behavioral Medicine, 4*, 381-406.

Schulz, R., Tompkins, C. A., & Rau, M. T. (1988). A longitudinal study of the psychosocial impact of stroke on primary support persons. *Psychology and Aging, 3*, 131-141.

Smith, T. W., & Gallo, L. C. (1994). Psychosocial influences on coronary heart disease. Special issue: Heart disease: The psychological challenge. *Irish Journal of Psychology, 15*, 8-26.

Teri, L., & Wagner, A. W. (1991). Assessment of depression in patients with Alzheimer's disease: Concordance among informants. *Psychology and Aging, 6*, 280-285.

Timko, C., & Moos, R. H. (1991). A typology of social climates in group residential facilities for older people. *Journal of Gerontology: Social Sciences, 46*, 160-169.

Turner, R. J. (1992). Measuring Social Support: Issues of concept and method. In H.O.F. Veiel & U.B. Baumann (Eds.), *The Meaning and Measurement of Social Support* (pp. 217-233). New York: Hemisphere.

Wan, T. T. H. (1982). *Stressful life events, social support networks, and gerontological health: A prospective study.* Lexington, MA: Lexington Books (D.C. Heath & Co.).

Weinberger, M., Samsa, G. P., Schmader, K., Greenberg, S. M., Carr, D. B., & Wildman, D. S. (1992). Comparing proxy and patients perceptions of patients functional status: Results from an outpatient geriatric clinic. *Journal of the American Geriatrics Society, 40,* 585-588.

Wells, L., & Macdonald, G. (1981). Interpersonal networks and post-relocation adjustment of the institutionalized elderly. *The Gerontologist, 21,* 177-183.

Winemiller, D. R., Mitchell, M. E., Sutliff, J., & Cline, D. J. (1993). Measurement strategies in social support: A descriptive review of the literature. *Journal of Clinical Psychology, 49,* 638-648.

Zimmerman, S. I., & Magaziner, J. (1994). Methodological issues in measuring the functional status of cognitively impaired nursing home residents: The use of proxies and performance-based measures. *Alzheimer Disease and Associated Disorders, 8,* S281-S290.

Chapter 11

Measurement of Use of Formal Health Care Services

Jennie Jacobs Kronenfeld

Over the years, researchers in fields such as medical sociology and epidemiology have focused on the development of measures addressing use of health care services. Sociologists have emphasized the creation of models that explain use of health care services (Aday, 1993; Anderson, 1973; Andersen & Aday, 1978; McKinlay, 1972; Mechanic, 1978). Epidemiologists have studied the use of health care as an adjunct to the study of populations' health. Both sociologists and epidemiologists have developed specialized measures employed in surveys of health services use.

Many of the in-person utilization surveys have been conducted as part of large national data collection efforts, such as the Health Interview Survey (HIS), conducted under the auspices of the National Center for Health Statistics (NCHS), and published as part of the Vital and Health Statistics series of the federal government (Benson & Marano, 1994). The HIS, conducted for over 30 years, is a survey of the noninstitutionalized population of the United States. In 1984, the special supplement on aging (Longitudinal Study on Aging (LSOA), 1986), was added to the HIS. This 30-minute interview followed the general HIS interview format and was designed to obtain special information about people 55 and older.

The purpose of this paper is to identify and describe measures of health services use that can be applied in studies of elderly persons with dementing illness and/or a communication disorder. As part of this, it is important to understand how measures of health service use have been developed and applied in more general population settings. For example, Andersen and Aday (Aday, 1993; Andersen & Aday, 1978) discuss four principal dimensions of utilization: type, purpose, site, and time interval of use. "Type" refers to the category of service, e.g., physician-based, institution-based (hospital, long-term care), or community-based (home health, personal care). "Purpose" includes primary prevention (health maintenance in the absence of symptoms), secondary prevention (treatment of illness for the purpose of restoration to a previous state of each), and tertiary (rehabilitation or maintenance in the case of long-term care). "Site" or organizational unit refers to the place where services are delivered (inpatient, outpatient, or home). "Time interval" relates to a different set of measures including those of contact (whether the service was received during a particular time period), volume (the total number of units of service received during a given time period), and episodic patterns (typically based on the patterns of providers, referrals and continuity of care for a given occurrence or episode of illness). While identified individually, these dimensions are not mutually independent.

In a recent overview article examining health services utilization issues among older adults, Wolinksy (1994) uses slightly different terms to discuss dimensions of health services utilization. His terms are type, nature (whether or not use of care is discretionary, mixed or nondiscretionary), purpose and unit of analysis (which Andersen and Aday refer to as the time interval of care).

This paper reviews measures of several utilization dimensions. It will review some of the standard ways measures have been employed both in studies of the general population and in specialized studies of the elderly, particularly those with communication disorders. Topics such as dental care, eye care, and care for hearing problems are not discussed, given the relatively small attention accorded in the literature to such care. (Rovin & Nash, 1982; U.S. Department of Health and Human Services, 1980).

DIMENSIONS AND TYPES OF UTILIZATION OF FORMAL HEALTH CARE SERVICES

Using the Andersen and Aday definitions of service characteristics, this section will focus primarily on distinctions according to type and site of care, also including aspects of the "time" dimension described above. The traditional distinction between formal and informal care focuses on the identity of the care provider rather than on the type of care provided. Adhering to this distinction (DeFriese & Woomert, 1992), a range of types and sites of care are included as part of formal care systems.

Ambulatory Care Services

As ambulatory care has become more comprehensive and more complicated, so have its measures. Thirty years ago questions concerning ambulatory care were termed the "doctor visit questions." Now they would generally include not only physician visits but visits to emergency rooms, to outpatient clinics, and all other forms of health care visits, including visits for tests, immunizations, and procedures. Measurement areas include number and frequency of contact, as well as whether a person has a regular source of care.

An important but unresolved issue relating to ambulatory care is the proper time frame of questions. The HIS uses several different recall periods to facilitate the construction of estimates of individuals' use of health care services. While respondents may be asked questions concerning care over the prior 2 weeks, they also may be asked questions relating to the past 3 months (Benson & Marano, 1994). The 2-week questions are generally considered to give the most accurate results, with appropriate weighting of data obtained from subsamples throughout the year, the 2-week estimates can readily be annualized (Aday, 1989).

For most surveys, it is not possible to use continuous interviewing strategies and from this basis to annualize 2-week recall data. Most researchers have to use either a 3-month or year-long recall period, with some suggesting a 6-month recall period (Mechanic, 1989). Some research has found that a year-long recall period provides estimates similar to the annualized HIS 2-week data. (Aday, 1989; Andersen, Kasper, & Franker, 1979). While some researchers have successfully used 1-year recall among the elderly (Thomas & Kelman, 1990), others have argued that the ability or willingness to report utilization accurately may decline with age, perhaps due to decreasing physical and cognitive function, thus making the longer period of recall more suspect with the elderly (Shanas & Maddox, 1985). Several Swedish studies have reported that a 12-month period leads to problems in estimating the association between health care utilization, age and health status. A review of these studies concludes that there are greater problems for those over 65, not due to age itself, but because of the underlying visiting pattern among the elderly that makes the task of recall more complicated (Carsjo, Thorslund, & Warneryd, 1994). In one study that used a 6-month reporting period and compared self-reports of utilization of physician services among the elderly with records obtained from a health maintenance organization (HMO), contact with a physician over the past 6 months was reported quite accurately while volume of visits revealed more discrepancy between the two sources, with underreporting of an average of .35 visits per person (Glandon, Conte, & Tancredi, 1992). This rate of underreporting (10.4%), while not small, is lower than that reported in other studies conducted in a general population (Jobe et al., 1990).

Besides the issue of time frame, questions about specific wording are important, as are considerations of how to combine data from various questions. In the HIS survey, the 2-week doctor visit question is worded as shown in Table 11.1 (Benson & Marano, 1994). This question focuses on visits to a doctor but broadens the definition of doctor, e.g., to include ophthalmologists and psychiatrists. It is followed with another question, also shown in Table 11.1, that broadens the definition of ambulatory care to include a doctor's office, a clinic, and a hospital, and includes care provided by a nurse or anyone working with or for a medical doctor. A third item covers advice or prescriptions provided over the phone. The entire schedule of the HIS is included in the back of the Benson and Marano report, as are other reports from the CDC/VHS series. A researcher can modify the time frame to fit his or her own study. Often, the three separate questions (especially 1 and 2) may be combined into one item by further explaining what a doctor visit could represent. Interestingly, in contrast to other areas of health measurement,

TABLE 11.1 Wording of Items About Ambulatory Care Utilization in the HIS Survey, 1993

Item 1   During these 2 weeks, how many times did ... see or talk to a medical doctor? (Include all types of doctors, such as dermatologists, psychiatrists, and ophthalmologists, as well as general practitioners and osteopaths.) (Do not count times while an overnight patient in a hospital).

Item 2   (Besides the time(s) you just told me about), during those 2 weeks, did anyone in the family receive health care at home or go to a doctor's office, clinic, hospital or some other place? Include care from a nurse or anyone working with or for a medical doctor. (Do not count times while an overnight patient in a hospital). How many times did ... receive this care during that period?

Item 3   (Besides the time(s) you already told me about), during those 2 weeks, did anyone in the family get any medical advice, prescriptions, or test results over the phone from a doctor, nurse anyone working with or for a medical doctor?

Source: Benson and Marano, 1994, pp. 149.

many of the questions used by national data gathering groups for decades have received only limited psychometric analysis.

In addition to such basic questions on use of ambulatory care, there are issues about how to combine and analyze the data. For example, the basic questions can be combined into a measure of total number of ambulatory care visits (volume) or whether or not an individual had any visits (contact). Depending on the amount of detail obtained about the actual place of care, some researchers differentiate between visits to clinics or ambulatory care centers and visits to private physician offices (Thomas & Kelman, 1990). However, with the growth of managed care, people are apt to see their physician—or nurse practitioner or physician's assistant—in more diverse settings. Most currently-used measures are not capturing these distinctions.

Another important measure linked to ambulatory care is information as to regular source of care. Here, the typical approach is to begin with a question asking "Is there a particular person or place that . . . usually goes to when . . . is sick or needs advice about health?" If the answer is yes, the person is then asked a (potentially lengthy) series of questions, e.g., what kind of place and person it is, the last time the person went there, and many other possible questions about waiting time, satisfaction with overall care, and distance and convenience of the place. This series of questions is included in many of the HIS surveys (Benson & Marano, 1994, pp. 169-174). Penning (1995) uses a different approach to collection of data on formal outpatient services. Respondents are asked how often they have seen or used each of a list of providers such as a medical specialist, medical laboratory, chiropractor, occupational or physical therapist, etc., in the past 6 months. This more simplified approach may be useful in many settings.

Another source of ambulatory care data resides in the records maintained by managed care organizations, themselves a rapidly growing coordinator/provider of care. It is true that not all plans maintain visit-specific information, and may record only visits to plan doctors, but not those to out-of-plan specialists. However, managed care records increasingly represent an important source of health care utilization data.

Hospital-Based Services

As with ambulatory care, hospital care can be examined with contact or volume measures, and most studies will typically obtain both types of data. Again, the HIS has developed a consistent approach to asking questions regarding hospital use; this approach is used by many researchers. As compared with ambulatory care, there are fewer questions about appropriate time frame (most people ask about hospitalizations over the past 12 months) and fewer concerns about recall. Hospitalizations have always been uncommon events for most people, and this is even truer today as more and more procedures are performed on an outpatient basis and more surgery is done as 1-day outpatient surgery. However, while most people recall hospital episodes with high accuracy, there may be more variability in accuracy of reporting the length of stay for each hospital episode. A recent study that examined hospital utilization profiles among both survivors and decedents of the LSOA cohort found that there are very few consistently high users of hospital services (Wolinsky, Stump, & Johnson, 1995). Even among those with one or more hospital episodes in this cohort, only one in six decedents and one in 50 survivors were consistently high users, reinforcing the belief that hospitalization is rare for most people and thus remembered with accuracy.

TABLE 11.2 Wording of Items About Use of Hospital Care in the HIS Survey, 1993

Hospital Probe Items

Since (13 month hospital date) a year ago, was ... a patient in a hospital overnight?

If yes, how many different times did ... stay in any hospital overnight or longer since (date) a year ago?

Other Hospital Items

You said earlier that ... was a patient in the hospital since (date) a year ago. On what date did ... enter the hospital the last time, the time before that, etc.?)

How many nights was ... in the hospital?

For what condition did ... enter the hospital?

Did ... have any kind of surgery or operation during this stay in the hospital, including bone settings and stitches?

Was there any other surgery or operation during this stay?

Source: Benson and Marano, 1994, pp. 144, 155.

However, some complications have developed during the last decade. For example, there is growing use of outpatient surgery and other procedures in which a patient goes to the hospital but does not remain overnight. Generally, hospitalization focuses on overnight stays, and the wording of the HIS questions reflects this. The term "beds" in ambulatory surgery units in which a patient might spend a night but often not a 24-hour period also complicates definitions of what constitutes a length of stay.

In the HIS, a hospital probe question is used first to find out if a person was in the hospital during the last year; if positive, subsequent questions determine frequency of use, as shown in Table 11.2 (Benson & Marano, 1994). To ensure that the respondent does not exclude a hospitalization started more than a year prior but finished during the preceding 12 months, the HIS uses a 13-month period, later correcting the data to reflect the 12-month period. Some researchers simplify that aspect of the question by stipulating a 12-month period, followed by a simple probe question.

Typically these data are reported as (a) a contact measure of any hospitalizations, (b) a volume measure of the number of times a person is hospitalized, and (c) a volume measure of the number of days that a person spent in the hospital. Sometimes reports also include the average numbers of days per episode of hospital care, and the proportions of hospital episodes that involve surgery. The episode approach, discussed below, can be applied to many types of services. For example, once a researcher finds out in a survey that a hospital stay has occurred, the health problem that necessitated the hospitalization may become a trigger leading to a series of episode of care questions.

National hospital data are also collected through the National Hospital Discharge System (Graves, 1994). Hospitals maintain and report data to outside sources more completely than do ambulatory care sources; even for patients who are not HMO members, it may be possible to obtain records from hospitals while for HMO members, there will probably be complete records of hospital visits. If measures are collected in a small area with only a few hospitals, it may be possible to obtain all necessary information by simply contacting all such facilities. In larger areas and for people with declining cognitive function, even if the person does not recall details of a visit, they or a caregiver may remember which facilities were used and more complete records may be available from the facility.

Pharmaceutical Services

Many studies have not included questions on pharmaceutical services. Studies of cost of care often focus more sharply on this area than do studies that are only counting utilization, because drug costs constitute an important part of total health care costs. This is especially true for Medicare recipients, since basic Medicare does not cover outpatient drugs (Rubin, Koelln, & Speas, 1995). If a person has a Medicare supplemental policy or uses an HMO, drug costs are usually covered. If a researcher hopes to collect this information, two different techniques are often used. One is to ask people to show the researcher all current medications, providing information about the types of drugs being used. Another approach is to ask the questions within the context of episodes of care, and follow-up with a question about whether there are any medications the person takes routinely.

Long-Term-Care Services (Nursing Home, Home Health Care and Other Types of Health Care Services)

There are fewer research data available with respect to long-term-care services than relating to ambulatory and hospital care. Additionally, the issue is complicated by the fact that the range of long-term-care services available has been undergoing even more change over the last few decades than have ambulatory and hospital services. Provision of formal home health services has increased greatly, partially due to increased public funding of the Medicare and Medicaid programs (Applebaum & Phillips, 1990). In 1974, 16 of every 1,000 Medicare enrollees received home health services, versus 65% in 1991 (Silverman, 1990). The introduction of Medicare's Prospective Payment System for hospitals in the mid-1980s accelerated these trends, because it increased the need for postacute care in the community as Medicare patients were discharged more quickly from hospitals. Medical technology has been changing so that many new therapies (parenteral therapies, oxygen therapies, and home dialysis) are now commonly performed in the home with the help of home health services (Keenan & Fanale, 1989). The changing trajectories of care make it more difficult to collect data on utilization of these services, because there are many more different discrete kinds of services that may be delivered as part of long-term care. Distinctions among levels of care are changing and, within long-term care, most researchers now focus on a continuum of services, of which more than 80 distinct services have been identified as constituting a complete continuum of care (Evashwick, 1993). The use of informal care further complicates interpretation of long-term health care data, as it has been estimated that 80% to 90% of long-term-care services are provided by family and friends (Evashwick, 1993).

Many of the data on use of nursing homes and use of home health care services at the national level come from studies conducted of facilities or from analysis of large national datasets (Wolinksy, Callahan, Fitzgerald, & Johnson, 1993) rather than from studies of individuals (Hing, 1994; Jones, 1994), although some local studies also have collected fairly comprehensive data (Tennstedt, Dettling, & McKinlay, 1992a). In the institutional surveys, many of the available data come from the National Health Provider Inventory (NHPI), which is a replacement for earlier surveys called the National Master Facility Inventory (Jones, 1994) and the Inventory of Long-Term Care Places, respectively. Data also are provided by the National Home and Hospice Care

Survey which is a stratified, staged sample that first uses the sampling frame of the NHPI and then randomly selects patients served by agencies currently and patients discharged within the last 12 months to answer more detailed questions (Hing, 1994). Because these surveys use institutions and their employees as data sources, very detailed information on use can be gathered from patient records. For patients currently in nursing homes (which will be true for a subset of the cognitively impaired), chart and record audits are probably the most reasonable sources of data about the nursing home care. An important factor to remember in a study of nursing home patients is that hospitalizations do occur, with estimates of frequency ranging widely (30% of NH residents hospitalized in the first year, Freiman & Murtaugh, 1993; 16% to 63% across different facilities within a single state, Teresi, Holmes, Bloom, Monaco, & Rosen, 1991). A review of this literature (Castle & Mor, 1996) underlines the need to obtain information on transfers from nursing homes, whether nursing home records are used or surveys are conducted with residents or proxies. Another potential source of data lies in the linking of Medicare databases with administrative databases (Hawthorne, 1994). This may be particularly fruitful among patients in nursing homes, because functional and cognitive impairments often make the resident's own reports problematic (Hawes et al., 1995).

Several different approaches have been used in surveys of home health care recipients (Hing, 1994). Agency records are one useful data source; if available they may provide the most complete and detailed information. Information from payers of care is another option, especially for home health services delivered through Medicare or Medicaid (Health Care Financing Administration, 1995). An important question for any researcher is to decide whether the study will focus only on skilled care (such as nursing care, physical, occupational or speech therapy, respiratory therapy, medical social service and nutrition counseling) or also on homemaker/home health aide care (personal care, bathing and grooming, meal preparation, shopping, transportation, and household chores). In general, Medicare limits participation to home care agencies that are primarily engaged in providing skilled nursing services and therapeutic services. Thus Medicare claims data will not include information about personal care services in most cases.

Another approach is to collect data from surveys with individuals, thus providing information which may not be available from administrative sources. Additionally, survey items can collect information about services performed by relatives or neighbors, i.e., informal services. In the studies using the national survey datasets, such as the LSOA, the information on use of nursing home and home health care services is often quite general (Wolinsky et al., 1993). For nursing homes, a contact measure of any use versus no use in a year was used. For home health services, a 4-item scale created by an aggregate of dichotomous indicators of whether a person used meal delivery programs, visiting nurses, home health aides and homemaker services was the measure of home health services use. In a study of Latino elderly conducted by the Commonwealth Fund Commission on Aging, use of home health services was assessed by determining whether or not a person used or did not use a home health nurse, a home health aide and/or a homemaker during the prior 12 months (Wallace, Campbell, & Lew-Ting, 1994). As Wallace and his colleagues note, this means that a single RN visit and 12 weeks of nurse visits were both coded as use of home health services. Penning (1995) used a more specific item in a Canadian home survey, asking about use and number of hours of service for a list of home health services: nursing services, visits by a social worker, homemaker, exercise/physiotherapist, sitter attendant, Meals-on-Wheels, drop-in visitor, bath help, medication help, foot care, meal preparation, social relief, orderly or other services. Between these approaches, researchers have a range of options from which to choose.

Episodes of Care

Episodes of care include ambulatory care, pharmaceutical services, hospital-based services, and long-term care. One approach to the collection of such data is to frame all questions in the context of a specific illness episode (Kosa & Robertson, 1975; Kronenfeld, 1980; Shortell, Richardson, & LoGerfor, 1977). Thus, this approach attempts to secure data about the whole stream of services associated with a particular episode (Wolinsky, 1994). For example, if a person mentions having sought treatment for a heart problem, this would trigger a sequence of questions dealing with number of physician visits, the nature of specialist involvement, outpatient diagnostic procedures, hospital visits, medications, and rehabilitation services. One advantage of this approach is that it helps people to recall the whole set of services associated with a specific problem. It may be easier for cognitively impaired respondents to answer questions about episodes of care that are episode-specific than it is to answer broader questions about various categories of services. Such organization is also particularly helpful among persons who have used many health care services during the time period under study, and for the occurrence of specific new problems requiring a series of treatments. However, the approach may not be suitable with respect to a continuing chronic problem unless there had been an acute attack which would provide an organizing context. Alternatively, episodes of care questions can be contextualized by a focus on groups of providers.

SPECIAL ISSUES OF VALIDITY

Overall Concerns and Special Concerns of Obtaining Information from the Cognitively Impaired and Those with Communication Difficulties

The validity of data on use of formal health care services is of particular concern when the subjects of interest are elderly, and particularly those elderly with cognitive impairment and communication difficulties. This section will review the few studies that have examined the validity of service use data with respect to the elderly. One important issue with health care utilization data is the relevance and validity of information drawn from administrative records generally and, in the changing health care delivery system, from managed care data records. Another issue lies in the use of proxy respondents, often necessary in collecting data regarding persons with cognitive impairments and/or communication difficulties.

General criticisms of health care data pertaining to older adults focus on lack of breadth and depth of the data, and the number of intervals at which the data have been recorded (Wolinsky, 1994). However, more of these concerns reflect limitations of survey design and data collection approaches than they do restricted ability of respondents. For example, several studies argue that self-report data can be gathered from older and younger patients without significant decrements in data quality (Boult, Boult, Pirie, & Pacala, 1994; Carsjo et al., 1994; Sherbourne & Merideth, 1992). There is some evidence that underreporting is greater for elderly persons with higher levels of utilization, and that elderly persons in poor health may overreport physician visits (Glandon et al., 1992), the inaccuracy is linked to the recency, frequency, and saliency of the event (Bradburn, 1993; Carsjo et al., 1994). Overall, the consensus appears to be that accuracy of self-report information is a function of the task or nature of the information requested rather than of the population from which the data are obtained. However, this observation may not be true for populations of cognitively impaired individuals.

There are several approaches used to improve accuracy of recall in surveys (Aday, 1989). These include bounded recall, aided recall, consultation of records, and use of diaries. Bounded recall procedures seek reduction of overreporting due to telescoping of health events across time periods. While originally developed for use with nationally funded panel surveys, the method has been adapted for cross-sectional surveys (Sudman, Finn, & Lannom, 1984). One approach is first to ask respondents about health behaviors in the previous month, giving dates, and then the current calendar month as a way to eliminate telescoping. Examples of aided recall techniques are the specific listing of types of doctors in Table 11.1, item 1. Another method recommended to reduce the underreporting of health events is to ask respondents to consult their own records, such as checkbooks, doctor bills, or appointment books. Diaries have had great success in situations where people are asked to record fairly constant events (such as food frequency diaries) but less success in asking people to note all health care events. Many study participants find diary-keeping to be burdensome and time consuming (Aday, 1989).

One alternative to asking people about use of health care services is to rely on administrative records, more available than heretofore due to the availability of automated information systems, the improved record keeping of programs such as Medicare, and the growth of HMOs. In fact, some studies that involve issues of accuracy of physician utilization reports use, as the comparison, HMO records (Dunham, 1994; Glandon et al., 1992); this is also true of the HIS (Edwards et al., 1994). One limitation of HMO records is that out-of-plan use is not necessarily recorded by the HMO. Depending on the structure of an HMO, records may be very specific and detailed about numbers of visits and care received (especially in a group model, staff HMO) or very cursory (in a Preferred Provider Organization (PPO) in which most of the specialists are referrals and the records only may reflect the fact that a referral was made, and a payment given, without details on numbers of visits and specifics of services). Moreover, Edwards and colleagues (1994) argue that idiosyncratic sources of error occur in records so that, while they have a different error structure from surveys, errors do occur. Glandon and colleagues (1994) found that older people had more visits and people with more visits underreported the amount of care compared to records. They concluded that declining cognitive function might be one factor explaining these results. On the other hand and contrary to these findings, Edwards and colleagues (1994) argue that people with more health problems are more accurate reporters of care if any care is used, possibly because of the presence of chronic problems and salience of health-related issues. Dunham (1994) argues that HMO databases are often less reliable for long-term-care services, and may not capture data on nursing home stays, especially stays of less than 30 days. Additionally, mental health service use is generally not included in the databases. She argues that checking with Medicare data may often improve the quality of utilization data obtained from administrative records.

One of the most important issues in collecting data from people with declining cognitive ability and communication skills is the use of proxy respondents. If a person cannot answer questions, and if adequate administrative records are not available, proxy respondents are often used. A number of difficulties can arise with the use of proxy respondents. One issue is when to use a proxy respondent. Several recent studies have argued that the capacity for self-observation is partially preserved in Alzheimer's patients and that the person with dementia has too often been relegated to the status of object rather than legitimate contributor to the research process (Cotrell & Schulz, 1993; Kiyak, Teri, & Borson, 1994). One study found strong correlations between retirees and their proxies' overall health and functional status and moderate correlations with satisfaction with care (Hall, Epstein, & McNeil, 1989). A newer study found somewhat lower correlations among a sample of patients with some cognitive dysfunction (Kiyak et al., 1994). Researchers need to remember that the caregiver's view may be biased by depression or a poor relationship with the relative (Cotrell & Schulz, 1993). Some consideration of when it may be possible to obtain information about use of services directly from the person with Alzheimer's disease may be particularly important to obtain a complete picture of use of care for people at earlier stages of the disease. A recent study has estimated that between 10% and 25% of those with the disease are living alone, a figure close to the 20% from a California study (Webber, Fox, & Burnette, 1994). While there is often a surrogate decision maker available who might provide health care utilization data, it can be difficult to identify the most knowledgeable surrogate. In some studies simple research questions focusing on contact with services rather than quantity of services are important. For example, in one study of the effects of living alone on the use of health-related services for persons with Alzheimer's disease, investigators found that those living alone were more likely to use home-delivered meals, homemaker chores, and case management, and that living alone was a barrier to use of nursing home, physician, hospital, and adult day care services (Webber et al., 1994).

A very important initial issue among impaired population is the readiness of proxies to provide informed consent on behalf of the impaired person. Refusal rates are often higher among proxies than among people responding for themselves (Tennstedt, Dettling et al., 1992a). Within a nursing home setting, the cooperation of the nursing home administration and staff is important in obtaining consent of proxies for interviews (Rapp, Topps-Uriri, & Beck, 1994).

Studies comparing the validity of data from proxies have been conducted with people with Alzheimer's disease, stroke patients, and people with AIDS. Many of these studies have focused on questions of patient management and health status (Berk, 1995; Korner-Bitensky, & Wood-Dauphinee, 1995; Korner-Bitensky, Wood-Dauphinee, Siemiatycki, Shapiro, & Becker, 1994; Magaziner, Basset, Hebel, Gruber-Baldini, 1996; Segal & Schall, 1994, 1995). Less research has been reported using older populations and nursing home residents, and focusing on use of health care services (Tennstedt, Skinner, Sullivan, & McKinley, 1992b). In a study of persons with previous strokes or orthopedic conditions, Korner-Bitensky and colleagues (1994, 1995) found that proxy respondents gave fairly detailed information on health and functional status because, by definition, a proxy was someone in contact at least 3 times weekly with the patient. They argue that selection of proxies should be made on the basis of frequency of exposure and not on kinship type. Studies of stroke survivors have also found proxy reports to be accurate for assessing functional/health status (Segal & Schall, 1994, 1995). One study dealing with community-dwelling elderly found proxy data dealing with chronic conditions, health symptoms, and physical and instrumental functioning to be generally accurate, although accuracy varied with the specific item being measured (Magaziner et al., 1996). Some studies of the health care needs of AIDS patients have reported good results using proxy interviewees (Berk, 1995). Tennstedt, Skinner and colleagues (1992b) dealt specifically with the question of who the best proxy respondent is in a nursing home setting. They argue that proxy selection should be based on the type of data needed and time period of interest, and perhaps should even be item specific. Family members gave more complete information about the patient prior to admission to the nursing home, but there was less agreement between family members and staff proxies regarding types of informal care and formal services used.

SUMMARY AND CONCLUSIONS

This paper has reviewed many different areas of health services utilization and addressed situations in which a patient can be interviewed personally, those in which a proxy respondent is required, and situations requiring use of administrative and health plan (including Medicare and Medicaid) records. Although use of health care services appears straightforward, there are many complexities involved which become more important as one deals with people with cognitive impairments and even more important if these people also have other serious health problems. One growing possibility for obtaining accurate information is to use administrative databases maintained by HMOs and care providers and to use Medicare databases. As computerization of medical records grows, linkages between administrative and clinical databases should increase, making these sources more useful, especially for measuring service use in long-term-care settings. Additionally, as the proportion of elderly receiving care through managed care systems grows, HMO plans may provide another source of data concerning health care utilization. This paper has discussed various approaches to direct assessment regarding various aspects of health services utilization, and issues to consider in the use of proxy respondents for those individuals with cognitive disorders and communication problems.

REFERENCES

Aday, L. A., (1989). *Designing and conducting health surveys*. San Francisco, CA: Jossey-Bass.
Aday, L. A. (1993). Indicators and predictors of health services utilization. In S.J. Williams & P.R. Torrens (Ed.), *Introduction to health services*, 4th ed. (p. 46-70). Albany, NY: Delmar.
Anderson, J. G. (1973). Health service utilization. *Health Services Research, 8,* 184-199.
Andersen, R., & Aday, L. A. (1978). Access to medical care in the United States: Realized and potential. *Medical Care, 16,* 533-546.

Andersen, R., Kasper, J. & Franker, M. R. (1979). *Total survey error: Applications to improve health surveys.* San Francisco, CA: Jossey-Bass.

Applebaum, R., & Phillips, P. (1990). Assuring the quality of in-home care: The other challenge for long-term care. *The Gerontologist, 30,* 444-450.

Benson, V., & Marano, M. A. (1994). *Current estimates from the National Health Interview Survey, 1993.* National Center for Health Statistics, Vital Health Statistics, 10 (190).

Berk, R. A. (1995). Use of primary caretakers as proxies to measure the health care needs of patients with AIDs. *Public Health Nursing, 12,* 109-116.

Boult, L., Boult, C., Pirie, P., & Pacala, J. T. (1994). Test-retest reliability of a questionnaire that identifies elders at risk for hospital admission. *Journal of the American Geriatrics Society, 42,* 707-711.

Bradburn, N. M. (1993). Response effects. In P.H. Rossie, J. D. Wright, & A. B. Anderson (Eds). *Handbook of survey research.* Orlando, FL: Academic Press.

Carsjo, K., Thorslund, M., & Warneryd, B. (1994). The validity of survey data on utilization of health and social services among the very old. *Journal of Gerontology: Social Sciences, 49,* S156-S164.

Castle, N. G., & Mor, V. (1996). Hospitalization of nursing home residents: A review of the literature, 1980-1995. *Medical Care Research and Review, 53,* 123-148.

Cotrell, V., & Schulz, R. (1993). The perspective of the patient with Alzheimer's disease: A neglected dimension of dementia research. *The Gerontologist, 33,* 205-211.

DeFriese, G. H., & Woomert, A. (1992). Informal and formal health care systems serving older persons. In M.G. Ory, R.G. Abeles, & P.D. Lipman (Ed.), *Aging, health and behavior.* Newbury Park, CA: Sage.

Dunham, M. L. (1994). Prospects and problems in using data from HMOS for the study of aging populations and their health care needs. *The Gerontologist, 34,* 481-485.

Edwards, W. S., Winn, D. M., Kurlantzick, V., Sheridan, S., Berk, M. L., Ratchin, S. & Collins, J. G. (1994). *Evaluation of National Health Interview Survey: Diagnostic reporting series 2, no. 12.* Hyattsville, MD: National Center for Health Statistics.

Evashwick, C. J. (1993). The Continuum of long-term care. In S.J. Williams & P.R. Torrens (Ed.), *Introduction to health services,* 4th ed. (p. 177-218). Albany, NY: Delmar.

Freiman, M .P., & Murtaugh, C. M. (1993). The determinants of the hospitalization of nursing home residents. *Journal of Health Economics, 12,* 349-359.

Glandon, G. L., Conte, M. A., & Tancredi, D. (1992). An analysis of physician utilization by elderly persons: Systematic differences between self-report and archival information. *Journal of Gerontology: Social Sciences, 47,* S245-S252.

Graves, E. J. (1994). *National Hospital Discharge Survey: 1992 Summary, Advance data from vital and health statistics.* No. 253. Hyattsville, MD: National Center for Health Statistics.

Hall, J. A., Epstein, A. M., & McNeil, B. J. (1989). Multidimensionality of health status in an elderly population. *Medical Care, 27,* 5168-5177.

Hawes, C., Morris, J. N., Phillips, C. D., Mor, V., Fries, B. E., & Nonemaker, S. (1995). Reliability estimates for the minimum data set for nursing home resident assessment and care screening (MDS). *The Gerontologist, 35,* 172-178.

Hawthorne, V. M. (1994) Aging, health and health care—Issues and data for secondary analysis: A interdisciplinary approach. *The Gerontologist, 34*, 447-448.

Health Care Financing Administration. (1995). Medicare and Medicaid statistical supplement. *Health Care Financing Review Statistical Supplement.* Washington, DC.

Hing, E. (1994) Characteristics of elderly home health patients: Preliminary data from the 1992 National Home and Hospice Survey. *Advance Data for Vital and Health Statistics,* No. 247.

Jobe, J., White, A., Kelley, C., Mingay, D., Sanchez, M., & Loftus, E. (1990). Recall strategies and memory for health care visits. *The Milbank Quarterly, 68*, 171-189.

Jones, A. J. (1994). Hospices and home health agencies: Data from the 1991 National Health Provider Inventory. *Advance Data for Vital and Health Statistics,* Number 257.

Keenan, J. M, & J. E. Fanale. (1989). Home care: Past and present, problems and potentials. *Journal of the American Geriatric Society, 37*, 1076-1083.

Kiyak, H. A., Teri, L., & Borson, S. (1994). Physical and functional health assessment in normal aging and in Alzheimer's disease: Self-reports vs. family reports. *The Gerontologist, 34*, 324-330.

Korner-Bitensky, N., & Wood-Dauphinee, S. (1995). Barthel Index information elicited over the telephone: Is it reliable? *American Journal of Physical Medicine and Rehabilitation, 74*, 9-18.

Korner-Bitensky, N., Wood-Dauphinee, S. Siemiatycki, J. Shapiro, S., & Becker, R. (1994). Health-related information postdischarge: Telephone versus face-to-face interviewing. *Archives of Physical Medicine and Rehabilitation, 75*, 1287-96.

Kosa, J., & Robertson, L. S. (1975). The social aspects of health and illness. In J. Kosa & I.K. Zola (Eds.), *Poverty and health: A sociological analysis.* Cambridge, MA: Harvard University Press.

Kronenfeld, J. (1980). Sources of ambulatory care and utilization models. *Health Services Research, 15*, 3-20.

Longitudinal Study of Aging. (1986). The National Center for Health Statistics. DHHS, Washington, DC: U.S. Government Printing Office, 1986.

McKinlay, J. B. (1972). Some approaches and problems in the study and use of services—An Overview. *Journal of Health and Social Behavior, 13*, 115-152.

Magaziner, J., Basset, S. S., Hebel, J. R., & Gruber-Baldini, A. (1996). Use of proxies to measure health and functional status in epidemiologic studies of community-dwelling women aged 65 years and older. *American Journal of Epidemiology, 143*, 283-292.

Mechanic, D. (1978). *Medical sociology: A comprehensive text.* New York: The Free Press.

Mechanic, D. (1989). Medical sociology: Some tensions among theory, method and substance. *Journal of Health and Social Behavior, 30*, 147-160.

Miller, B., Campbell, R. T., Davis, L., Furner, S., Giachello, A., Prohaska, T., Kaufman, J. E., Lin, M., & Perez, C. (1996). Minority use of community long-term care services: A comparative analysis. *Journal of Gerontology: Social Sciences, 51B*, S70-S81.

Penning, M. J. (1995). Health, social support, and the utilization of health services among older adults. *Journal of Gerontology: Social Sciences, 50B*, S330-S339.

Rapp, C. G., Topps-Uriri, J., & Beck, C. (1994). Obtaining and maintaining a research sample with cognitively impaired nursing home residents. *Geriatric Nursing, 15,* 193-196.

Rovin, S., & Nash, J. (1982). Traditional and emerging forms of dental practice: Cost, accessibility, and quality factors. *American Journal of Public Health, 72,* 656-662.

Rubin, R. M., Koelln, K., & Speas, R. K. (1995). Out-of-pocket health expenditures by elderly households: Change over the 1980s. *Journal of Gerontology: Social Sciences, 50B* S291-S300.

Segal, M. E., & Schall, R. R. (1994). Determining functional/health status and its relation to disability in stroke survivors. *Stroke, 25,* 2391-2397.

Segal, M. E., & Schall, R. R. (1995). Assessing handicap of stroke survivors: A validation study of the Craig handicap assessment and reporting technique. *American Journal of Physical Medicine and Rehabilitation, 74,* 276-286.

Shanas, E., & Maddox, G. (1985). Aging, health and the organization of health resources. In R. Binstock & E. Shanas (Eds.), *Handbook of aging and the social sciences.* New York: Van Nostrand Reinhold.

Sherbourne, C. D. & Meredith, L. (1992). Quality of self-report data: A comparison of older and younger chronically ill patients. *Journal of Gerontology: Social Sciences, 47,* S204-S211.

Shortell, S., Richardson, M., & LoGerfor, W. C. (1977). The relationship among dimensions of health services in two provider systems: A causal model approach. *Journal of Health and Social Behavior, 18,* 139-159.

Silverman, H. A. (1990). Use of Medicare covered home health agency services. *Health Care Financing Review, 12,* 113-126.

Sudman, S., Finn, A., & Lannom, L. (1984). The use of bounded recall procedures in single interviews. *Public Opinion Quarterly, 48,* 520-524.

Tennstedt, S. L., Dettling, U., & McKinlay, J. B. (1992a). Refusal rates in a longitudinal study of older people: Implications for field methods. *Journal of Gerontology, 47,* S313-S318.

Tennstedt, S. L., Skinner, K. M. Sullivan, L. M., & McKinlay, J. B. (1992b). Response comparability of family and staff proxies for nursing home residents. *American Journal of Public Health, 82,* 747-749.

Teresi, J., Holmes, D., Bloom, H. G., Monaco, C., & Rosen, S. (1991). Factors differentiating hospital transfers from Long-Term Care facilities with high and low transfer rates. *The Gerontologist, 31,* 795-806.

Thomas, C., & H. R. Kelman. (1990). Gender and the use of health services among elderly persons. In M.G. Ory & H.R. Warner (Ed.), *Gender, health and longevity: Multidisciplinary Perspectives.* New York: Springer Publishing Co.

U.S. Department of Health and Human Services. (1980). *A decade of dental service utilization, 1964-74.* (DHHD Publication No. (HRA) 80-56). Washington, DC: Government Printing Office.

Wallace, S. P., Campbell, C., & Lew-Ting, C. (1994). Structural barriers to the use of in-home services by elderly latinos. *Journal of Gerontology: Social Sciences, 49,* S253-S263.

Webber, P. A., Fox, P., & Burnette, D. (1994). Living alone with Alzheimer's disease: Effects on health and social service utilization patterns. *The Gerontologist, 34,* 8-14.

Wolinsky, F. D. (1994). Health services utilization among older adults: Conceptual, measurement and modeling issues in secondary analysis. *The Gerontologist, 34*, 470-475.

Wolinsky, F. D., Callahan, C. M., Fitzgerald, J. F., & Johnson, R.J. (1993). Changes in functional status and the risks of subsequent nursing home placement and death. *Journal of Gerontology: Social Sciences, 48*, S93-S101.

Wolinsky, F. C, Stump, T. E., & Johnson, R. J. (1995). Hospital utilization profiles among older adults over time: Consistency and volume among survivors and decedents. *Journal of Gerontology: Social Sciences, 50B*, S88-S100.

Chapter 12

Assessing Environments for Older People With Chronic Illness

M. Powell Lawton, Gerald D. Weisman, Philip Sloane, and Margaret Calkins

Although this volume is concerned with the assessment of people, this article turns toward the assessment of environments. The logic is that the person-environment transaction constitutes an event where person and environment are often inseparable in their relationship to well-being. On the other hand, for heuristic reasons, we must make that separation if we are to describe how people use their environments. The range of environments which potentially impact the lives of older persons is substantial and includes the dwelling, neighborhood, and community as well as work, transportation, education, entertainment, commercial, and natural settings. There are, however, few instruments presently available for the assessment of environments utilized by elders and these focus virtually without exception on residential settings. In this article we discuss the assessments of the residential environments inhabited by frail elders. As will be seen, most of the literature deals with institutions for the frail elder. That is thus necessarily the focus of the content. Nonetheless, an effort will be made to note other settings in which environmental assessment for frail elders is needed.

The instruments reviewed in this article deal primarily with two forms of living environments for older people. *Group residential environments* are planned to serve specific user groups, for example the poor, the ill, the elderly, or children. Some of the more important group residential environments for older people include assisted living facilities, board and care homes, and nursing homes. *Individual residential environments* refer to homes and apartments, not planned to be age-specific or to serve a particular user group scattered in ordinary neighborhoods and communities. Such residences accommodate an estimated 85%-87% of all people age 65 and over.

It must also be noted that a great proportion of people 65 and over are fully capable of maintaining everyday activities and do not require special design or special assessment tools; one estimate from the National Center for Health Statistics (Dawson, Hendershot, & Fulton, 1987) suggests that only about 20% of all elders experience any limitation of activities in their everyday lives. This might lead one to question the necessity of an emphasis on the design of individual and group residences for older people that places particular emphasis on the frailties and disabilities that are more likely in older users. The position taken here is that many presently vigorous, healthy people will eventually pass through a phase of compromised ability during which

193

previously well-matched home environments become less and less functional. To the extent that specialized design can serve the needs of the presently healthy without conveying a message of disability, serve the intact as they become more frail, and finally provide a supportive residential environment for those experiencing disability, the effort to create and assess environments responsive to the special needs of frail or chronic-diseased elders would seem to be well justified.

Given the paucity of existing measuring instruments, this article will begin with a brief notation of conceptual issues in environmental assessment and desiderata for the development of needed instruments. Recognition of these dimensions enables us to characterize better what each instrument does and does not do. A critical review of existing instruments and gaps in suitable instruments composes the majority of the article. The article ends with the recognition of the desirability of moving toward the use of generic environmental assessment dimensions wherever possible, but a present need to apply environment-specific modules where necessary. Such a combinatory strategy will be seen as applying to the types of assessment instruments now available for use in several types of residential environments.

APPROACHES TO RESIDENTIAL ENVIRONMENTAL ASSESSMENT

Dimensions by Which Environment May be Described

The literature on environmental assessment shows several dimensions by which researchers have attempted to characterize environment. Several such dimensions are particularly relevant to the task of measuring environments for the chronically ill and are described below.

Social Versus Physical Environment. The social realm itself may be represented in terms of single significant individuals, primary groups, the suprapersonal environment, and the megasocial environment (Lawton, 1982).

Objective Versus Subjective Quality. Common metrics such as number, length, width, time and so on, refer to the objective, as compared to subjective judgments such as rating scales estimated by a person.

Descriptive Versus Evaluative Quality. Any quality that can be described may also be evaluated, first in terms of the liking, satisfaction, or preference by a user, or second, in terms of some demonstrated good versus bad quality according to a specifiable criterion.

Global Versus Discrete Quality. Items to be measured may represent large or complex environments, or single attributes (Weisman, Calkins, & Sloane, 1994).

There are also a number of purposes for environmental assessment. This article emphasizes the research purpose. As will be seen, however, some instruments were designed to evaluate and improve individual environments, while others serve to evaluate for the purpose of regulating quality.

Sources of Data for Residential Environmental Assessment

Archival sources include, but are not limited to, technically measured information, architectural plans, licensure and regulatory data bases, self-monitoring reports, and special survey data files. Because such data have often been produced for or subjected to public scrutiny, they often include objectively determinable items.

Observational sources also start with the presence of the objective reality and their objectivity is increased to the extent that the measure deals with the physical environment, uses description, and focuses on discrete rather than global quality. Clear definition of terms and training in what to observe are the main contributors to high quality of the data. The *user* has the advantage of direct experience and insider knowledge and the disadvantage of a lack of systematic background. The *expert* (researcher, design professional) may observe with a broader and more precisely defined range of comparison standards but lacks the insider perspective. Sometimes a researcher may seek reports from an *informant*, who may be either a user or a person with intimate knowledge of the way direct users judge the environment.

Consensual data are individual perceptions in aggregate form, that is, the averages, modes, or majority-opinion judgments of many users or experts, while individual perception is a characteristic of a single person. It is argued that consensual data are characteristics of an environment, based on the reasoning that the judgments of multiple individuals will converge on the actual properties of the environment.

Individual perceptions may be based either on direct observation or cognitive representations of the observable reality but will use criteria that go clearly beyond the countable and centimeters-grams-seconds approaches. Individual perceptions are typically evaluative ("good-bad," "prefer," "satisfied") or request that more global and abstract qualities be judged ("colorful," "bright," "complex," "stimulating"). Considerations regarding differences between users and experts discussed earlier apply here.

Each of the measures to be described in this article may be characterized in terms of its location on the four dimensions and the sources of data. Each focus will be shown to have its specific uses, but there are gains and losses involved in choosing one focus over another. Each measure will be discussed in terms of such strengths and weaknesses.

GROUP RESIDENTIAL ENVIRONMENTS

Perhaps because of the ease of performing research in locations where potential subjects are geographically clustered and public spaces easy for the researcher to enter, group residential environments have been the locus of much the greatest portion of all research involving environmental assessment. Although some of the measures to be described are not limited to institutions such as nursing homes, all may be used for this purpose. The discussion will begin in historical order, with the attempt to integrate the conceptual and empirical aspects of the measures' development and uses.

Early Conceptions

What appears to have been the first attempt to conceptualize the dimensions of residential environments for older people was Kleemeier's (1959) suggestion that such residences could vary along the dimensions of segregation (extent to which residents are separated from nonresidents), congregation (extent to which all residents perform same activities at the same time), and control (extent to which decisions are made by residents versus staff). Kleemeier did not develop measures, but this original conception was both elaborated and operationalized by several groups with roots at the University of Chicago Committee on Human Development. Although measures resulted from each, none has been widely used. They are very worthwhile consulting for contemporary ideas, however. All share the characteristics of representing primarily the social environment, being more subjective than objective, falling midway on the descriptive-evaluative focus, and being clearly global. Pincus (1968) and Pincus and Wood (1970) applied individual judgments and consensual judgment methods to dimensions of privacy, freedom (structured versus unstructured), resources (sparse to rich), integration (Kleemeier's segregating dimension reversed), and personalization.

Several major multi-institutional studies reported in integrated form by Lieberman and Tobin (1983) expanded greatly the environmental dimensions subjected to formal assessment: Achievement-Fostering, Individuation, Dependency-Fostering, Warmth, Affiliation-Fostering, Recognition, Stimulation, Physical Attractiveness, Cue Richness, and Tolerance for Deviance. The criteria for ratings are spelled out in detail in Lieberman and Tobin (1983, pp. 381-413). Their global and evaluative quality is enhanced by the broad mix of subjective and objective characteristics; the majority of criteria are social as compared to physical environmental. Although the content of these scales appears readily usable in all planned residential environments, psychometric data are not presented. Therefore an investigator would need to perform this phase in contemporary use of the scales.

A direct descendant of the Kleemeier typology is one developed by Kahana (1982) for assessing nursing homes on dimensions of segregate, congregate, control, structure, stimulation, affect, and impulse control, as rated by multiple staff members. The scale definitions are almost exclusively in the social realm. Although psychometric data were presented (Kahana, Liang, & Felton, 1980), they do not appear to have been used by later researchers. These dimensions have an almost completely social focus; they are subjective, global, and midway on the descriptive-evaluative continuum. As in the case of the Lieberman and Tobin measures, psychometric data other than predictive validities do not seem to have been published.

The Multiphasic Environmental Assessment Procedure

The most extensive and best-developed battery of environmental assessment instruments is that developed by Moos and his colleagues (Moos & Lemke, 1994), the Multiphasic Environmental Assessment Procedure (MEAP). These measures were designed for use in group residential environments for older people, specifically including nursing homes, veterans facilities, and several forms of service-rich housing; it is important to note that independent housing was not included, and the data were gathered before the genre termed "assisted living" came on the scene. Furthermore, the MEAP was not designed specifically for use with frail, chronically ill, or impaired elders. It will be described in detail, however, because all components of the MEAP contain content that is clearly salient for this target population.

Moos began with a structural model suggesting that four major classes of variables were necessary to assess such environments: Physical and architectural features, policy and program factors, suprapersonal factors (characteristics of the aggregate of people; Lawton, 1970), and social climate. Construction of measures representing these classes were guided by both a priori conceptions of the structure of each class and by the inductive use of the literature to assemble indicators of the classes and subclasses.

The *Physical and Architectural Features Checklist* (PAF; Moos & Lemke, 1980) is composed of 153 items distributed unequally among subscales termed Community Accessibility, Physical Amenities, Social-recreational Aids, Prosthetic Aids, Orientational Aids, Safety Features, Staff Facilities, and Space Availability. The content is mainly physical environmental, objective, and discrete. Although nominally descriptive, a majority of the items have normatively desirable or undesirable connotations. It is designed for use by a single observer walking through an environment. With training, any observer could complete the PAF.

The *Resident and Staff Information Form* (RESIF; Lemke & Moos, 1981) organizes information that describes the normative characteristics of residents, staff, and the behaviors that occur in the facility. Subscales of Resident Social Resources, Resident Heterogeneity, Resident Activity Level, Resident Activities in the Community, and Staff Resources are indexed by 69 items which are obtained by a researcher from various sources such as administrative, medical, and activities records and residents' histories. Many items may be counted if records are adequate but the greater proportion are items of the type, "What proportion of residents need assistance with activities of daily living (ADL)?" or "How many residents go into the community regularly?" It is likely that such items will typically be estimated by a single informant rather than counted. The content of the RESIF is exclusively in the suprapersonal sector of the social environment, ideally objective (but estimated as necessary), descriptive and discrete on the individual level but more global as individuals are aggregated. The data source is an amalgam of an individual (e.g., a researcher) eliciting aggregate estimates of individual characteristics from either archival or informant sources.

The *Policy and Program Information Form* (POLIF; Lemke & Moos, 1980) consists of 130 items falling into subscales named Expectations for Functioning, Acceptance of Problem Behavior, Policy Choice, Resident Control, Policy Clarity, Provision of Privacy, Availability of Health Services, Availability of Daily Living Assistance, and Availability of Social-Recreational Activities. The items represent rules, regulations, practices, and normative behaviors falling mainly in the social realm, but a number of observable physical features and services that may be counted or indexed archivally also make up some of the content of the POLIF. Although it is nominally descriptive, like the PAF there is an obvious valence to many of the items. Items range widely on the global-to-discrete continuum. The source of POLIF information includes archives, observations, and individuals, but it is completed by a researcher using best-available source.

The *Sheltered Care Environment Scale* (SCES; Lemke & Moos, 1987) is the measure of "social climate," which expresses the broadest attitudes, values, and care philosophies that appear to be evidenced in seven subdimensions: Cohesion, Conflict, Independence, Self-Exploration, Organization, Resident Influence, and Physical Comfort (70 items). The items refer to interpersonal processes, apparent affective communications, and judged environmental qualities. The content is mainly social, with a few physical environmental items, and deliberately subjective. Because the SCES is designed to be administered to large numbers of staff and residents in a single facility, individual differences in perceived social climate are minimized when aggregated. It is also highly evaluative and global. The SCES is the prototype of an individual-perception measure that is useful as an individual measure but also, when aggregated across individuals in a single environment, as a characteristic of the consensual environment.

Finally, the *Rating Scales* (Lemke & Moos, 1986) consist of generalized evaluative ratings of Physical Attractiveness (9 items), Environmental Diversity, Resident Functioning, and Staff Functioning (5 items each). The first two are physical environmental measures, the last two social. The Rating Scales lend themselves to completion by users (residents or staff), informants, and experts and they aggregate easily to form a composite picture of an environment.

Separate manuals are available for the MEAP as a whole and for each of the five components separately (Moos & Lemke, 1992a; 1992b; 1992c; 1992d; 1992e; 1992f). They are models of clarity and completeness. For full psychometric data the book (Moos & Lemke, 1994) only partially fulfills that need since it concentrates particularly on applications of the MEAP in residential and caregiving situations. Full psychometric information is presented on the PAF (Moos & Lemke, 1980), the RESIF (Lemke & Moos, 1981), the POLIF (Lemke & Moos, 1980), and the SCES (Lemke & Moos, 1987). All measures are presented with internal consistency and retest reliability. Interobserver agreement is not always reported. Rater reliability was excellent for the Rating Scales, and clearly convergent among multiple raters for the SCES. For the POLIF, the RESIF, and the PAF it is simply recognized that more reliable estimates are likely if more than one person completes the scales.

THE EVOLUTION OF DESIGN GOALS FOR THE CHRONICALLY ILL OLDER PERSON

Most of the scales reviewed thus far were developed by 1980. This date conveniently marks the beginning of a period of quiescence in the development of formal assessment technology for group residential environments. During this period, the conceptual advances underlying this area became diffused among design practitioners and elicited further focus on the goals and the practice of design for the chronic-care population.

The dimensions of assessment chosen by the early researchers implied some overall conception of appropriate care goals. Such goals might be based on either a catalog of the major deficits for which an environmental antidote might be sought (Lawton, Fulcomer, & Kleban, 1984), preferences or needs of older users (Kahana, Liang, & Felton, 1980), or positively stated goals. Attempts to match design specifications with users' goals are a generic issue in environmental psychology. For example, Brill and Krauss (1970) specified a series of "performance concepts" toward which design specifics should contribute: Communality versus Privacy; Sociopetality versus Sociofugality; Informality versus Formality; Familiarity versus Remoteness; Accessibility versus Inaccessibility; Ambiguity versus Legibility; Diversity versus Homogeneity; Adaptability versus Fixity; and Comfort versus Discomfort. Although the authors applied these concepts to the analysis of community mental health centers, theoretically one could imagine a set of generic goals, some of whose features would be tailored to specific contexts and users.

In fact, since 1980 much of the development of design goals was focused on the chronically ill older person, beginning with the nursing home or highly protected residential environment and more recently converging on care settings for elders with dementing illness. With the general sensitization of the public and the scientific community to the existence of Alzheimer's disease and related conditions has come a major concentration of interest in the design of dementia-specific environments (Calkins, 1988; Cohen & Day, 1993; Cohen & Weisman, 1991). The major measurement activity during this period of time was the shaping of the important conceptual dimensions of person-environment interaction. Defining such dimensions constitutes a necessary beginning point for effective measurement.

Table 12.1 shows several attempts to organize a set of central dimensions explicitly describing the person-environment interactions of chronically ill and demented elders. There is considerable consensus across investigators. Few dimensions with an exclusively environmental focus are included; most authors named dimensions with respect to needs of the person rather than characteristics of the environment. Zeisel, Hyde, and Levkoff (1994), in contrast, identified six of their eight dimensions in terms of environmental characteristics. A holistic view of person-environment transactions would emphasize the unity of person and environment and therefore not be particularly concerned about any surface appearance of ambiguity regarding whether the focus of the dimension is on person or environment. Nonetheless, at least in the early phases of the investigation of an area, there are gains in developing parallel pairs of person attributes (needs, disabilities, preferences) and environment attributes (physical and social features that serve or inhibit the personal goal). The choice of person or environment as dependent versus independent variable is usually made on the basis of a particular study's goals.

Contemporary Measures for Special Care Units for Dementia

During the decade of the 1990s, empirical advances were spurred by the emergence of the special care unit (SCU) for elders with dementing illness. Three assessment instruments for this purpose are available at the present time. In addition, several others are known to be under development and will be described conceptually. Those now available in published research reports are the Therapeutic Environment Screening Scale (TESS, Sloane & Mathew, 1990; 1991), the Professional Environmental Assessment Protocol (PEAP, Norris-Baker, Weisman, Lawton, & Sloane, in press), and the Nursing Unit Rating Scale (NURS; Grant, 1996).

The *TESS* began as a relatively short observational scale of physical features of dementia care units. Its original form consists of 12 items: floor surface, glare, lighting, noise, cleaning solution odor, bodily excretion odor, personal items in rooms, home-like public areas, access to outdoors, small group space, absence of continuous television, and kitchen in unit. An additive scale, the TESS yields scores from 0 to 24. A validation study found that TESS scores differentiated SCUs from non-SCUs (Sloane & Mathew, 1991).

The TESS underwent a series of revisions, resulting in the TESS-2+, which was developed for use as part of the National Institute on Aging Collaborative Research Project on Special Care Units (Ory, 1994). The TESS-2+ contains 37 questions and 128 variables, many of which were new items with untested psychometric properties. Domains covered included the following areas of environmental design and function: general design, maintenance, space and seating, lighting, noise, resident rooms, privacy and personalization, and programming orientation. The TESS-2+ also includes three global ratings: staff interaction with residents, resident involvement in planned activities, and overall physical environment.

Use of the TESS-2+ by the 10 NIA study sites and by several related studies has generated considerable data on the psychometric properties of the instrument. Numerous items were identified that demonstrated little or no variation, and others that had poor interrater reliability (Sloane, Mitchell, Long, & Lynn, 1995). A composite score of 17 items, including floor safety, lighting, cleanliness, maintenance, cueing, visual stimulation, and resident appearance in public areas, yielded excellent interrater reliability (Cronbach's alpha = .825). In addition, several subscales proved reliable and

TABLE 12.1 Age-Specific Environmental Dimensions Suggested by Several Researchers

Generic Dimension	Moos (1980) Physical & Architectural Features	Lawton (1980/1986) Nursing Home Design Objectives	Calkins (1988) E/B Issues	Cohen & Weisman (1991) Therapeutic Goals	Regnier & Pynoos (1992) E/B Principles	Weisman, Lawton, Sloan, Calkins, & Norri-Baker (1996) PEAP Dimensions
Safety	Safety Features	Safety	Safety & Security	Safety & Security	Safety & Security	Safety & Security
Orientation	Orientation Aids	Orientation	Wayfinding & Orientation	Awareness & Orientation	Orientation & Wayfinding	Awareness & Orientation
Functionality	Prosthetic Aids	Negotiability (Increase Autonomy in ADLs)	Competence in Daily Activities	Support Functional Abilities	Accessibility & Functioning	Support Functional Abilities
Stimulation		Aesthetics		Stimulation & Change	Stimulation & Challenge; Sensory Aspects; Aesthetics & Appearance	Regulation & Quality of Stimulation
Personal Control	Architectural Choice	Personalization	Personalization	Autonomy & Control	Control, Choice & Autonomy; Personalization; Privacy	Opportunities for Personal Control; Provision of Privacy
Social Interaction	Social & Recreational Aids	Social Interaction	Privacy & Socialization	Social Contact & Privacy	Social Interaction	Facilitation of Social Contact
Continuity				Ties to the Healthy & Familiar	Familiarity	Continuity of the Self
Change				Adapt to Changing Needs	Adaptability	

valid: floor safety (4 items; Cronbach's alpha = .836), lighting (5 items; alpha = .692), cleanliness (4 items; alpha = .789), and maintenance (4 items; alpha = .872). Studies of the TESS are ongoing, and a revised instrument is in preparation.

The *PEAP* was originally designed to be used as a criterion against which the many TESS items could be validated. Its origin was also the NIA collaborative study. The goal was to construct a global, subjective, evaluative assessment of the physical environment of the SCU that could be performed by a trained professional (design or behavioral research) on the basis of an observational tour of the care unit. As it developed, it became evident that there would be a use for the PEAP independently of the TESS. Early pilot data gathering also made it evident that a walk-through observation would be an insufficient basis for rating the PEAP. It was then amended to include a brief open-ended interview with the administrator or care supervisor, primarily to learn more about how the care environment was used or regulated and to ascertain a few features that were not always evident to an observer.

The designers of the PEAP used their predecessors' constructs as displayed in Table 12.1. The PEAP dimensions were chosen to be individually assessed (each rated in terms of 14 scale points, with 5 of the points specified in words and the intermediate points as + or _) (Weisman, Lawton, Sloane, Calkins, & Norris-Baker, 1996). Reliability (kappa) for individual dimensions ranged from .69 to .85 in 20 sites surveyed independently by two trained raters (Norris-Baker et al., in press). In process is the item analysis of the enlarged TESS against the separate dimensions and total score of the PEAP.

The *NURS* was designed by Grant (1996) for one of the NIA collaborative studies, which involved a survey of a statewide sample of 390 care units, located in 59 facilities that each reported having one or more SCUs and 64 facilities without an SCU. Using the constructs developed by earlier investigators, Grant began with six a priori dimensions, but rather than rating them directly, he assembled 158 indicators (reduced to 81 by item analysis) assigned among six dimensions: Separation (of dementia residents from nondementia residents), Stability, Stimulation, Complexity, Control/Tolerance, and Continuity. Although the indicators are described as reflecting "policy and program features that are not easily observed," a number of the items reflect physical environmental attributes. Nonetheless, the items are primarily social. They are derived from the interview of the nurse in charge of each unit. The questions are framed, variously, in terms of "How often...," "To what extent...," or "How many...." Although many items refer to objectively determinable features, almost all require on-the-spot estimates, clearly a subjective process. Most items are descriptive and discrete. Although internal consistencies were in an acceptable range, interobserver agreement is not reported and thus one is uncertain about this critical psychometric characteristic. Five of the six scales showed significant differences between SCUs and non-SCUs.

Resource for Evaluation and Modifications Optimizing Dementia Environments for Living (REMODEL; Calkins, 1996). In contrast with the other instruments reviewed earlier, the REMODEL was designed with the primary purpose of serving as a clinical tool for self-evaluation and facility improvement. REMODEL enables an environmental assessment and evaluation of a dementia unit without necessitating a site visit by an expert. Nonetheless its design also will eventually make it usable as a quantitative instrument. The instrument affords an in-depth picture of a dementia care setting, using information provided by the site (over 800 questions responded to by knowledgeable staff informants and their individual perceptions, observations, and archival sources).

This material is used by an expert as the basis for recommendations for enhancing the supportiveness of the environment for people with dementia. Like the MEAP, the REMODEL includes the social and the organizational environment and systematically provides parallel assessment of person and environment. The REMODEL is based on a set of 15 empirically derived therapeutic goals. Each of these sections begins with an inquiry on the person side to characterize the target population. This person-level inquiry is then followed by sets of questions that represent the organizational policies, care practices, and physical and social environmental features relevant to each goal. Full psychometric analysis is in process to determine reliability, validity, and clinical usefulness of the instrument.

Finally, the *Nursing Home Surveyor* assessment performed as part of the regulation of Medicaid and Medicare by the U.S. Health Care Financing Administration represents one of the quality-control measures specified in the Omnibus Budget Reconciliation Act of 1987 (OBRA 87). Monitoring quality of care, with the power to decertify and close facilities, is an extremely demanding task. Historically, the physical environmental aspects of such surveys have been of the "white glove" type, that is, concerned with identifying cleanliness and hygienic aspects of the care environment. OBRA 87, however, was the occasion to consider whether some of the physical design principles identified in the work of environment and behavior research could be incorporated into the survey process. The trade-off principle, that is, allowing positive features above minimum levels to be recognized, rewarded, and possibly offset other negative features, was considered in the revision of the survey process. The present survey forms (HCFA, July 1995) include observational and both resident- and family-generated indicators such as provisions for privacy, homelike surroundings, support of activities, physical comfort, and room personalization. These characteristics are not systematically rated, however, and the survey information now being accumulated does not lend itself to formal data analysis.

SUMMARY OF THE PRESENT STATE OF RESIDENTIAL CARE ENVIRONMENTAL ASSESSMENT

To conclude this section on group environmental assessment instruments, it should be clear that environmental assessment for chronically ill elders under residential care is an area under development, with very little to show beyond the conceptual basis for assessment. The MEAP is by far the best developed. It has the disadvantage of being very long if administered in its entirety, particularly if, as recommended, multiple staff and multiple residents are to be tested. In fact, the target group of residents most important in the care of the chronically ill is very likely to be unable to complete the SCES because of cognitive impairment. The standardization group for the MEAP included many care settings of the 1970s and 1980s that may have been fairly similar to those serving the chronically ill and cognitively impaired of the present. It might be worthwhile to go back to those data to construct subgroups of units of this type. As far as physical environment measures go, the content of the PAF, two of the Rating Scales, and the Physical Comfort factor of the SCES are highly relevant to the environmental assessment task on which this article is focused. It would be extremely useful to determine the relationship of these measures to basic structural features of care environments (whether it was an SCU, assisted living, its size, sponsorship, etc.). Frances Carp (personal communication, June 19, 1996) has suggested that housing originally planned for the fully independent now accommodates an increasing number of elders with compromised health. Thus measures relevant to these housing environments and particularly to person-environment fit within them, deserve to be developed and used in these settings.

Among the other measures, only the TESS qualifies as an established measure, and its final form is yet to be determined. At present, it seems overloaded with descriptive features whose relevance to quality or basic functions of the care environment is yet to be established. Analysis currently under way should trim the TESS to become a more efficient technique. It has the great advantage of being usable by observers with a modest level of training and experience with person-environment concepts. All the other measures require more use and reporting of psychometric characteristics to warrant recommendations regarding their general application.

INDIVIDUAL RESIDENTIAL ENVIRONMENTS

Planned residential environments serve the special needs of a very important subpopulation of elders. Nonetheless, only 5% reside in nursing homes, and only an estimated 7% to 8% live in other forms of planned living residences. Thus the great majority of elders live in scattered, unplanned community residences. Because of the high rate of home ownership among the population 65 and over (75%, U.S. Bureau of the Census, 1995) and the low rate of residential mobility even among renters (5% annually, BOC, 1995), the majority may be said to have "aged in place," that is, grown into old age in long-occupied residences (Tillson, 1990). In addition to the 20% who experience disability in performing activities of daily living, an estimated 5% to 6% are characterized by some form of moderate to severe dementing illness (Office of Technology Assessment, 1982). It is therefore clear, first, that the sheer number of physically and cognitively frail elders living in the community (7 to 8 million) greatly outnumbers those in nursing homes (perhaps 1 million) and, second, that they live in homes unlikely to have been constructed with features designed to enhance the functioning of a frail or chronically ill person.

Community Surveys. The environmental needs of frail community residents have been less salient in national housing policy. In similar fashion, the development of assessment devices for home environments has lagged far behind that of planned residences. An excellent review of this small literature was provided by Carp (1994), necessarily focusing primarily on the community housing of the elderly population in general. It should be noted that the most extensive contributions to this literature have been by Carp herself, reporting from community surveys on instruments assessing objective, physical features (Carp & Carp, 1982a) and evaluative judgments (Carp & Carp, 1982b) of neighborhood features and parallel physical (Carp & Carp, 1984) and perceived (Carp & Christensen, 1986a; 1986b) characteristics of the dwelling unit. These instruments have not been published in a form easy to obtain. Although their psychometric treatment was of very high quality, a manual organizing that information is lacking. The frail elderly were not a focus of this research but the measures clearly lend themselves to the investigation of the person-environment transactions of frail elders living in their community residences.

American Housing Survey. A few other sources of information on the characteristics of community housing occupied by elders may be noted briefly. The biennial American Housing Survey (AHS; Office of Policy Development and Research, 1989) is the largest such data file, containing basic objective, descriptive, physical environmental information on housing type, tenure, and financial characteristics, as well as a list of housing deficiencies. A small group of subjective, evaluative questions on perceived quality of the neighborhood and community services is included. The virtual absence of health data blocks one's ability to relate these housing characteristics to physical functions. Although the survey is done by the U.S. Department of Housing and Urban Development, few regularly published reports dealing with the elderly are available (but see Gaberlavage & Sloan, 1993). Lawton (1980), Struyk and Turner (1984), and Christensen, Carp, Cranz, and Wiley (1992) have utilized multi-item indices of housing quality from the AHS to relate to other data on older householders.

The 1978 AHS contained a supplement on disability, which afforded a survey of home modifications and assistive devices which could be linked to functional disability (Struyk, 1987). This included a checklist of features which disabled elders who did not have the feature thought would be helpful to them (Gilderbloom & Markham, 1996). Reschovsky and Newman (1990) used similar data from other HUD surveys. Another more modest source of such data is the National Long Term Care Survey, which has yielded informative data on the adaptation of older people over time to changing health conditions (Manton, Corder, & Stallard, 1993).

Nonetheless, the AHS and the other surveys include simply lists of basic housing characteristics; lists whose relevance to the chronic care population is difficult to probe because of the unfortunate separation of housing data and health-related data in different surveys. Even on a smaller scale, gerontological researchers have moved hardly at all into the development of formal environmental assessment for ordinary housing relevant to frail or cognitively impaired elders. What does exist can only be characterized as a collection of lists, assembled by service-delivery and design professionals seeking to identify problematic features of ordinary homes. Without attempting to be exhaustive in reviewing such lists, several useful attempts to specify problematic household features may be noted. Moleski, Saperstein and Lawton (1985) compiled a category list of potentially problematic features of the homes of older recipients of in-home services, coupled with a section on problems and solutions. The latter were organized under categories of ADL, senses, safety, security, thermal comfort, maintenance, communication, and enrichment.

Home Environment Checklist. A very useful home environment checklist was provided by Trickey, Maltais, Gosselin and Robitaille (1993); Canada Mortgage and Housing Corporation (1989), where the physical characteristics are organized around the necessary ADLs. This is perhaps the most complete home checklist. This assessment procedure and several others (Brent, Phillips, Brent, & Gupta, 1993; Olsen, Ehrenkrantz, & Hutchings, 1993; Pynoos & Cohen, 1990) are geared primarily to service use with older clients, caregivers, and agencies. They do not attempt to be either theoretically driven or psychometrically treated. Further, the content emphasis of these checklists is on safety, security, access, and competence in performing basic ADLs. Perhaps because more complex needs in such areas as time use, social behavior, and aesthetics are so individual and preference-driven, little attempt has been made to include such higher-order functions in home-oriented checklists and self-inventories.

Home Environment Assessment Test. Because of the absence of psychometrically derived measures in this area, one under development may be noted, the Home Environmental Assessment Test (HEAT, Laura Gitlin, Thomas Jefferson University, personal communication, June, 1996). The HEAT is designed to assess the physical environment of the home of family members caring for an individual with dementia. The assessment involves a walk-through of the rooms and areas of a home that are used by an individual with dementia. The assessment combines direct observation and caregiver query to assess each area of the home along 6 dimensions: the presence of safety hazards, visual cues (color coding, signs, drawings), assistive devices, home alterations, and the level of clutter and comfort. The HEAT is currently undergoing psychometric testing. Guidelines for use, reliability and evaluation, and sensitivity to detect environmental changes over time are under investigation.

Suggestions for Future Research on Assessing Individual Residences

In concluding this section on community residential assessment, one is forced to the opinion that a technology of assessment has hardly begun. A model for future development may be found in the work of Frances and Abraham Carp. A brief summary (Carp, 1994) will lead the reader to the many technical reports from this research. Their approach is notable because they have followed a three-point rational strategy. First, the residential unit and the local environs have been systematically and separately measured. Second, both the objective physical environment and users' perceptions and evaluations of them have been separately measured (both dwelling unit and neighborhood). Third, the person-environment transaction has been captured by choosing carefully the personal characteristics to be assessed. These choices were derived from clear hypotheses about which personal characteristics would be relevant to which environmental characteristics. The main limitation of the Carps' work is that, while cognitive and functional competencies enter into their study of person-environment transactions, there was no focus on the frail or chronically ill and no attempt to identify such a subgroup within their large community samples. The potential for using their measures to evaluate the outcomes of frail elders living in residences not planned to accommodate their impairments is great, however. For the future one can hope that a conceptual beginning as strong as that around which the Carps's work was built can then lead future researchers to the tasks of inventorying and organizing the environmental attributes of this user group.

CONCLUSION

In both areas reviewed, planned residences and community residences, the strongest body of assessment research in each has been criticized for its inattention to the chronically ill as a target group. At this point it seems worthwhile to examine the assumption that special user groups require their own assessment instruments. Must there be separate theory-technology combinations for each new group?

As far as we are aware, no one has attempted to analyze and integrate the higher-order dimensions that have been used to address en masse the person-environment issues dealing with infants, schools, adolescents, prisons, hospitals, or older people. A short list of dimensions generic across both settings and users analogous to those shown in

Table 12.1 might well be the result. For example, "orientation" occurs in most lists. It may well be that "environmental knowledge" is the most general descriptor for this class; orientation is a member of the class which represents a range of knowledge affordance which is relatively low on the total continuum of environmental cognition. Thus one way to move in the future would be to select subdimensions for assessment based on the range of competence over which the person-environment transaction is critical for a particular user group. Safety is a universal person-environment requirement. Access to safe and unsafe areas is quite different in practice for the fully functioning person and the victim of Alzheimer's disease, however. The goal of the ideal environmental assessment battery might thus be to represent with user- and context-specific content limited ranges in each generic dimension.

Finally, to what extent do the measures reviewed here successfully address such targeted ranges of each dimension? To be sure, nursing homes, assisted living, and community dwelling units have different spaces, thus forming one essential and necessary source of uniqueness. Stripping away references to these unique physical features, however, perusal of the PEAP Manual (Weisman et al., 1996) reveals references to many features that seem specific to users with dementing illness. To cite just a few, the observer is asked to note whether there is clear visual differentiation of key activity areas (orientation); whether exits are disguised to discourage egress (safety); whether there is an overabundance of artifacts, wall hangings, etc. (regulation of stimulation). It is easy to see how each of these indicators is relevant to dementia. Yet, denotation of the appropriate activity for a setting by environmental markers is a universal principle, as is control of dangerous places for even the most competent and the reduction of excessive complexity and busyness in home decor for the aesthetically sensitive. The chronic-illness specificity of the environmental assessment task is thus only partial, more a matter of the surface physical features than of the dimensions of person-environment interaction.

With this uncertainty of the user-specific nature of environmental assessment, it would seem worthwhile to take another look at the assessment models provided by Moos and Lemke and the Carps. It is likely that there is something in these present systems ready to be applied to chronic-care people, and more which could be applied if the descriptors were altered to reflect the setting specificities of this target population.

REFERENCES

Brent, R., Phillipa, R., Brent, E., & Gupta, M. (1993). Validating a computer assessment of housing for older adults. *Housing and Society, 20,* 23-29.

Brill, M., & Krauss, R. (1970). Planning for community mental health centers. In H. Sanoff & S. Cohn (Eds.), *Proceedings of the Environmental Design Research Association 1.* Oklahoma City: EDRA.

Calkins, M. (1988). *Design for dementia.* Owings Mills, MD: National Health Publishing.

Calkins, M. (1996). Manuel for Resource for Evaluation and Modification Optimizing Dementia Envioronments for Living (REMODEL). Cleveland Heights, OH: IDEAS Incorporated.

Canada Mortgage and Housing Corporation (1989). *Maintaining seniors' independence: A guide to home adaptations.* Montreal: CMHC.

Carp, F. M. (1994). Assessing the environment. In M.P. Lawton & J.A. Teresi (Eds.), *Annual review of gerontology and geriatrics*, Vol. 14 (pp. 302-323). New York: Springer Publishing Company.

Carp, F. M., & Carp, A. (1982a). A role for technical assessment in perceptions of environmental quality and well-being. *Journal of Environmental Psychology, 2,* 171-191.

Carp, F. M., & Carp, A. (1982b). Perceived environmental quality of neighborhoods. *Journal of Environmental Psychology, 2,* 4-22.

Carp, F. M., & Carp, A. (1984). A complementary congruence model of well-being or mental health for the community elderly. In I. Altman, M.P. Lawton, & J.F. Wohlwill (Eds.), *Elderly people and their environment* (pp. 279-336). New York: Plenum.

Carp, F. M., & Christensen, D. L. (1986a). Technical environmental assessment predictors of residential satisfaction. *Research on Aging, 8,* 269-287.

Carp, F. M. & Christensen, D. L. (1986b). Older women living alone: Technical environmental assessment of psychological well-being. *Research on Aging, 8,* 407-425.

Christensen, D. L., Carp, F. M., Cranz, G. L., & Wiley, J. A. (1992). Objective housing indicators as predictors of the subjective evaluations of elderly residents. *Journal of Environmental Psychology, 12,* 225-236.

Cohen, U., & Day, K. (1993). *Contemporary environments for people with dementia.* Baltimore, MD: Johns Hopkins University Press.

Cohen, U., & Weisman, G. D. (1991). *Holding on to home.* Baltimore, MD: Johns Hopkins University Press.

Dawson, D., Hendershot, G., & Fulton, J. (1987). Functional limitations of individuals age 65 years and older. Advance Data, *Vital and Health Statistics,* No. 133. Hyattsville, MD: USPHS.

Gaberlavage, G., & Sloan, K. S. (1993). *Progress in elderly housing: Who's left behind?* Washington, DC: American Association of Retired Persons.

Gilderbloom, J. I., & Markham, J. P. (1996). Housing modification needs of the disabled elderly. *Environment and Behavior, 28,* 512-535.

Grant, L. A. (1996). Assessing environments in Alzheimer special care units: The Nursing Unit Rating Scale. *Research on Aging, 18,* 275-291.

Kahana, E. (1982). A congruence model of person-environment interaction. In M.P. Lawton, P.G. Windley, & T.O. Byerts (Eds.), *Aging and the environment: Theoretical approaches* (pp. 97-121). New York: Springer Publishing Company.

Kahana, E., Liang, J., & Felton, B. J. (1980). Alternative models of person-environment fit: Prediction of morale in three homes for the aged. *Journal of Gerontology, 35,* 584-595.

Kleemeier, R. W. (1959). Behavior and the organization of the bodily and the external environment. In J. E. Birren (Ed.), *Handbook of aging of the individual* (pp. 400-451). Chicago: University of Chicago Press.

Lawton, M. P. (1970). Ecology and aging. In L.A. Postalan & D.H. Carson (Eds.), *Spatial behavior of older people,* (pp. 40-67). Ann Arbor, MI: Institute of Gerontology, University of Michigan.

Lawton, M. P. (1980). Residential quality and residential satisfaction among the elderly. *Research on Aging, 2,* 309-328.

Lawton, M. P. (1982). Competence, environmental press, and the adaptation of older people. In M.P. Lawton, P.G. Windley, & T.O. Byerts (Eds.), *Aging and the environment: Theoretical approaches,* (pp. 33-59). New York: Springer Publishing Company.

Lawton, M. P. (1986). *Environment and aging.* Second printing. (orig. 1980). Albany, NY: Center for the Study of Aging.

Lawton, M. P., Fulcomer, M. C., & Kleban, M. H. (1984). Architecture for the mentally impaired elderly: A post-occupancy evaluation. *Environment and Behavior, 16,* 730-757.

Lemke, S., & Moos, R. H. (1980). Assessing the institutional policies of sheltered care settings. *Journal of Gerontology, 35,* 96-107.

Lemke, S., & Moos, R. H. (1981). The suprapersonal environments of sheltered care settings. *Journal of Gerontology, 36,* 233-243.

Lemke, S., & Moos, R. H. (1986). Quality of residential settings for elderly adults. *Journal of Gerontology, 41,* 268-276.

Lemke, S., & Moos, R. H. (1987). Measuring the social climate of congregate residences for older people: The Sheltered Care Environment Scale. *Psychology and Aging, 2,* 20-29.

Lieberman, M. A., & Tobin, S. S. (1983). *The experience of old age.* New York: Basic Books.

Manton, K. G., Corder, L., & Stallard, E. (1993). Changes in the use of personal assistance and special equipment from 1982 to 1989. *The Gerontologist, 33,* 168-176.

Moleski, W. H., Saperstein, A., & Lawton, M. P. (1985). Determining housing quality: A guide for home-health care. *Pride Institute Journal, 4,* 41-51.

Moos, R. H. (1980). Specialized living environments for older people: A conceptual framework. *Journal of Social Issues, 36,* 75-94.

Moos, R. H., & Lemke, S. (1980). Assessing the physical and architectural features of sheltered care settings. *Journal of Gerontology, 35,* 571-583.

Moos, R. H., & Lemke, S. (1992a). *Multiphasic environmental assessment procedure: User's guide.* Palo Alto, CA: Center for Health Care Evaluation, Department of Veterans Affairs.

Moos, R. H., & Lemke, S. (1992b). *Physical and architectural features checklist manual.* Palo Alto, CA: Center for Health Care Evaluation, Department of Veterans Affairs.

Moos, R. H., & Lemke, S. (1992c). *Resident and staff information form manual.* Palo Alto, CA: Center for Health Care Evaluation, Department of Veterans Affairs.

Moos, R. H., & Lemke, S. (1992d). *Policy and program information form manual.* Palo Alto, CA: Center for Health Care Evaluation, Department of Veterans Affairs.

Moos, R. H., & Lemke, S. (1992e). *Rating scale manual.* Palo Alto, CA: Center for Health Care Evaluation, Department of Veterans Affairs.

Moos, R. H., & Lemke, S. (1992f). *Sheltered Care Environment Scale manual.* Palo Alto, CA: Center for Health Care Evaluation, Department of Veterans Affairs.

Moos, R. H., & Lemke, S. (1994). *Group residences for older adults.* New York: Oxford University Press.

Norris-Baker, L., Weisman, J., Lawton, M. P., & Sloane, P. (in press). Assessing special care units for dementia: The Professional Environmental Assessment Protocol. In E.A. Steinfeld & G.S. Danford (Eds.), *Measuring enabling environments.* New York: Plenum.

Office of Policy Development and Research (1989). *The American Housing Survey: General.* Washington, DC: U.S. Department of Housing and Urban Development.

Office of Technology Assessment (1992). *Special care units for people with Alzheimer's and other dementias.* OTA-H-543. Washington, DC: U.S. Government Printing Office.

Olsen, R. V., Ehrenkrantz, E., & Hutchings, B. (1993). *Homes that help: Advice from caregivers for creating a supportive home.* Newark, NJ: New Jersey Institute of Technology Press.

Ory, M. G. (1994). Dementia special care: The development of a national research initiative. *Alzheimer's Disease and Associated Disorders, 8* (Suppl. 1), S389-S404.

Pincus, A. (1968). The definition and measurement of the institutional environment in homes for the aged. *The Gerontologist, 8,* 207-210.

Pincus, A., & Wood, V. (1970). Methodological issues in measuring the environment in institutions for the aged and its impact on residents. *Aging and Human Development, 1,* 117-126.

Pynoos, J., & Cohen, E. (1990). *Home safety guide for older people.* Washington, DC: Serif Press.

Regnier, V., & Pynoos, J. (1992). Environmental interventions for cognitively impaired older persons. In J.E. Birren, B. Sloane, & G. Cohen (Eds.), *Handbook of mental health and aging,* 2nd ed. New York: Academic Press.

Reschovsky, J. D., & Newman, S. J. (1990). Adaptations for independent living by older frail households. *The Gerontologist, 30,* 543-552.

Sloane, P. D., & Mathew, L. J. (1990). The therapeutic environment screening scale. *American Journal of Alzheimer's Care and Research, 5,* 22-26.

Sloane, P. D., & Mathew, L. J. (Eds.) (1991). *Dementia units in long-term care.* Baltimore, MD: Johns Hopkins University Press.

Sloane, P. D., Mitchell, C. M., Long, K., & Lynn, M. (1995). TESS 2+ Instrument B: Unit Observation Checklist - Physical Environment. A report on the psychometric properties of individual items, and initial recommendations on scaling. Chapel Hill, NC: Unpublished.

Struyk, R. J. (1987). Housing adaptations. In V. Regnier & J. Pynoos (Eds.), *Housing the aged* (pp. 259-276). New York: Elsevier.

Struyk, R. J., & Turner, M. (1984). Changes in the housing situation of the elderly: 1974-1979. *Journal of Housing for the Elderly, 2,* 3-20.

Tillson, D. (Ed.) (1990). *Aging in place.* Glenview, IL: Scott-Foresman.

Trickey, F., Maltais, D., Gosselin, C., & Robitaille, Y. (1993). Adapting older people's homes to promote independence. *Physical and Occupational Therapy in Geriatrics, 12,* 1-14.

U.S. Bureau of the Census (1995). *Current Population Reports,* C.M. Taueber. Sixty-five plus in America. Washington, DC: U.S. Government Printing Office.

Weisman, G. D., Calkins, M., & Sloane, P. (1994). The environmental context of special care. *Alzheimer's Disease and Associated Disorders Journal, 8,* (Suppl.1), S308-S320.

Weisman, J., Lawton, M. P., Sloane, P. S., Calkins, M., & Norris-Baker, L. (1996). *The professional environmental assessment protocol.* Milwaukee, WI: School of Architecture, University of Wisconsin at Milwaukee.

Zeisel, J., Hyde, J., & Levkoff, S. (1994). Best practices: An environment-behavior (E-B) model for Alzheimer special care units. *American Journal of Alzheimer's Disease, 9*(2), 4-21.

Chapter 13

Assessing Health-Related Quality of Life in Chronic Care Populations

Steven M. Albert

Quality of life (QOL) assessment can be based on measures from a variety of conceptual domains, with varying levels of depth or breadth in any particular domain. This is its strength and weakness. For example, even with broad consensus among investigators on the necessity of including indicators of functional health in QOL assessment, there are no clear guidelines on how many indicators of functioning are sufficient. Certainly one should include the activities of daily living, but should one also assess upper and lower extremity function because these, too, are independently associated with risk of death and other health outcomes (Johnson & Wolinsky, 1993)? Similarly, if social functioning is a necessary part of health-related QOL, what about its component elements, such as cognitive status and communicative ability? These clearly affect social functioning but also represent potentially distinct QOL domains.

The challenge to health-related QOL assessment, then, is to develop a wide range of indicators of patient functioning and well-being; however, for taxonomic and practical purposes investigators must specify a series of basic domains that summarize (and presumably show the effect of) impaired competencies in component domains. This review follows Schipper and assesses the content of generic, health-related QOL (HRQL) instruments according to their coverage of four intermediate domains of QOL: physical and occupational function, psychological function, social interaction, and somatic symptoms (Schipper, Clinch, & Olweny, 1996).

A further consideration in the measurement of QOL is the extent to which features of chronic care populations, e.g., the institutional setting of care, constrain HRQL assessment. Additionally, given the high prevalence of cognitive impairment in the old-old, how might assessment instruments need to be altered to capture HRQL in this group? This review adopts the position that cognitive impairment poses a fundamental challenge to QOL assessment, because cognitive impairment directly compromises the ability of patients to perceive internal states and make judgments regarding QOL.

Acknowledgments. The author would like to thank the editors and the reviewer for their helpful comments and also the quality of life researchers who kindly supplied unpublished material for this review. Research was supported by the Alzheimer's Association (FSA-93-026).

Even with this delimitation of the domain of HRQL, we are forced to be selective. Spilker's recent compendium of HRQL measures for *clinical trials*, for example, runs to some 1250 pages (Spilker, 1996). Readers are referred to this source and also to Bowling (1994) for recent, indeed encyclopedic, overviews of QOL assessment strategies.

CONCEPTUAL MODEL OF HEALTH-RELATED QOL

Health-Related and General QOL. HRQL represents one component of general quality of life, which encompasses other determinants of QOL besides health. These other determinants include features of the physical and social environment (e.g., water quality, noise level, community cohesion, educational opportunity, access to health and social services), as well as personal resources (e.g., receptivity to the arts, spirituality, capacity to form friendships). Health conditions are a central determinant of general QOL; indeed, some features of the physical or social environment are relevant to general QOL because they increase the risk of disease or disability.

Generic and Disease-Specific HRQL Measures. With HRQL we focus on the effects of health limitation on functioning and well-being. The effects of health limitation may be specific to a disease, as in the case of social restrictions resulting from the chronic diarrhea typical of bowel disorders or activity limitation due to uncontrolled epileptic seizures. Other effects of health limitation are more diffuse and represent the generalized impact of poor health. These generic indicators of impaired functioning are applicable across disease conditions and are valuable for assessing the degree of health limitation typical of different diseases.

The difference between disease-specific and generic measures is largely a matter of detail. Social limitations related to bowel disorders or restrictions on activity related to epilepsy should be detected by generic HRQL measures. Disease-specific measures of HRQL offer the advantage of assessing the effects of particular symptoms and are thus likely to be more precise indicators of disease severity than generic measures (Patrick & Deyo, 1989). A disadvantage in the use of disease-specific measures is that there is less potential for comparison to other chronic disease populations. The current recommendation is to combine generic and disease-specific measures when assessing particular patient populations (Aaronson et al., 1991), allowing both population comparisons and a finer understanding of disease-specific impacts on patient functioning.

One other approach to the choice of disease-specific or generic measures is to incorporate common somatic symptoms, such as pain, dyspnea, fatigue, and nausea, into generic HRQL measures. Such symptoms are a common component of many diseases and are thus appropriate in generic HRQL measures. This is the approach of Kaplan and Bush (1982) and others and will be adopted in this review.

A Four-Factor Model of HRQL. Spilker (1996) views HRQL as a kind of pyramid, with a global assessment of functioning and well-being at the peak, a series of broad but discrete QOL domains at the center, and a much broader and diverse series of indicators for each domain at the base. Global indicators include self-perceived health, the Karnofsky rating of physical function (Karnofsky, Abelmann, Burehencal, & Craver, 1948), and Spitzer index (Spitzer et al., 1981). The intermediate domains of HRQL include relatively discrete, coherent areas of functioning and well-being that individuals presumably draw upon in making global ratings. Much of the debate regarding assessment of HRQL revolves around specification of these domains: how many (and which) of these domains need to be included in a measure for it to be considered a valid indicator of HRQL?

A review of HRQL measures shows quite a range of such intermediate domains. The theoretical minimum appears to be two domains, a physical function and mental health domain, because factor-analytic studies show that items designed to assess health in chronic disease populations form separate, only moderately correlated factors corresponding to these content domains (Hays & Stewart, 1990; Ware & Keller, 1996). (We exclude Gill and Feinstein's [1994] one-factor approach, in which HRQL is simply a person's satisfaction with his or her state of health. This is simply an alternative phrasing of a global rating.) The two-factor approach has shown its value in population-based surveillance of HRQL, as in the use of Health Interview Survey measures of self-rated health and activity limitation to construct a composite HRQL measure (Erickson, Wilson, Seitz, & Shannon, 1993), and CDC efforts to combine days of poor mental health and days of poor physical health in the Behavioral Risk Factors Surveillance System (Hennessy, Moriarty, Zack, Scherr, & Brackbill, 1994).

The two-factor HRQL approach, however, is probably inadequate for assessment of chronic disease populations. Given the impaired health of these populations, it is important to employ finer measures of physical health, for example, measures of somatic symptoms (such as pain), physical impairment, and activity limitation. The same argument can be made for indicators of mental health, for example, inclusion of an indicator of social involvement. Finally, in the presence of severe disease and its unquestionable association with impaired physical function and activity limitation, it is important to assess compensating factors, e.g., positive emotional health and social activity, that may elevate QOL.

For these reasons, surveillance of HRQL in chronic disease populations has typically involved measures with three to five such intermediate domains. Table 13.1 indicates the major domains, along with component indicators, used in a number of the most common HRQL assessment instruments. We limit instruments to *generic, HRQL measures*, recognizing that many of the disease-specific measures (such as those assessing the quality of life impact of cancer or arthritis) may also be valuable for general HRQL assessment.

Assessment instruments were considered HRQL measures and included in the table if they (a) minimally included measures of both physical function and mental health, or (b) were explicitly developed as generic QOL indicators (as opposed to more general health assessment tools; see Lawton & Lawrence [1994] for a review of such measures), or (c) have come to be used as generic HRQL measures despite other origins. The table identifies four broad QOL domains as well as a global indicator.

Table 13.1 differs from other tabulations of features of generic HRQL measures (such as those of Patrick and Deyo [1989] and Ware and Keller [1996]) in a number of ways. First is its decomposition of major QOL domains into component elements; in other tabulations, these subcomponents may be elevated to the level of independent, separate domains (as in role function vs. physical function in the Medical Outcomes Study SF-36) (Steward & Ware, 1992). Second, Table 13.1 also leaves out other domains assessed in some of the instruments. Some of these domains (i.e., financial security, access to health services, spirituality) are defined here as part of more general

QOL rather than HRQL; others represent allied but distinct elements of well-being (i.e., life events, coping ability, optimism, life satisfaction, relationship to physician, etc.). Still, others index cross-cutting capacities that are not easily accommodated in any particular domain or component (e.g., the manual dexterity item in the Health Utilities Index Mark III [Feeny, et al., 1996]). Finally, it should be noted that terms for QOL domains vary across instruments. For example, what Kaplan and Bush (1982) in the Quality of Well-Being (QWB) assessment call "social function" is actually a measure of role function as defined here, the ability to perform activities more general than ADL and IADL (e.g., work and "usual activities"); we reserve "social function" in Table 13.1 for measures of social interaction and satisfaction with such interaction.

The absence of indicators of cognitive function in virtually all the generic measures (barring perhaps the SIP alertness and communication domains (Bergner, et al., 1976), the FIM social cognition domain, (Granger, 1984) and the Minimum Data Set (MDS) (Morris, et al., 1990) is worth comment. Administration of these measures, all of which rely on self-report or a combination of clinician and patient judgments, presumes intact cognitive function in respondents. Hence the absence of a distinct cognitive function domain. In the case of the cognitively impaired subject, an entirely different assessment system is required, described below.

Table 13.1 shows that no assessment scale covers every component listed in the table. At a higher level of inclusiveness, most assessment systems tap at least one component in each of the larger domains. Social functioning is not assessed in the Quality of Well-Being scale, the EuroQoL, the Health Utilities Index, or the Functional Independence Measure (FIM). Direct assessment of mental health is not included in the FIM, and so this measure may not truly belong in the class of HQRL measures. We include it here because of its growing popularity and use in defining "function-related groups" (on the analogy of Diagnosis-Related Groups) in medical rehabilitation (Stineman et al., 1994). Global respondent ratings are obtained in under half the instruments. While somatic symptoms are assessed quite variably across the assessment batteries, pain seems to be most frequently assessed, and, indeed, is the only symptom assessed in a number of the measures (e.g., EuroQOL, COOP, MOS SF-36, Rosser Index of Health-Related QOL).

The narrowest definition of HRQL is evident in the Health Utilities Index Mark III. Feeny and colleagues explicitly restrict their assessment to an approach "that focuses on physical and emotional dimensions of health status and excludes social interaction because it takes place 'outside the skin'" (Feeny, Torrance, & Furlong, 1996). Consistent with this "within the skin" approach, they also exclude ADL and IADL abilities, which involve social- or role-bound functions, and stress instead dexterity and mobility. So narrow a definition of HRQL, however, seems inappropriate for chronic care populations, when what is of most interest is the degree to which health limitation has undercut the ability to perform socially defined roles and interfered with daily social contact. For this population, limitations in dexterity and mobility are extremely common; what one wants to know is the degree to which they compromise more general competencies.

At the other pole of inclusiveness are measures that are based on far more expansive notions of HRQL. For example, the WHOQOL definition of HRQL is "an individual's perception of their [sic] position in life in the context of the culture and value systems

TABLE 13.1 Component Domains in Generic HQOL Assessment Instruments

	SIP	NHP	MOS	QWB	MHIQ	Rosser	WHO	EuroQ	COOP
Physical Function									
Mobility	X	X	X	X	X	X	X	X	--
IADL	X	--	X	X	X	X	--	--	--
ADL	X	--	X	X	X	X	X	X	--
Strength	--	--	X	--	X	X	--	--	X
Leisure Activity	X	X	--	--	X	--	X	--	--
Role	X	X	X	X	X	X	X	X	X
Mental Health									
Negative Affect	X	X	X	X	X	X	X	X	X
Positive Affect	--	--	X	--	X	X	X	--	--
Symptoms									
Nausea	--	--	--	X	--	--	--	--	--
Dyspnea	--	--	--	X	--	--	--	--	--
Pain	X	X	X	X	X	X	X	X	X
Fatigue	X	X	X	X	--	--	X	--	--
Alertness	X	--	X	X	X	--	X	--	--
Communication	X	--	--	X	--	--	X	--	--
Sleep	X	X	--	X	--	--	X	--	--
Appetite	X	--	--	X	--	--	--	--	--
Bowel	X	--	--	X	--	--	--	--	--
Sexual	X	X	--	X	--	--	X	--	--
Social Function									
Contact	X	X	X	--	X	--	X	--	X
Quality	--	--	--	--	--	--	--	--	--
Patient Global Rating	--	X	X	--	X	--	--	X	X
Total Items[1]	136	45	36	30	172	175	231	6	6

	HUI	FIM	MDS	FSQ
Physical Function				
Mobility	X	X	X	--
IADL	--	X	--	X
ADL	--	X	X	X
Strength	--	--	--	--
Leisure Activity	--	--	X	X
Role	--	--	X	X
Mental Health				
Negative Affect	--	--	X	X
Positive Affect	X	--	--	X

(Continued)

TABLE 13.1 *(Continued)*

	HUI	FIM	MDS	FSQ
Symptoms				
Nausea	--	--	--	--
Dyspnea	--	--	--	--
Pain	X	--	--	--
Fatigue	--	--	--	--
Alertness	--	X	X	--
Communication	X	X	X	--
Sleep	--	--	--	--
Appetite	--	--	X	--
Bowel	--	--	X	--
Sexual	--	--	--	X
Social Function				
Contact	--	--	X	X
Quality	--	--	X	X
Patient				
Global Rating	--	--	--	X
Total Items[1]	8	18	284	34

Legend for Table 13.1
SIP, Sickness Impact Profile (Bergner,Bobbit, Kressel, Pollard, Gilson & Morris, 1976)
NHP, Nottingham Health Profile (Hunt, McEwen & McKenna, 1986)
MOS, Medical Outcomes Study SF-36 (Ware & Stewart, 1992)
QWB, Quality of Well-Being Scale (Kaplan & Bush, 1982)
MHIQ, McMaster Health Index Questionnaire (Chambers, MacDonald, Tugwell, Buchanan, Kraag, 1982)
Rosser, Index of Health-Related QOL (Rosser & Kind, 1978)
WHO, World Health Organization QOL (WHOQOL, 1994)
EuroQ, EuroQOL, European QOL Assessment (EuroQOL Group, 1990)
COOP, Dartmouth Functional Health Assessment Charts (Nelson, Wasson & Kirk, 1987)
HUI, Health Utilities Index Mark III (Feeny, Torrance & Furlong, 1996)
FIM, Functional Independence Measure (Granger, 1984)
MDS Minimum Data Set (Morris, Hawes, Fries, Phillips, Mor, Katz, et al, 1990)
FSQ, Functional Status Questionnaire (Jette, Davies, Cleary, Calkins, Rubenstein, Fink, et al., 1986)

in which they live and in relation to their goals, expectations, standards, and concerns" (WHOQOL, 1994).

Finally, Table 13.1 does not reflect the different scaling systems required by the measures. Some of the measures simply rely on categorical scales, without weighting of states for severity of dysfunction or health impact (MOS, WHOQOL, COOP, MDS, MHIQ, FSQ, FIM); others combine item-level information to generate composite health states (EuroQOL); still others use formal judgment analysis techniques to weight item-level responses by severity of impact, as derived from community consensus or the judgments of health professionals (SIP, NHP, QWB, HUI).

SPECIAL CONSIDERATIONS IN ASSESSING HQRL
IN CHRONIC CARE POPULATIONS

Constraints on QOL Assessment in Chronic Care Populations. The health conditions typical of chronic care population make QOL assessment in this group different from assessment in other populations. Patients in residential care settings, for example, are constrained in the activities they can perform and their ability to demonstrate independence. Also, the special interpersonal setting of nursing home care may introduce new sources of positive and negative QOL, with new challenges for interpreting behaviors. For example, is the resident who retreats from common areas to a private room (or who does not participate in scheduled activities) demonstrating autonomy and an understandable attempt to secure privacy (i.e., an indicator of positive QOL), or rather poor mental health and a retreat from activities perceived as overly taxing? These questions can only be answered with microbehavioral investigations.

Assessing HRQL Among People With Cognitive Impairments. Even moderate memory impairment may entail loss of insight on one's condition, making QOL reports unreliable; for the most advanced states of dementia, cognition is impaired to the point that it is almost impossible to know how patients experience the world at all except for extremely primitive behaviors, such as obvious agitation or eye movements that may indicate awareness. Assessment of HRQL in the case of demented patients poses special problems. This area of assessment has only recently received attention, and at this point it is still unclear when in the course of dementing disease a patient loses the capacity to report on his or her quality of life (Stewart, Sherbourne, & Brod, 1996).

Among people with severe dementia, HRQL assessment must be based on ratings by clinicians or observers (such as family members or others in daily contact with elders), in addition to, or perhaps in the absence of, patient self-reports. The loss of cognitive capacity is also associated with major restrictions in activity, leading to "floor effects" for most indicators of HRQL in standard assessment tools. In such circumstances, HRQL must be based on recognition of behavioral states that are likely to be informative about a patient's subjective experience.

A number of assessment instruments have been developed to capture HRQL in demented subjects, though research in this area is still in its earliest phase. Table 13.2 lists plausible indicators of HRQL in demented people, grouping such indicators by valence. This list was generated from a review of the literature but also from detailed discussions with home health care agency staff who have had experience in care for demented people.

A first point to note in Table 13.2 is the context-specific valence (i.e., potentially positive or negative) applied to some behaviors, such as excessive vocalization, perseveration, wandering, null time, and delusions. These behaviors are almost always considered indicators of negative HRQL in research on QOL in people with dementia. Yet in the absence of other indicators of poor quality, such as anxiety or reduction of activities normally enjoyed by patients, the behaviors should not, *ipso facto,* be presumed to be negative. Excessive vocalization is disturbing to caregivers and nursing home staff, but may represent a demented person's attempt at self-stimulation in unsatisfying environments, with attendant benefit from such stimulation (Hallberg, Norberg, & Erickson, 1990). Wandering for some nursing home residents is clearly associated with positive affect (and with other benefits as well, e.g., improved sleep). Perseveration may represent a patient's attempt to orient himself and to establish

TABLE 13.2 Indicators of QOL in Dementia

Negative:

Agitation
Psychoses
Functional dependence
Negative affects: anger, anxiety, sadness

Context-Specific (Positive or Negative):

Wandering
Perseveration
Vocalization
Delusions
Null time use

Positive:

Positive affects: happy, contentment, interest
Extent and diversity of activity, including
  activity guided by cueing and supervision;
  initiation of activity, i.e., food choice
Continued attachment to premorbid interests,
  objects, activities
Territoriality behavior

contact with caregivers. An increase in null time (time spent without any obvious activity) must be considered an aspect of good quality of life if it represents a reduction in such obviously negative behaviors as agitation. Finally, even delusions can be a positive component of daily experience if accompanied by positive affect.

From this it follows that one must consider not just the effect of such behaviors on caregivers (which are, on the whole, negative), but the potential benefits of such behavior to patients. Similarly, attention to the context of such behaviors (such as accompanying affect) forces a reconsideration of the standards by which one judges these behaviors.

A further point is the need to consider not just negative elements of quality of life in this population (agitation, negative affect, discomfort), but also the contribution of factors that may enhance quality, the positive behaviors of Table 13.2. Lawton and colleagues have demonstrated this point well with behavioral stream investigations that have shown a reduced but still impressive prevalence of positive affect among demented nursing home patients relative to nondemented residents (Lawton, Van Haitsma, & Klapper, 1996).

Finally, Table 13.2 suggests additional behaviors that may contribute to positive quality of life among demented elders. We really know very little about demented patients' continued attachment to premorbid interests, objects, and activities. Recently, Albert and colleagues showed that patients who had completed a high school education were more likely to read, or be read to, throughout the course of dementia, compared to patients who had not completed high school (Albert et al., 1996). Thus, premorbid interests may be maintained in dementia, even if the quality of such interests is altered.

PSYCHOMETRIC PROPERTIES OF HRQL INSTRUMENTS

QOL Instruments Relying on Self-Report. Table 13.3 returns to the instruments listed earlier and provides information regarding content areas specified by developers of the instrument, the primary reference for the measure, the sample on which the measure was developed, and psychometric indices of reliability and validity (when available).

The content areas shown in Table 13.3 should be compared to those shown in Table 13.1. It is evident that many of the instruments extend or recategorize the domains included in the basic four-factor conceptualization of HQRL.

While many measures of validity are available, Table 13.3 stresses construct validity, a positive correlation between the measure and an alternate measure designed to assess the same domain. The range of such coefficients is presented, with subscale information when available. Validity based on differences between known groups (patient vs. nonpatient, patients with varying severity of disease) is harder to summarize in table form, but when only this indicator is available, we include it as well. For reliability estimates, alpha coefficients (range for subscales), test-retest *r*, and kappa for interrater reliability are presented.

Table 13.3 shows that the HRQL instruments have by and large undergone extensive refinement and psychometric assessment. Only the WHOQOL remains in the pilot stage; other instruments have long histories and continue to be refined. Many have been used in cross-cultural research. There is considerable overlap among a number of the measures, since in some cases the measures have drawn on common item pools. The cancer-specific measures are included in the table because all have adopted the "core plus module" approach, in which a generic HQRL core is included with additional disease-specific add-on measures. The Health Utilities Index-Mark III is included, even though it has not been used in chronic care populations, because of its careful psychometric development and likely extension to such populations.

A major divide in the instruments listed in the table is their provenance, that is, whether they were developed in the general population or among patient groups. In fact, only a few were developed in the general population (for example, the HUI Mark III and QWB); the others were first developed among patient populations (or at least clinic users, as in the case of the MOS SF-36) and later extended to community populations. For the assessment of HQRL among chronic care populations, which is, after all, a patient population, there is no clear advantage of one over the other except that one would like to see measures that travel well across patient groups and that allow comparison to nonpatient community populations.

The psychometric data show that the measures, on the whole, meet standards for acceptable reliability and demonstrate reassuring validity. Measures of construct validity are usually higher than validity estimates based on correlations between the measures and either clinician ratings or physiologic indicators. This is not a weakness of the measures and, in fact, should be expected. By design, the HQRL indicators assess a much broader domain than clinician-assessed function or physiologic status. For HRQL measures, construct validity is probably more important. Not included in the table are indicators of predictive validity, that is, the ability of the measures to predict

TABLE 13.3 Summary of HQRL Assessment Instruments that Rely on Patient Self-Report

Measure and Subscales	Primary Sources	Development Samples (n)	Psychometrics
Sickness Impact Profile (SIP) Sleep and Rest Emotional Behavior Body Care and Movement Home Management Mobility Social Interaction Ambulation Alertness Behavior Communication Work Recreation and Pastimes Eating	Bergner, et al. 1976	n = 1100, elicitation of health states n = 25 health care staff, scaling of health states n = 246 patients, n = 278 rehab n = 696 HMO, 199 clinic patients	*Reliability* retest r, .73-.96 α, .63-.90 *Validity* clinician-ratings, r, .27-.49 HIS survey, r, .61 Physiologic indicators, r, .41-.91
Nottingham Health Profile (NHP) Energy Level Emotional Reactions Physical Mobility Pain Social Isolation Sleep Activities	Hunt, et al., 1986	n = 768, elicitation of health states n = 215 weighting of health states n = 2176 postal survey	*Reliability* test-retest r, .77-.85 *Validity* Known groups differences
Medical Outcomes Study (MOS SF-36) Physical Function Role Function-Physical Pain Mental Health Role Function-Emotion Social Function Health Perception	Stewart & Ware 1992	n = 22,000, HMO norming sample	*Reliability* α, .76-.94 *Validity* .27-1.0 physical .31-.43 mental (Rel precision)
Quality of Well-Being (QWB) Mobility Physical Activity Social Activity Symptom-Problems	Kaplan & Bush 1982	n = 866, random sample, scaling of health states	*Reliability* r, .94 *Validity* Known groups

(Continued)

TABLE 13.3 *(Continued)*

Measure and Subscales	Primary Sources	Development Samples (n)	Psychometrics
McMaster Health Index (MHIQ) Physical Activities Mobility Self-Care Communication Role Performance Social Function Emotional Function	Chambers, et al. 1982	n = 70 patients	*Reliability* Retest r, .48.-.70 (physiotherapy) Retest r, .66.-.95 (psychiatry) κ, .80 *Validity* Known groups
Rosser Index of Health-Related QOL (IHQOL) Functional Disability Emotional Distress Pain	Rosser & Kind 1978	n = 20 patients n = 20 non-patients n = 30 health staff	*Reliability* retest agreement: 97%; inter-observer agreement: 88% *Validity* Known groups
WHOQOL Physical Function Psychological Function Independence Social Relationships Environment Spirituality	WHOQOL Group, 1994	n = 250 patients n = 50 non-patients	*Reliability* Unavailable *Validity* Unavailable
EuroQOL Mobility Self-Care Usual Activity Pain/Discomfort Anxiety/Depression	EuroQoL Group, 1990	n = 592 postal survey, 3 sites	*Reliability* Unavailable *Validity* Unavailable
COOP Physical Fitness Emotional Status Daily Activities Social Activities Pain Social Support Overall Health Overall QOL	Nelson, et al. 1987	n = 2000 patients, 4 clinical settings	*Reliability* retest: r, .73-.98 *Validity* r = .62 MOS

(Continued)

TABLE 13.3 *(Continued)*

Measure and Subscales	Primary Sources	Development Samples (n)	Psychometrics
Health Utilities Index-Mark III (HUI) Vision Hearing Speech Ambulation Dexterity Emotion Cognition Pain	Ontario Ministry of Health, 1993 Feeny, et al. 1996	n = 506, general population sample	*Reliability* retest: r, .77 *Validity* Unavailable for chronic care populations
Functional Independence Measure (FIM) Self-Care Continence Mobility Locomotion Communication Social Cognition	Granger 1984 Hamilton et al. 1987	n = 263 patients, 21 hospitals	*Reliability* Interrater r, .97 κ, .54 *Validity* Known groups
Minimum Data Set (MDS) Cognition Communication Vision Physical Function Continence Psychosocial Well-Being Mood Activity Pursuit Health Conditions	Morris et al. 1990	n = 383 nursing home residents, 10 sites	*Reliability* α, .75 ADL; .73 cognition .61 social *Validity* r = .94 cognition
Functional Status Questionnaire (FSQ) Physical Function Psychological Function Social Function Role Function	Jette et al. 1986	n = 1153 ambulatory patients	*Reliability* α, .64-.82 *Validity* r = .15-.33 bed disability

onset of clinical endpoints, either in natural history studies or clinical trials; but these, too, are impressive.

Self-Report Assessment Instruments With Variations in Elicitation of HRQL Information. Not included in Table 13.3 are a series of newly developed measures that either rely on alternative techniques for the elicitation of HRQL information or have not been fully developed. We describe three such measures here.

One such measure is the *Perceived Quality of Life* scale (Patrick, Danis, Southerland, & Hong, 1988; Danis, Patrick, Southerland, et al., 1988). Originally developed in the context of intensive care, the PQOL consists of 20 items scored in a 10-point format. It incorporates SIP domains and yields summary measures of perceived physical, social, and cognitive function. The measure was used in the recent Women's Health and Aging Study [WHAS] (Guralnick, Fried, Simonsick, Kasper, & Lafferty 1995), so that population-based norms on perceived QOL among disabled women are now available.

The Schedule for Evaluation of Individual QOL (O'Boyle, McGee, Hickey, O'Malley, & Joyce, 1992) differs from the other QOL instruments in that it asks respondents to nominate important domains of QOL and examines QOL within this framework. Five such domains are elicited. Once respondents have nominated the domains, they rate each on a visual analogue scale (ranging from "as good as could possibly be" to "as bad as could possibly be").

The Smith-Kline Beecham QOL scale (Stoker, Dunbar, & Beaumont, 1992) uses 23 predetermined 10-point visual analogue scales. A unique aspect of the measure is its use of three different reference points: "self now" (current condition), "ideal self" (the best patients have been), "sick self" (the worst patients have been). Use of these additional referents "provides a personal frame of reference for the individual and recognizes the highly idiosyncratic and subjective nature of the experience which constitutes QOL."

Instruments Not Relying on Self-Report: Assessment Tools for People with Dementia. Table 13.4 lists current instruments explicitly designed to assess HRQL in dementia patients. The list is small, though new instruments are currently under development. For the most part, the instruments stress affect and activity.

Some measures assess only negative features of QOL (Cohen-Mansfield Agitation Index, [Cohen-Mansfield, Marx, & Rosenthal, 1989] Discomfort scale [Hurley, et al., 1992]), defining high QOL only by low frequency of negative features. Others stress positive elements only. For example, Teri and Logsdon's Pleasant Events Schedule (AD) defines high QOL in terms of maximum preservation of premorbid patterns of activity and substitution of independent activity by assisted activity (through caregiver cueing and supervision) (Logsdon & Teri, 1996; Teri & Logsdon, 1991).

Other instruments assess both positive and negative aspects of QOL. The Progressive Deterioration Scale notes the frequency of positive and negative activities, such as "interest in doing household tasks" and "confusion in familiar settings," but is redundant with components of cognitive and functional assessment (DeJong, Osterlund, & Roy, 1989). The Withdrawal subscale of the MOSES (Multidimensional Observational Scale for Elderly Subjects) obtains staff ratings of whether subjects prefer solitude, initiate social contact, respond to social contact, make friends, are interested in events, keep occupied, and help others (Helmes, Csapo, & Short, 1987). While the breadth of behaviors is admirable, many are inappropriate for patients with advanced dementia. Lawton's Affect Rating Scale (ARS) assesses the frequency of both positive (pleasure, interest, contentment) and negative (anger, anxiety/fear, sadness) affects. In a sample of nursing home patients, Lawton and colleagues found that behavior stream observations of affect in these patients were correlated with staff and family ratings of a variety of indicators of patient behavior (such as extraversion and task assertiveness), as well as other measures of dementia (Lawton, Van Haitsma, & Klapper, 1996).

One final point about these measures is worth noting. Because patients cannot report on HRQL, researchers have had recourse to both reports by others about patient

TABLE 13.4 Instruments for Assessing QOL in Patients with Dementia

Measure	Development Sample (n)	Psychometrics
Cohen-Mansfield Agitation Index (Cohen-Mansfield, 1989)	Nursing Home, n = 408	*Reliability* 88-92% agreement *Validity* Unavailable
Discomfort Scale (Hurley, 1992)	AD Special Care Units, n = 82	*Reliability* α = .86-.89 *Validity* Known groups
Pleasant Events Schedule-AD (Teri & Logsdon, 1991)	Community sample, n = not stated	*Reliability* .86-.90 *Validity*, r = .57, MMSE
MOSES: Withdrawal Subscale (Hermes, 1987)	Hosp/NH n = 2391	*Reliability* α = .78 *Validity*, r = .30-.78 mental health
Affect Rating Scale (Lawson, 1996)	Nursing Home, n = 253	*Reliability* α =.76-.89 *Validity* r = .25 depression .32 agitation .37 irritability
Progressive Deterioration Scale (DeJong, 1989)	Caregivers, community AD patients, n = 53	*Reliability* test-retest r, .78-.90 *Validity* Discrimination between AD severity levels

behaviors and microbehavioral recording (as in behavior stream observations). At this point, microbehavioral investigation remains essential for establishing the texture of daily life among demented patients. It is this sort of attention to detail that will establish how often wandering or excessive vocalization truly reflects negative patient QOL. Thus, behavioral records of patient behavior (such as Burgio's research on vocalization in nursing homes [Burgio et al., 1994]) are valuable even if they do not directly assess patient QOL. Reliance on subjective reports by caregivers alone may underestimate potentially positive features of such behavior.

RECOMMENDATIONS FOR ASSESSING QOL IN CHRONIC CARE POPULATIONS

As should be evident from this review, picking the best QOL measure for chronic disease populations depends on the particular population and, most critically, on the cognitive status of patients. In addition to such standard bearers as the SF-36, SIP, and QWB, measures for nursing home populations (MDS) and patient populations with different symptom complexes (cancer, rheumatoid disease, stroke and neurologic disease) are now available.

On the other hand, this review has shown the inadequacy of some HRQL measures for chronic disease populations. The HUI Mark III, though impressive in its strict "within the skin" approach to HRQL, does not have significant breadth because of its absence of functional health measures. Similarly, the FIM, while appropriate in predicting rehabilitation outcomes, lacks a mental health component, making it inappropriate for general HRQL assessment.

For cognitively impaired elders, QOL assessment is more complicated. Here choices of instruments are more limited, and most instruments continue to evolve or have not yet left the pilot stage. A measure specifically designed for the mildly demented elder is still lacking (though preliminary results for such a measure have recently been presented [Brod & Stewart, 1995]). Lawton's Affect Rating Scale and other microbehavioral measures have given the first detailed picture of the everyday lives of demented people, an essential beginning for understanding QOL in this population. More than likely, a combination of observed and reported behaviors will be required for adequate QOL assessment of demented elders.

In short, good measures for assessing QOL in elderly chronic care populations are not lacking. Better QOL instruments will emerge as we pay closer attention to the texture of daily life in such populations and better understand the ways elders adapt to states of health limitation.

REFERENCES

Aaronson, N. K., Meyerowitz, B. E., Bard, M., Bloom, J. R., Fawzy, F. I., Feldstein, M., Fink, D., Holland, J. C., Johnson, J. E., & Lowman J. T. (1991). Quality of life research in oncology. Past achievements and future priorities. *Cancer, 67,* 839-843.

Albert, S. M., Castillo-Castaneda, C., Sano, M., Jacobs, D. M., Marder, K., Bell, K., Bylsma, F., Lafleche, G., Brandt, J., Albert, M., & Stern, Y. (1996). Quality of life of patients with dementia as rated by proxies. *Journal of the American Geriatrics Society, 44,* 1-7.

Bergner, M., Bobbit, R. A., Kressel, S., Pollard, W. E., Gilson, B. S., & Morris, J. R. (1976). The Sickness Impact Profile: Conceptual formulation and methodology for the development of a health status measure. *International Journal of Health Services Research, 6,* 393-415.

Bowling, A. (1994). *Measuring illness: A review of disease-specific quality of life measurement scales.* Philadelphia: Open Society Press.

Brod, M., & Stewart, A. (1995). Quality of life of persons with dementia. *The Gerontologist, 35,* 114 (abstract).

Burgio, L. D., Scilley, K., Hardin, J. M., Janosky, J., Bonino, P., Slater, S. C., & Engberg, R. (1994). Studying disruptive vocalization and contextual factors in the nursing home using computer-assisted real-time observation. *Journal of Gerontology: Psychological Sciences, 49,* P230-P239.

Chambers, L. W., MacDonald, L. A., Tugwell, P., Buchanan, W. W., & Kraag, G. (1982). The McMaster Health Index Questionnaire as a measurement of quality of life for patients with rheumatoid arthritis. *Journal of Rheumatology, 9,* 780-784.

Cohen-Mansfield, J., Marx, M. S., & Rosenthal, A. D. (1989) A description of agitation in the nursing home. *Journal of Gerontology: Medical Sciences, 44,* M77-M84.

Danis, M., Patrick, D. L., Southerland, L. I., & Green, N. (1988) Patients' and families' preferences for medical intensive care. *Journal of the American Medical Association, 260,* 797-802.

DeJong, R., Osterlund, O. W., & Roy, G. W. (1989). Measurement of quality-of-life changes in patients with Alzheimer's disease. *Clinical Therapeutics, 11*, 545-554.

Erickson, P., Wilson, R. W., Seitz, J. F., & Shannon, I. (1993). Years of healthy life: A measure of healthy life span for *Healthy People 2000. Proceedings of the 1993 Public Health Conference on Records and Statistics.* U.S. Department of Health and Human Services, Washington, DC, pp. 21-27.

EuroQOL Group. (1990). EuroQOL—A new facility for the measurement of health-related quality of life. *Health Policy, 16*, 199-208.

Feeny, D. H., Torrance, G. W., & Furlong, W. J. Health utilities index. In Spilker, 1996. pp. 239-252.

Gill, T. M., & Feinstein, A. R. (1994). A critical appraisal of the quality of quality of life measurements. *Journal of the American Medical Association, 272*, 619-626.

Granger, C. V. (1984). A conceptual model for functional assessment. In C.V. Granger & G.E. Greshem (Eds.). *Functional assessment in rehabilitation medicine.* Baltimore: Williams & Wilkins.

Guralnick, J. M., Fried, L. P., Simonsick, E. M., Kasper, J. D., & Lafferty, M. E. (1995). *The women's health and aging study: Health and social characteristics of older women with disability.* Bethesda, MD: National Institute on Aging.

Hallberg, I. R., Norberg, A., & Erickson, S. (1990). Functional impairment and behavioral disturbances in vocally disruptive patients in psychogeriatric wards compared to controls. *International Journal of Geriatric Psychiatry, 5*, 53-61.

Hays, R. D., & Stewart, A. L. (1990). The structure of self-reported health in chronic disease patients. *Psychological Assessment, 2*, 22-20.

Helmes, E., Csapo, K. G., & Short, J. A. (1987). Standardization and validation of the Multidimensional Observation Scale for Elderly Subjects (MOSES). *Journal of Gerontology, 42*, 395-405.

Hennessy, C. H., Moriarty, D. G., Zack, M. M., Scherr, P. A., & Brackbill, R. (1994). Measuring health-related quality of life for public health surveillance. *Public Health Reports, 109*, 665-672.

Hunt, S. M., McEwan, J., & McKenna, S. P. (1986). *Measuring health status.* Beckenham: Croom Helm.

Hurley, A. C., Volicer, B. J., Hanrahan, P. A., Houde, S., & Volicer, L. (1992). Assessment of discomfort in advanced Alzheimer patients. *Research in Nursing and Health, 15*, 369-377.

Jette, A. M., Davies, A. R., Cleary, P. D., Calkins, D. R., Rubenstein, L. V., Fink, A., Kosecoff, J., Young, R. T., Brook, R. H., & Delbanco, T. L. (1986). The Functional Status Questionnaire: Reliability and validity when used in primary care. *Journal of General Internal Medicine, 1*, 143-149.

Johnson, R. J., & Wolinsky, F. D. (1993). The structure of health status among older adults: Disease, disability, functional limitation, and perceived health. *Journal of Health and Social Behavior, 34*, 105-121.

Kaplan, R. M., & Bush, J. W. (1982). Health-related quality of life measurement for evaluation research and policy analysis. *Health Psychology, 1*, 61-80.

Karnofsky, D. A., Abelmann, W. H., Burehencal, J. H., & Craver, L. F. (1948). The use of nitrogen mustards in the palliative treatment of cancer. *Cancer, 1*, 634-656.

Kind, P. The EuroQoL Instrument: An index of health-related quality of life. In Spilker, 1996, p. 191-201.

Lawton, M. P. (1994). Quality of life in Alzheimer disease. *Alzheimer Disease and Associated Disorders, 8*(Suppl. 3), 138-150.

Lawton, M.P., Lawrence, R. H. (1994). Assessing health. *Annual Review of Geriatrics and Gerontology,* 14, 23-56.

Lawton, M. P., Van Haitsma, K., & Klapper, J. (1996) Observed affect in nursing home residents with Alzheimer's disease. *Journal of Gerontology: Psychological Sciences, 51B,* P3-P14.

Logsdon, R. G., & Teri, L. (1996). The Pleasant Events Schedule-AD: Psychometric properties and relationship to depression and cognition in Alzheimer's disease patients. *The Gerontologist 37,* 40-45.

Ministry of Health, Ontario. (1993). *Ontario Health Survey 1990. User's Guide. Vol I: Documentation.* Toronto: Ministry of Health, Ontario and Premier's Council on Health, Well-Being, and Social Justice.

Morris, J. N., Hawes, C., Fries, B., Phillips, C. D., Mor, V., Katz, S., Murphy, K., Drugovich, M. L., & Friedlob, A. S. (1990). Designing the national resident assessment instrument for nursing homes. *The Gerontologist, 30,* 293-307.

Nelson, E. C., Wasson, J., Kirk, J. (1987). Assessment of function in routine clinical practice: Description of the COOP chart method and preliminary findings. *Journal of Chronic Disease, 40*(Suppl. 1), S55-S63.

O'Boyle, C. A., McGee, H., Hickey, A., O'Malley, K., & Joyce, C. R. B. (1992). Individual quality of life in patients undergoing hip replacement. *Lancet, 339,* 1088-1091.

Patrick, D. L., Danis, M., Southerland, L. I., & Hong, G. (1988). Quality of life following intensive care. *Journal of General Internal Medicine, 3,* 218-223.

Patrick, D. L., & Deyo, R. A. (1989). Generic and disease-specific measures in assessing health status and quality of life. *Medical Care, 27,* S217-S232.

Rosser, R. M. , & Kind, P. (1978). A scale of valuations of states of illness: Is there a social consensus? *International Journal of Epidemiology, 7,* 347-358.

Schipper, H., Clinch, J. J., & Olweny, C. L. M. (1996). Quality of life studies: Definitions and conceptual issues. In Spilker, 1996, pp. 11-24.

Spilker, B., (Ed.). (1996) *Quality of life and pharmacoeconomics in clinical trials.* Philadelphia: Lippincott-Raven.

Spitzer, W. O., Dobson, A. J., Hall, J., Chesterman, E., Levi, J., Shepard, R., Battista, R. N., & Catchlove, B. R. (1981). Measuring the quality of life of cancer patients: A concise QL-Index for use by physicians. *Journal of Chronic Disease,* 34, 585-597.

Stewart, A., & Ware, J. (1992). *Measuring functioning and well-being: The medical outcomes study approach.* Durham, NC: Duke University Press.

Stewart, A., Sherbourne, C. D., & Brod, M. (1996). Measuring health-related quality of life in older and demented populations. In Spilker, 1996, pp. 819-830.

Stineman, M. G., Escarce, J. J., Goin, J. E., Hamilton, B. B., Granger, C. V., & Williams, S. V. (1994). A case mix classification system for medical rehabilitation. *Medical Care, 32,* 366-379.

Stoker, M. J., Dunbar, G. C., & Beaumont, G. (1992). The SmithKline Beecham quality of life scale: A validation and reliability study in patients with affective disorder. *Quality of Life Research,* 1, 385-395.

Teri, L., & Logsdon, R. G. (1991). Identifying pleasant activities for Alzheimer's disease patients: The Pleasant Events Schedule - AD. *The Gerontologist, 31,* 124-127.

Ware, J. E., & Keller, S. D. (1996) Interpreting general health measures. In Spilker, 1996, pp. 445-460.

WHOQOL Group. (1994). The development of the WHO Quality of Life assessment instrument (WHOQOL). In Orley, J., Kuyken, W., (eds.), *Quality of life assessment: International perspectives.* Berlin: Springer-Verlag, pp. 41-60.

Chapter 14

Measurement of Personal Care Inputs in Chronic Care Settings

Douglas Holmes, Jeanne Teresi,
David A. Lindeman, and Gerald L. Glandon

The measurement of personal care inputs warrants detailed attention because in settings serving persons with chronic conditions such as dementing illness, personal care costs, i.e., inputs made by caregivers, are both the major and the most malleable cost center. While capital costs are relatively invariant, staffing patterns can be changed, and constitute at least 80% of total costs of care in long-term residential health care facilities (Palmer & Cotterill, 1982). Similarly, Mehr and Fries (1995) and Fries, Mehr, Schneider, Foley, and Burke (1993) note that staff time expenditures constitute the largest component of cost of care that relates directly to the characteristics of individual residents. (See also Glandon, Lindeman, and Holmes in this issue.)

Fifteen years ago, McCaffree, Baker, and Perrin (1979) initiated an assessment of the case-mix approach to reimbursement, focusing on differences in personnel inputs among different categories of patients. However, almost a decade later, Hu, Huang, and Cartwright (1986), observed that nursing home care costs were still usually based on the assumption of a homogeneous population.

More recently, methods of differentiating among resident subgroups have become relatively commonplace. New York State was one of the first states to use a case-mix approach; Medicaid payment for nursing homes is based on empirically derived Resource Utilization Groups (RUGS) (Anderman, 1990; Mills, Fetter, Riedel, & Averill, 1976). There are 16 RUGS, each with distinct clinical characteristics and different costs of care. These groups were identified primarily on the basis of associated staff inputs measured initially through traditional time and motion study (Schneider, 1993) and, most recently, recalibrated using the barcode technique (Holmes, Lindeman, Ory, & Teresi, 1994) described later in this paper. A number of states now use a case-mix approach; recent implementation by the Health Care Financing Administration (HCFA) of the Minimum Data Set (MDS: Morris et al., 1990) will probably reinforce this trend.

Despite the importance of measuring service inputs made on behalf of persons with chronic illness, there are relatively few available approaches, most of which are seriously flawed. Generally speaking, inputs are cast in terms of (a) numbers of providers or provider occasions (e.g., number of staff on a particular shift in a nursing home, or number of nursing visits), (b) the *charges,* rather than the *costs* of service inputs, and/or (c) the variety of different services received. The difference between *charge* and *cost* is often overlooked and, therefore, bears some discussion. Most important, in economic terms the cost of a particular item to an individual reflects the amount of sacrifice which must be made in order to obtain the item. In order to obtain a new car, for example, the purchaser sacrifices certain amounts of present and future resources. Now, it is true that one person's cost can be another person's charge: the "cost" to the car purchaser is the "charge" made by the car dealer. Or, in the present context, the "cost" claimed by the nursing home becomes the "charge" to the reimbursement source which may, in turn, become a "cost" to the government, i.e., through Medicaid reimbursement. The essential notion, however, is that cost and charge be brought into alignment. In the case of automobiles the assumption is that a free market economy will guarantee such alignment, i.e., the purchaser can select among a variety of cars, from an elastic group of providers (dealers). However, when dealing with public reimbursement to quasi monopolistic service providers, this assumption can break down in relation to either payer or payee. There is only one principal payer (the state Medicaid intermediary), and the number of nursing home beds is not elastic, so that competitive forces are attenuated. It therefore becomes essential to measure and document true cost as a basis for charge. In this instance, given that the greatest source of nursing home costs is personal service costs, the task becomes that of measuring as precisely as possible the specific personnel inputs made on behalf of each care recipient so that the claimant can justify reimbursement requests.

The actual data may take the form of (a) administrative records (e.g., numbers of staff), (b) direct observations (e.g., time and motion study usually conducted by trained observers with stopwatches, and work sampling, in which random work *occasions* are timed), (c) diaries or logs (maintained by the service providers), and (d) retrospective recall by key informants.

Although these several approaches remain in use, the collection of individual patient service data remains problematic because fundamental measurement requirements are not fulfilled (Fox, 1989; Hidalgo, 1989; Scitovsky, 1989; Seage 1989). For example, the presence of an observer is almost bound to influence or bias work performance; diary data and retrospective reports of key informants may be inaccurate. Ironically, despite the availability of computerized database management systems dealing with the general aspects of care in nursing homes (e.g., pharmacy, census, multidisciplinary care plans), virtually nothing has been developed for use in long-term-care facilities relating to automated collection and manipulation of valid service delivery data.

There remains the need to develop and implement a more accurate, routine method for measuring personal care inputs among chronic care populations. Taking special dementia care as an example, opinions vary widely regarding the need for additional reimbursement for demented residents. Nursing home staff and administrators are convinced that demented residents require relatively more staff effort (Wagner, 1987), while investigators responsible for rate establishment argue that no meaningful differences exist (Schneider, 1993). Thus, the issue of whether or not to develop a separate category for demented residents becomes critical. Reimbursement—which affects the willingness of nursing homes to accept demented residents, and the general quality of care given to demented residents—hinges directly on this decision. However, the differentiation between demented and cognitively intact residents in terms of staff inputs has received relatively little attention.

TRADITIONAL METHODS OF MEASURING SERVICE INPUT

Administrative Data Sets

Administrative data sets, i.e., data that are used for administrative or reimbursement purposes, are apt to reflect inputs as a basis for charges or for various forms of administrative classification, e.g., a resident/staffing ratio, or number of full-time equivalent hours of therapeutic recreation. Pursuing this example, attribution of input according to staff/patient ratios is problematic because actual resident-staff ratios are apt to fluctuate, given irregular patterns of absence common among nursing aides (despite use of "floaters," i.e., staff persons who are not permanently assigned to any one unit, instead covering the absences of other regularly assigned staff). More generally, such administrative data do not reflect service inputs made on an individual recipient level.

Direct Observation

Direct observation, as noted previously, requires the presence of an "other" person or, as in the case of video technology (Connell, 1994), a technological presence. Time and motion studies, usually involving timed observations by an observer with a stopwatch, have been the staple of service input data collection efforts.

An example of direct observation methodology is found in a study by Roddy, Liu, & Meiners (1987), who applied both work sampling and time and motion (T&M) study (both forms of direct observation) in the evaluation of a nursing home incentive reimbursement study. However, for practical reasons T&M data were not collected with respect to nursing aides, who are responsible for most of the routine "hands-on" care of demented residents (aide data from other studies were incorporated; however, the interplay between site-specific aide/nurse input could not be addressed). The work sampling method was found problematic with respect to "impromptu activities," which are particularly those which occur frequently among demented patients (e.g., quelling aggressive behavior). Further, the logistics of the T&M approach required that all staff inputs be reduced to a limited number of categories; the authors make note of the large standard deviations associated with the average scores for each of the categories, observing that the costs required for a larger sample with concomitant reduced standard errors would be prohibitive. An alternative approach is to effect far finer distinctions among residents, including demented/nondemented, and to collect data with fewer categorization constraints.

Maintenance of Diaries or Logs

Both diaries and logs involve concurrent recording of events, usually via pencil-and-paper. A principal difference is in the nature of information recorded: often diaries involve narrative description of activities and/or inputs, while logs involve only summary or checklist recording. Use of diaries is exemplified in a study by Hu et al. (1986), who estimated cost based on measures of labor inputs made on behalf of 25 residents of three facilities, obtained through diaries maintained by nursing staff over a 2-week period. Conclusions were based on a comparison between diary data relating to demented residents with average facility-wide data obtained through examination of resident/staff ratios. More recently, Manton, Cornelius, and Woodbury (1995) used logs to measure nurse and aide time spent performing nursing tasks as well as care planning, charting, breaks, and off-unit time. Staff time spent in group activities was allocated equally across all residents participating in each group. No data on reliability of the measures are reported. The authors report that study staff performed frequent checks and that items were checked following each shift. However, no data are presented regarding the convergence of these data with staff logs. Diary and, to a lesser extent, log data require verbal and writing skills; some formal caregivers, e.g., personal care workers or nursing home aides, may be only marginally literate, making the task both arduous and subject to recording error. Moreover, in some settings, e.g., cluster care, day care, or nursing homes, aides may be involved in caring for several persons simultaneously. This will result in inaccurate time allocations, unless time of "overlapped" services is also included, which is a nigh-on impossible task for a busy service provider. Schwartz and colleagues (1991) note that in diary data there is a tendency toward high autocorrelations, and to the influence of subject heterogeneity, both of which must be taken into account in study design and analysis. Finally, because maintenance of logs and/or diaries becomes a competing task during the course of service delivery, distortion of both the aggregate and the task-relative time expenditures may occur. A recent overview of the diary approach to data collection is provided by Burman (1995).

Retrospective Recall by Key Informants

Recall by key informants has been the main method for collection of service inputs by formal and informal caregivers in the community (see Kronenfeld, this volume, and Newsom, Bookwala, & Schultz, 1996). In such surveys, caregivers are asked about whether they perform services in the areas of personal care and assistance with instrumental activities of daily living. Typically, caregivers are asked to report on frequency and duration (in gross units such as hours per week) of lists of services. For example, based on data collected through key informant recall, Harrow, Tennstedt, and McKinlay (1995) estimated costs associated with hours of formal and informal care provided in six areas: personal care, housekeeping, meals, managing finances, arranging services, and transportation.

Retrospective data are embodied in efforts such as the National Long Term Care Survey (Stone, Cafferata, & Sangi, 1987) in which caregivers to the sample of impaired persons were interviewed regarding the types and amounts of support services they provided, and in the White-Means and Chollet (1996) analysis of these data in interpreting the cost of in-home elder care. Similarly, in a study of support services provided to impaired elderly persons, Holmes, et al. (1989) queried formal and informal caregivers in 52 Israeli kibbutzim as to the nature, frequency, and duration of services provided to elderly impaired persons. While there was a seemingly appropriate relationship between the types and levels of disability and the amounts of service inputs reported, it was impossible to (a) verify the informant reports, or (b) obtain information about the duration of each service *input,* as contrasted with each service. In other words, using this methodology only global, retrospective recall of hours per week is possible, rather than concurrent recording of seconds and minutes spent performing each task, for specific, identified persons. Other problems inherent in retrospective recall include (a) broad categories of services, (b) the need for proxy information because individuals with cognitive impairment cannot reliably report service inputs (see Zimmerman &

Magaziner, 1994), (c) unavailable proxy reporters when there are no caregivers present (Brock, Holmes, Foley, & Holmes, 1992), and (d) recall bias. Recall bias (Chouinard & Walter, 1995; Herrman, 1995; Mancuso & Charlson, 1995) often may be a particularly important source of error, because relatively complex information about service patterns may be required. Recent analyses of studies using complex questions, such as those required to obtain detailed information on patterns of service use, have shown that such questions can result in bias due to unreliable reporting (see Lessler, 1995, for a review). This is particularly true when the respondent is of marginal cognitive competence. More generally, research on cognitive processes involved in responding to questionnaire items has shown that the comprehension process, itself, will influence response, e.g., recall distortion can occur when unfamiliar or inappropriate terminology is used (Herrman, 1995; Jobe & Mingay, 1991).

Clearly, given both the centrality of personal service input measurement to the definition and monitoring of care and the estimation of cost associated with different forms of care, a method for measurement is required which:

a) Minimizes bias due to recording process;
b) captures the majority of interventions;
c) captures the maximum of detail in each instance of service provision;
d) enables measurement of duration as well as act; and
e) is reproducible (reliable).

A MODERN METHOD FOR COLLECTING SERVICE INPUT DATA

Recently, barcode methodology has been used to measure service inputs. One such system is InfoAide© (see Holmes, Lindeman, Ory, & Teresi, 1994). Central to the system are barcoded service sheets and a portable barcode reader (DATAWAND©IIB[1]), with accompanying database management system. Because it becomes a part of the service-providing act, and because of internal monitoring routines, it self-identifies occasions in which an unrecorded action is likely to have occurred. It captures essential descriptors of every instance of care: What is provided, for whom, by whom, at what time. Through a simple internal calculation, the duration of every instance of care provision is provided automatically. Service inputs include: bathing, grooming, feeding, toileting, and walking; indirect service inputs include charting, preparing supplies, training, and care plan development.

The file generated by the barcode reader includes five data points for each intervention: the Resident ID, the Service provider ID, the designation of the service provided, and the date and time of service delivery. At the end of each specified period, the portable scanner data are downloaded into a desktop computer in under four seconds.

A database management system intrinsic to InfoAide then scrubs, stores, and backs up the data, developing reports and producing graphics. Prior to generating reports, this software calculates durations of service provision (the wand automatically time and

---

[1] DATAWAND © IIB is a product of Symbol Technologies, Inc. The wand has 8K storage, sufficient for approximately 2 weeks' data storage. Mean time between overnight recharging appears to be in excess of 2 weeks, although this has not been determined definitively.

date stamps the beginning and ending of each service so it is possible to compute the amount of time associated with each service). This duration of each "transaction" is particularly important in the measurement of service inputs.

Extensive checking and error-correcting algorithms have been applied to such missing data as "start" with no "end," duplicate entries. For example, each service delivery unit requires two sweep cycles: one for initiation, one for termination. Occasionally, one or the other (initiation or completion, respectively) are forgotten. In such instances, prior and subsequent "scores" of the service provider—*relative to that service for that patient*—are averaged automatically and the individualized average value is used to provide a pseudo termination time. If there is no history of that particular service for that particular patient, then the average of that service for *all* patients is substituted. The fact of the omission is recorded; a report of such omissions is generated and used for individualized supervision.

Moreover, service providers provide some services for different residents simultaneously. For example, at meals one service provider may assist two or three residents at the same time. A sizable distortion of labor cost could arise from this. However, because the datawand automatically records the time on/off of all activities, the DBMS package includes routines which check each service provider's entries for such simultaneity, and provide a "score" for each patient which takes this into account.

Applications of the system include service provision by nursing staff as well as recording of physician visits and preparation of data for direct billing for Medicare Part B. The system has been used in several different applications: The New York State RUGS update, involving service data collection from 60 residents in each of 80 New York State nursing homes; a study of pediatric AIDS case management in six New York City hospitals; a study of emergency room interventions in 26 New York State hospitals; and studies of the inputs and costs of inputs associated with special care for dementia residents in California and in New York State.

RELIABILITY AND VALIDITY OF SERVICE INPUT METHODOLOGIES

Throughout the various studies cited, there is virtually no information given regarding the reliability of measures. In some, reference is made to ongoing checking and monitoring of data inputs but, again, reliability studies are usually not conducted, and no reliability estimates are provided. Clearly such data are necessary as a basis for evaluating the relative merits of any of the methods discussed. While internal consistency and test-retest reliability estimates would probably not be appropriate for service input measures, inter-rater reliability analysis could and should be established.

The barcode methodology is subject to error associated with items and with data collectors, i.e., to error borne of not capturing all relevant information. If some categories of service are not captured, or captured too broadly (services collapsed into one category), it is possible that important service inputs may be missed. Limitations of the method include motivation of the "raters" which might influence the recording. While various monitoring subroutines built into the InfoAide system provide online safeguards which, at the very least, minimize such error, this source of potential error should be examined in new applications by conducting inter-rater reliability studies.

SUMMARY AND CONCLUSIONS

Technology changes from day to day. For example, the datawands used in developing the InfoAide system have been replaced by wands which permit greater programming flexibility and control, reflected in evolving system applications. Despite these changes, the basic premise will continue to apply: that, through the application of evolving technology, it will be possible to make direct service measurement an intrinsic part of any clinical information system. Thus, while the datawand methodology embodied in InfoAide is well advanced with respect to research applications, much remains to be developed from the administrative and clinical perspectives. That is, it remains to define clinical practice—and administrative function—in such terms as to permit the use of objective data in their application. For example, the routine collection of MDS+ data is a federal/state requirement. Care plans triggered by MDS data should be defined in terms of critical service paths, further defined in terms of discrete activities which should be carried out on behalf of the patient. Currently, barcode methodology is being used to input MDS data; it also would be possible for each service "activity" to be recorded routinely by a system such as InfoAide, which then would generate reports with "flags" indicating under- or overprovision of specific services.

A major lesson to be learned is that there exists an abundant technology, waiting only for imaginative application. Historically, health-care information systems have lagged systems used in commerce and industry. Within health care, systems used in long-term residential health care have lagged those used in hospitals. Cost-reduction imperatives, involving better targeting and tailoring of services, mandate the collection of valid resident/patient-level service data. Effective targeting and tailoring, in turn, mandate the creation of an automatic link among service need, comprehensive care plan, and actual provision of care. The technological potential for such linkages exists; it remains for emerging application software to fulfill this potential.

REFERENCES

Anderman, S. (1990). Development of AIDS resource utilization groups. *Proposal/ ACHPR*, Albany, N.Y.

Brock, D., Holmes, M., Foley, D., & Holmes, D. (1992). Methodological issues in a survey of the last days of life. In R. Wallace, & R. Woolson (Eds.), *The epidemiologic study of the elderly* (pp 315-332). New York: Oxford University Press.

Burman, M. (1995). Health diaries in nursing research and practice. *Image Journal Nursing School, 27,* 147-152.

Chouinard, E., & Walter, S. (1995). Recall bias in case-control studies: An empirical analysis and theoretical framework. *Journal of Clinical Epidemiology, 48,* 245-254.

Connell, B. (1994). *Using video technology in studies of naturally-occurring behavior in long term care setting.* Paper presented at the 1994 Annual Meetings of the American Gerontological Society, Atlanta, GA.

Fox, D. (1989). What are the costs of AIDS: Alternative methodological approaches. *Health services research methodology: a focus on AIDS.* Conference Proceedings.

National Center for Health Services Research and Health Technology Assessment, Public Health Service, U.S. DHHS.

Fries, B., Mehr, D., Schneider, D., Foley, W., & Burke, R. (1993). Mental dysfunction and resource use in nursing homes. *Medical Care, 31,* (10), 898-920.

Harrow, B., Tennstedt, S., & McKinlay (1995). How costly is it to care for disabled elders in a community setting? *The Gerontologist, 35,* 803-813.

Herrman, D. (1995). Reporting current, past, and changed health status. What we know about distortion. *Medical Care, 33,* AS89-AS94.

Hidalgo, J. (1989). Collecting statewide data on HIV costs and financing: Pitfalls and payoffs. *New Perspectives on HIV-Related Illnesses: Progress in Health Services Research.* (W. LeVee, Ed.) Report No. (PHS) 89-3449, Springfield, VA: NTIS.

Holmes, D., Lindeman, D., Ory, M., & Teresi, J. (1994). Measurement of service units and costs of care for persons with dementia in special care units. *Alzheimer Disease and Associated Disorders, 8*(Suppl. 1), S328-S340.

Holmes, D., Teresi, J., Holmes, M., Bergman, S., King, Y., & Bentur, N. (1989). Informal versus formal supports for impaired elderly: Determinants of choice on Israeli kibbutzim. *The Gerontologist, 29,* 195-202.

Hu, T., Huang, L., & W. Cartwright (1986). Evaluation of the costs of caring for the senile demented elderly: A pilot study. *The Gerontologist, 26,* 158-163.

Jobe, J., & Mingay, D. (1991) Cognition and survey measurement: History and overview. *Applied Cognitive Psychology, 5,* 175.

Lessler, J. (1995). Choosing questions that people can understand and answer. *Medical Care, 33,* AS203-AS208.

Mancuso, C., & Charlson, M. (1995). Does recollection error threaten the validity of cross-sectional studies of effectiveness? *Medical Care, 33,* AS77-AS88.

Manton, K., Cornelius, E., & Woodbury, M. (1995). Nursing home residents: A multivariate analysis of their medical, behavioral, psychosocial, and service use characteristics. *Journal of Gerontology, Medical Sciences.* 50A, M242-M251.

McCaffree, K., Baker, J., & Perrin, E. (1979). Long-Term Care Case Mix Compared to Direct Care Time and Costs. *Final Report* on Contract No. HRA-230-76-0285. Seattle, WA: Battelle Human Affairs Research Centers.

Mehr, D., & Fries, B. (1995). Resource use on Alzheimer's special care units. *The Gerontologist, 35,* 179-184.

Mills, R., Fetter, R., Riedel, D., & Averill, R. (1976). AUTOGRP: An interactive computer system for the analysis of health care data. *Medical Care.* XIV, 603-615.

Morris, J., Hawes, C., Fries, B., Phillips, C., Mor, V., Katz, S., Murphy, K., Drugovich, M., & Friedlob, A. (1990). Designing the National Resident Assessment Instrument for Nursing Homes. *The Gerontologist, 30,* 293-307.

Palmer, H., & Cotterill, P. (1982). Studies of nursing home costs. In R. Vogel & H. Palmer (Eds.), *Long term care: Perspectives from research and demonstrations* (pp. 665-722). Washington, DC: Health Care Financing Administration, DHHS.

Roddy, P., Liu, K., & Meiners, M. (1987). Resource requirements of nursing home patients based on Time and Motion studies. *Long Term Care Studies Program Research Report.* DHHS Publication No. (PHS) 87-3408. USDHHS, NCHSR, April.

Schneider, D. (1993). *Report on the impact of updating the base year and updating case mix indices used in the Resource utilization Groups Nursing Home Payment*

System. (Draft report) submitted to the NYS Department of Health Division of Health Care Financing.

Scitovsky, A. (1989) Past lessons and future directions: The economics of health services delivery for HIV-related illnesses. *New Perspectives on HIV-Related Illnesses: Progress in Health Services Research.* (W. LeVee, Ed.). Report No. (PHS) 89-3449. Springfield, VA: NTIS.

Schwartz, J., Wypij, D., Dockery, D., Ware, J., Zeger, S., Spengler, J. & Ferris, B. (1991). *Environment Health Perspectives, 90,* 181-187.

Seage, G. (1989). Discussion Paper: *New perspectives on HIV-related illnesses: Progress in health services research.* (W. LeVee, Ed.) Report No. (PHS) 89-3449. Springfield, VA: NTIS.

Stone, R., Cafferata, G., & Sangi, J. (1987). Caregivers of the frail elderly: A national profile. *The Gerontologist, 27,* 616-626.

Wagner, L (1987). Nursing homes develop special Alzheimer's units. *Modern Healthcare.* April 24, 40-46.

White-Means, S., & Chollet, D. (1996) Opportunity wages and workforce adjustments: Understanding the cost of in-home elder care. *Journals of Gerontology: Social Sciences,* S82-S90.

Zimmerman, S., & Magaziner, J. (1994). Methodological issues in measuring the functional status of cognitively impaired nursing home residents: The use of proxies and performance-based measures. In D. Holmes, M. Ory, & J. Teresi (Eds.) Special Care Units: New Models of Residential Dementia Care. *Alzheimer's Disease and Associated Disorders: An International Journal,* 8(Suppl. 1), S281-S290.

Chapter 15

Issues in Measuring Costs in Institutional Settings

Gerald L. Glandon, David A. Lindeman, and Douglas Holmes

The rising costs of health care services have been of major concern for a number of years and will likely continue as a policy issue into the future. Nursing home expenditures constitute a large and rapidly growing component of those overall expenditures. In 1993, the U.S. spent approximately $70 billion on nursing home care or about 8.0% of total health care expenditures (DuNah, Harrington, Bedney, & Carrillo, 1995). By 2030, estimates are that this spending will rise to $1,477.4 billion or 9.25% of the estimated $15,969.6 billion to be spent in total health care expenditures (Burner, Waldo, & McKusick, 1992). While many disease processes lead to the use of nursing home services, persons with Alzheimer's disease and related dementias make up more than 50% of the nursing home population and are likely to contribute, at a minimum, 20% of total nursing home expenditures (Ernst & Hay, 1994; Maslow, 1994). In fact, when psychiatric diagnoses are used instead of staff reports, between 67% and 87% of nursing home residents have clinically diagnosable dementia (Maslow, 1994).

To help control the costs of treating these patients, it is crucial to consider alternative treatment methodologies. Identification and measurement of costs of care provided to Alzheimer's patients in specialized care settings such as nursing home special care units, is a first step in trying to determine and improve the cost effectiveness of alternative care delivery processes. With the advent, improvement and now widespread application of cost effectiveness studies, analysts and providers are in a position to identify optimal care strategies which are also most cost-effective, and to determine which types of patients benefit most from innovative treatments and alternative treatment settings. However, the initial steps, of measuring costs and developing a model to assist in determining the appropriate cost elements to consider, will influence how rapidly cost analysis proceeds and how quickly the "best" treatment options are identified and adopted. One question to consider is why a costing study is needed for these patients. We do not undertake cost studies for computers or automobiles; why, then, is this done for the treatment of Alzheimer's patients? As will be explained below, the interest and need for "costing studies" arises from many factors, but generally results from: the lack of reliability of the prices of health care services, the need for better cost control mechanisms internal to the firm (nursing home), and the importance of the costs associated with the consumption of nursing care services as they relate to the private and public sectors.

BACKGROUND

In 1987, Hay and Ernst published estimates of the cost of treating Alzheimer's patients. More recent studies have benefited from improved data sets, study locations with a greater number of clearly defined dementia patients, and generally better methodology. Even with these advantages, review of existing studies reveals little consensus as to what elements should be considered in the costs of care for Alzheimer's disease patients and, consequently, there is no consensus as to associated costs of care.

In order to provide a better understanding of costing, this section does two things. First, it presents the context of caring for persons with dementia in institutional settings by discussing the development of dementia-specific care settings and the special needs and characteristics of these clients. Second, this section reviews some of the recent cost studies with regard to methodology and findings.

Context of Dementia

In response to the increasing number of persons with Alzheimer's disease and other dementias, and to the need for optimizing their care, special care units for persons with dementia have proliferated in nursing homes and other residential care settings. Between 1991 and 1995 alone, the number of nursing homes with special care units increased by more than 114% with an accompanying almost doubling of capacity (Ory & Leon, 1996). While outcomes research concerning special care programs is just becoming available, market forces already have led to the expansion of specialized care by the nursing home industry, and to greater acceptance of these programs by nursing home and assisted living facility owners and staff as well as by the families of persons with Alzheimer's disease.

One aim of these programs is to reduce excess disability and improve the individual's functioning and quality of life through changes in the social and physical environment (Maslow, 1994). Data suggest that persons in special care units are younger, more likely to have a specific diagnosis of Alzheimer's disease, more cognitively impaired while less physically and functionally impaired, and have more behavioral problems than do other nursing home residents (Ory & Leon, 1996; U.S. Office of Technology Assessment, 1992). Partially in response to these characteristics, providers have argued that these units require increased staffing, staff training and activity programming, which in turn has led to calls for differential reimbursement for the care of persons with dementia (Holmes, Lindeman, Ory, & Teresi, 1994). Considering the demand for special care, ultimately the potential costs associated with providing care to persons with dementia in specialized settings is staggering.

Previous Costing Studies

Table 15.1 presents a brief summary of cost studies which examine either dementia care or relevant aspects of long-term care. Across these studies the absence of a common definition of cost is striking. The diversity primarily reflects different perspectives and objectives used in analysis. For example, only five of the 12 studies address Alzheimer's disease specifically. Of these, two (Collins & Stommel, 1991; Stommel, Collins, & Given, 1994) examine the costs to the family of caring for these patients and thus are not comparable to the institutional cost studies.

The most comprehensive analyses (Ernst & Hay, 1994; Rice et al., 1993) examined both direct and indirect costs specifically associated with the care of Alzheimer's

TABLE 15.1 Special Care Unit Literature Review

Author/Date	Primary Objective	Cost Items	Utilization Measurement	Price of Cost Weight	Findings	Inflation Adjustment Discount
Ernst & Hay, 1994	Economic/Social Cost of Alzheimer's Disease	Direct Costs: Diagnosis, nursing home, long-term mental hospital, paid home care, regular physician care, acute care hospital, and caregiver costs (medical)	Prevalence estimates from literature for example 20% of all nursing home patients with AD	Annual national expenditures except for MD fees of revenue per vistits	Total Direct $47,581	Adjusted using CPI to base year Discounted to base using 4%
Hay & Ernst, 1987		Indirect costs: Unpaid home care	Literature estimate of 52.5 hours per week	Equal to rate for paid home care ($9.40–$10.30)	Total unpaid caregiver costs $75,705	
		Indirect costs: Mortality and morbidity	Patient labor income from diagnosis to normal life expectancy	Age/Income profile from D. Rice	Total Mortality and Morbidity Costs $50,376	
Welch, Walsh & Larson, 1992	Cost of Institutional Care for AD Patients	Nursing home costs to patients	Measured entry estimates LOS	Two per diem rates for Western US in 1985 National Nursing Home Survey Medicaid ($58) and Private ($73)	Nursing Home Costs for 123 patients: $5.0 to $6.4 million	Adjusted to 1991 dollars using CPI at 4%
		Hospital Charges from Medicare Claims files	Diagnosis for Admissions files	Charges from claims files	Hospital charges for 123 patients: $460,000	

(Continued)

TABLE 15.1 (*Continued*)

Author/Date	Primary Objective	Cost Items	Utilization Measurement	Price of Cost Weight	Findings	Inflation Adjustment Discount
Stommel, Collins & Given, 1994	Costs of Family Caregiving to AD patients	Unpaid caregiver labor services	Hours spent on typical day	Home health aide market wage ($7.82) and informal household ($6.00) in Michigan	Total cash expenditures $1450	Too short for discounting
		Paid and unpaid family labor services	Caregiver list of time spent by other family members	Same as above	Total unpaid costs	
		Paid and unpaid services of non-family members	Caregiver list of time spent by all others	Actual charges or imputed wage as above		
		Cash for equipment and services	Survey Report	Dollars spent and not reimbursed		
Collins & Stommel, 1991	Out of Pocket Expenditures by Family Caregivers	Survey of caregivers regarding expenditures on separate categories	Total expense, no quantity or unit price	Hospital bills, hospital related Mds, temp nursing home placement, medications, skilled nursing care, home health aids/ companions, equipment, supplies	Total was $1149 for a three month period	No time frame given

(*Continued*)

TABLE 15.1 (*Continued*)

Author/Date	Primary Objective	Cost Items	Utilization Measurement	Price of Cost Weight	Findings	Inflation Adjustment Discount
Rice et al., 1993	Economic Burden of Alzheimer's Disease Care	Direct Costs: Hospital, nursing home, physician, social services, home care	Direct measurement and caregiver report	Facility charge for private patients, Medicaid, and Medicare	Total Direct $47,591	Adjusted using CPI to 1990
		Indirect Costs: Unpaid caregivers		reimbursement for skilled and intermediate care		
				Market wage for all unpaid caregivers		
Weinberger, Gold, Divine et al., 1993	Expenditures for Home Based Dementia Patients	Formal Services: MD visits, ER visits, Hospital stays, nursing home stays, legal services, adult day care, and visiting nurses	Caregiver report in	Actual Charges (60 per visit if not recorded), fixed ER charge of $120, $750 per day for Hospital for average daily revenue, $90 per day in NH, Fixed hourly for other		
		Informal Services: Respite care, Chores and meal preparation	Diary of time spent	$10 per hour for time spent		

(*Continued*)

TABLE 15.1 (*Continued*)

Author/Date	Primary Objective	Cost Items	Utilization Measurement	Price of Cost Weight	Findings	Inflation Adjustment Discount
Brodaty, Peters, 1991	Cost Effectiveness of training for Dementia Carers	Institutional and health services costs	Days in institution for up to 48 months post program. Chance being admitted times the average time in institution	Area specific cost per day of 92.23 A which includes a Memory fixed, variable (severity) and "other" cost component.	Dementia carers $19,918 Retraining $36,753 Wait list $27,375	No discounting or price adjustments mentioned
			Cost of health services from diary: medications, consults to health professionals, nights in a hospital, visits to day centers and admissions	No price estimates		
Chappel & Dickey, 1993	Decrease in cost of Hospital Care with Nursing Input	Hospital Admissions	Record review measured inpatient days for two samples	Per diem cost rates applied ($100-$1000)	Intervention lowered total hospital costs from $390,000 to $210,000	Two year pre/post intervention. No cost adjustment or discounting
		Emergency Room Costs	Number of returns	Not mentioned	Intervention lowered ER Costs from $34,000 to $28,000	

(*Continued*)

TABLE 15.1 (*Continued*)

Author/Date	Primary Objective	Cost Items	Utilization Measurement	Price of Cost Weight	Findings	Inflation Adjustment Discount
		Nurse Visits (Intervention)	Nurse Visit and Travel Time	Total Expenditures?	Nursing intervention was $7189	
		Nursing Home Costs not incurred	Nursing Home Costs Avoided while Hospitalized	Contract Cost per Diem	Intervention avoided nursing home costs of $199,000 while control avoided only $91,000	
Gertler & Waldman, 1992	Quality Adjusted cost functions for the Nursing Home industry	1980 survey of Total cost per day for long-term care facilities	NA, inputs used the nursing home as a whole	Cost per day $5320 per home included skilled labor, unskilled labor and supplies	Not relevant for average of 121 patients	
McCloskey, 1996	Nurses' Use and Delegation of Indirect Care Intervention	Caregiver and integrator role of Nurses i.e. direct, indirect and unit related activities	Survey of frequency and time spent Direct: all activities performed in presence of patient/family. Indirect: done away from patient but on a specific patient's behalf. Unit related: general maintenance of the unit but not specific to patient and personal time: breaks, meals, socializing with other worker	Not done	No cost findings	Not relevant

patients. Ernst and Hay used national prevalence, utilization and unit cost data in order to estimate direct costs of hospital, physician, formal home care, and nursing home resource elements for the nation. The indirect costs include a category for unpaid home care and cost of premature morbidity and mortality. Costs were incremental in that they comprised only costs that were greater than the normal or expected costs of living. All total estimates were for the patient's expected life post diagnosis and discounted to a common year, 1991. Total lifetime costs per case were $173,932. As it turns out, the direct care costs ($47,581) were the smallest and unpaid caregiver costs the largest ($75,705) of the three major components of costs. Disability and premature mortality costs were $50,376.

Rice et al. prospectively examined the costs of formal and informal care for persons with dementia residing in the community as well as nursing homes, including special care units. The sample was randomly drawn from five counties in northern California. Direct costs were identified for hospital, physicians, social services, medications and nursing care costs, while indirect costs were obtained using a "replacement cost approach" which valued the time spent by family caregivers at a wage equal to what it would cost to replace the caregiver's services with paid assistance. While incremental costs associated with caring for a demented person and attributed to the disease were measured, indirect productivity losses were not estimated. The annual total cost of caring for a person in an institution, in 1990 dollars, totaled $47,591. Informal services account for 12% ($5,542) of the total costs of care while 88% ($42,049) is attributable to formal services. This study accounted for variations in dementia severity in its findings.

These analyses establish basic standards by which all additional costing studies in this area can be measured. The recognition, estimation and valuation of both direct and indirect costs should not be ignored for dementia patients. Further, for valid comparisons all lifetime costs must be discounted to a common time period. It should be noted that neither Ernst and Hay nor Rice et al. obtained actual labor costs of facilities' staff, service unit data, or actual costs of all services.

Others of the studies reflected in Table 15.1 generally defined their purpose more narrowly in order to justify a less comprehensive costing methodology. For example, Welch, Walsh and Larson (1992) propose to estimate only the "cost of institutional care" and thus estimate only nursing home and hospital charges (direct costs). Their estimates are derived from "200 patients evaluated for symptoms of cognitive impairment" that were consecutively referred from a Geriatric and Family Service clinic affiliated with the host institution. Their cost estimates are greater than are the direct costs suggested by the Ernst and Hay study despite use of only two cost items (nursing homes and hospitalizations). Nursing home costs per resident ranged from $40,800 to $51,700 and hospitalizations were about $3,700 per patient.

In summary, cost estimates for Alzheimer's patients differ dramatically across existing studies. While many reasons exist for these differences, the most important include: computing annual versus lifetime costs; including paid home and other noninstitutional care givers; including implicit costs of unpaid caregivers; and using retrospective, macro cost estimates versus directly measured micro costs.

COSTING PARADIGM

Definition of Terms

Before we discuss approaches to cost analysis, it is important to have a common understanding of the terms that will be used. In the ensuing discussion, we will employ the following definitions:

Cost: The monetary value of resources used in the production or provision of goods or services.

Charge: The monetary value a supplier asks for in return for the delivery of goods or services.

Price: This term is used in two ways. One is essentially equivalent to charge in that it is the monetary value a supplier asks for in return for the delivery of goods or services. The second meaning is the actual monetary value received for the good or service. In this meaning, price is equivalent to the reimbursement received for the good or service. The charge for a good or service does not necessarily equal the reimbursement received.

Cost analysis: An analytical method that seeks to define, measure and value all of the resources used in the provision of a service.

Cost-benefit analysis: An analytical method that systematically measures the monetary value of the resources used by a program or technology and the monetary value of the benefits received from a program or technology.

Cost-effectiveness analysis: An analytical method that systematically measures the monetary value of the resources used by a program or technology and the benefits or effects of that program or technology.

Cost Analysis in Health Care

Cost analysis appears to be a relatively simple process but is, in fact, relatively complex. Thus, while it might appear that one need only add up the value of resources used to purchase or produce a good or service, economists include all of these readily apparent resources used and add the opportunity cost of resources foregone. Clearly, the latter are not as easy to identify, measure or value. Further, the resources must be classified as direct, indirect and/ or psychosocial (Hu & Sandifer, 1981). Direct costs are the resources consumed in the targeted activity (e.g., supplies and utilities used, equipment and machinery use, and provider time). These are usually observable, and can be easily counted with the help of a good accountant. Indirect costs are those for which no accounting is usually made but are important elements in the activity being examined. For health care services, a major indirect cost is the uncompensated time of the family or the lost income of the patient in receiving or recovering from the illness or treatment. Psychosocial costs are the value of "pain and suffering" associated with the illness or treatment and are usually not considered.

Pure cost studies can be considered a subset of the more comprehensive Cost-Effectiveness Analysis (CEA) and Cost-Benefit Analysis (CBA). As noted earlier, the primary difference in these techniques is that CBA translates all cost and benefit elements into dollars, while CEA leaves a single outcome or benefit in "real" terms. For example, CEA would report the cost of an intervention per life saved while CBA would estimate the dollar value of that life saved for comparison to the costs. Despite these apparent differences, many now regard these approaches as essentially equivalent in terms of the influence on policy (Phelps & Mushlin, 1991).

While some important differences exist between CEA and CBA, the analytical steps used in CEA can help one to understand cost analyses. As detailed nearly 15 years ago, CEA (Warner & Luce, 1982) has become a common technique applied to the special problems found in health care markets (Drazen, Feeley, Metzger, & Wolfe, 1980; Foote & Erfurt, 1991; Mauskopf, Bradley, & French, 1991; Trahey, 1991; Tsevat, Wong, Pauker, & Steinberg, 1991; Veluchamy & Saver, 1990; Weeks, Tierney, & Weinstein, 1991). CEA requires the analyst to follow a standard protocol as embodied in the following steps drawn from the literature (Glandon & Shapiro, 1988; Warner & Luce, 1982).

Identify Study Objectives. As with most evaluations, identifying the key objectives represents the crucial means of both limiting and defining the study. As the studies in Table 15.1 indicate, differences in objectives probably explain most of the differences in outcomes.

Specify Alternatives. A comprehensive list of alternatives must be developed to fully capture the costs associated with the relevant option relative to those associated with the best alternatives. While not as important for pure costing, examination of alternatives (home as opposed to institutional care) can provide better insight into all of the elements of cost.

Develop a Framework for Analysis. From the economist's standpoint, the health care delivery system can be viewed as a production process. This framework for analysis treats labor, machines, and supplies as specific inputs that, combined in a precise manner, produce measurable output. To cost the treatment of Alzheimer's patients the analysis must understand the relevant "production technologies." Economists call this modeling the production process.

Measure costs. The identification and measurement of costs will be discussed below.

Measure benefits. The measurement of benefits is not relevant for pure cost studies. However, benefits must be quantified for CEA, and both quantified and monetized for CBA.

Life cycle/discounting. Typically, projects have start-up costs which occur primarily in an early period, operating costs which continue over time and, possibly, major periodic maintenance or enhancement costs which should be anticipated at various points over time. In addition, analysts must discount measured costs to a common time period.

Uncertainty. By their nature, cost analyses require analytic inclusion of substantial uncertain events. The sensitivity of evaluation results to the accuracy with which such events are estimated should therefore be considered.

Equity. Applications should consider the equity of the distribution of costs. Because these analyses usually apply to social programs, the locus of burden can be as important to decision makers as is the total level of costs.

With this framework in mind, costing studies must *identify*, *measure* and *value* all of the relevant cost elements (Warner & Luce, 1982). Identification and measurement involves determining the most important cost elements and counting their use in the activity in question. *Identification* requires understanding the process required to produce or provide the resources. For example, caring for patients in nursing homes requires a major consumption of skilled and semiskilled labor. Nurses and aides provide a substantial portion of patient services. *Measurement* of these cost elements involves determining the amount of time spent by each category of labor in delivering the service. While this can involve many levels of complexity, it is still relatively direct.

Valuation for health care, however, is a major concern. In markets for most goods and services, prices serve as an effective mechanism for determining the relevant cost per unit of service used. Individual consumers and providers use prices as the signals to purchase more or less (consumers) or produce more or less (providers). Posted prices for health care services are highly unreliable indicators of the opportunity cost of resources used (Dranove, Shanley, & Wiley, 1992; Warner & Luce, 1982). Therefore, costing studies are needed as a basis for making decisions as to allocation and consumption.

In a broader context, health care prices do not reflect relative resource costs because insurance intervenes, shielding consumers from paying these prices. In total, private or government payers cover nearly 75% of all health expenditures. Out-of-pocket expenditures for direct elements of cost are relatively minor except for select services (nursing home care and dental services). As a result, the market for most health care services is unable to effectively enforce a true market price.

Yet even without the distortion introduced by insurance, the use of price still constitutes a potential problem. Because of the way health care providers have been paid by government payers, charges, reimbursement and costs may not be related. Stated prices for health care services often do not resemble either exchange prices or costs (Dranove, Shanley, & White, 1992). For example, a nursing home may charge $4,000 for a resident's stay, be paid (reimbursed) $3,200 and have estimated costs of $3,850. What is the "price" of care in this case and how does anyone interpret and respond to these confused price signals?

Another problem is that prices may not exist for some services. Many services and programs that are being evaluated are internal to the facility; however, because prices are rarely used to transact the internal transfer of goods and services, prices do not exist. Yet, management needs an analytic method to help it decide which investment decisions are beneficial to the facility, which programs should be expanded and which eliminated.

Finally, there are often substantial indirect costs, not reflected in prices which are, nevertheless, associated with the delivery of health care services. For example, the costs of surgery include not only the hospitalization expenses, physician fees, nurse time, etc., but also the opportunity-cost time spent by the patient in surgery (pre-op, admission and post-op time) and the time lost from work while in recovery.

Direct Costs

To fully capture costs of dementia care, it is crucial to specify objectives, understand the production process and identify all of the cost components as indicated above. Direct costs have been used most frequently in cost studies in health care because of their relative ease of identification, measurement and valuation (see Harrow, Tennstedt, & McKinley, 1995; Leon, 1994; Mehr & Fries, 1995). For institutional dementia care, there are many major elements of direct cost that must be considered. Even if some are found to contribute relatively little, all must be examined. For ease of presentation, these cost elements are grouped below in terms of their being either variable or semi-variable.

Variable costs are those that vary directly with the quantity of services provided. For example, if a resident requires an hour of nursing per day, each additional resident adds an hour of nursing time to the cost of care. Variable costs pick up differences in direct use of services and probably capture the most important elements of cost variation among delivery settings and patients. This class of costs can be traced or allocated directly to the individual resident. Long-term residential health care variable costs include: (a) nursing time and services, (b) LPN time and services, (c) nursing aide time and services, (d) other labor time and services (e.g., occupational therapy, physical therapy, recreation therapy, dietary, speech therapy, social work), (e) supply use, (f) equipment, (g) procedures and therapies, (h) physician visits, and (i) hospitalizations. Comments regarding these elements may help to clarify some of the elements. Labor is listed as "time and services" because there are two elements of services delivered by these labor components: time directly spent with the resident and services performed for the resident but not necessarily directly in the resident's presence. Supplies consist only of captured use of supplies that are not placed into "overhead," i.e., special billings for specific items used and assigned to a specific resident. The equipment category includes any special equipment that is used by a resident that is not part of the normal daily room rate. Even though some equipment might be provided by family and friends, it should be reflected in the cost analyses. Procedures and therapies consist of services provided for the patient which are not, however, included in the "normal" room services.

Fixed or semi-variable costs are elements that do not vary directly according to the number of residents being treated, or are elements that are allocated to the entire nursing unit or area but not to the individual resident. The economist considers true fixed costs as totally invariant to changes in volume of activity; all other costs are variable. In the real world, however, there are a host of cost elements that do not vary in immediate response to volume changes. These inputs will adjust only if volume changes endure for an extended period (changes either up or down). For example, an increase in census can cause severe overcrowding of a facility that will persist if the census is not perceived as having increased permanently. Building a new wing (more capital) will only occur after the census increase is truly deemed permanent. These semi-variable cost elements are important for the estimation of total costs of service but are not particularly important in most instances for an examination of the variation in costs between types of units. Semi-variable costs can include (a) indirect labor costs (i.e., health benefits, retirement, etc.), (b) unit management/administration, (c) unit-specific overhead, and (d) general overhead.

Indirect Costs

As suggested by Ernst and Hay (1994), the opportunity cost of lost work and function is particularly important for Alzheimer's patients. In addition, the time and effort expended on informal services provided by family and friends should be treated as a true cost of care when costing Alzheimer's residential care.

Measurement of these items is similar in that some direct or indirect method of estimation of lost time must be obtained. Ernst and Hay (1994) assumed that the Alzheimer's patient is completely disabled at the time of diagnosis, and that the lost wages resulting from disability persist until death. Because valuation of lost time is generally undertaken using market-based expected lost wages, the authors used estimates derived from the age/income profile of the U.S. Along the same lines, the authors monetized unpaid caregiver time by valuing it at the expected hourly cost of paid caregivers.

ISSUES RELATED TO SPECIAL CARE UNITS (SCU)

Elements of Direct Cost

A critical factor in determining costs of special care units is the extensive heterogeneity of the production process among SCUs. Differences in the production process can be attributed to scale of production (i.e., size of units), stage of learning (i.e., age of unit), type of physical plant, and type of care techniques and technology (e.g., program activities, staff training, and management style) (Miller, 1994). In addition, there is a lack of specificity in defining resident characteristics including diagnostic as well as functional, behavior and cognitive measurement of residents. These variations require careful assessment of what is measured, when measurement takes place and how cost measures are computed and interpreted.

As has been stated above, elements of cost for a pure costing study must determine what the costs are likely to be in the absence of the disease. Using data from a controlled clinical trial would appear to be directly applicable to cost comparisons. However, the sample sizes necessary to estimate significant differences in clinical outcome are not sufficient to determine significant differences in cost, because there is greater variability in patient cost than there is with respect to most clinical outcome measures. The difficulty of studying dementia care in nursing home settings is compounded by limited or missing diagnostic data, variations in clinical record keeping, and the impact of comorbidities on service utilization.

As the collection and reporting of direct costs are being contemplated, one must balance the relative "cost of measurement" with "value of the measurement." As identified by Holmes et al. (1994), there are significant strengths and weaknesses in different cost measurement techniques. In attempting to provide greater rigor to cost studies there is imperative need for more comprehensive and systematic cost measurement techniques.

Family Time and Other Indirect Costs

The contributions of unpaid family caregiver time and volunteers can be a primary source of indirect costs in specialized dementia care settings. There is an expanding body of empirical evidence documenting the continued role of family members in caring for their family member who is placed in a residential setting (Montgomery & Kosloski, 1994; Townsend, 1990). The relative magnitude of the contribution varies widely due to the variability of interest of both the family and the facility in having family caregivers provide assistance in special care settings. The attribution of cost is hampered by the difficulties associated with direct collection of caregiver time and task data.

Determining the cost of lost opportunity time or function for residents in special care settings is potentially complex. Lost opportunity costs may be relatively minimal for many persons due to their extended age at admission, which is often 80 or above. On the other hand, many special care residents are younger than the average nursing home resident and may reside in special care for an extended period of time, suggesting greater lost opportunity costs. The cost of lost opportunity time is especially relevant for family caregivers.

DISCUSSION

A primary limitation of cost analyses of special care settings conducted to date has been a general lack of clarity in the identification of production processes and measurement of staff time and services. In part, this is due to the confusion that arises over the lack of specificity in definitions and common units of measurement in costing for institutional dementia care. When inputs and costs are measured, there often is a lack of accurate measurement due to differences in measurement techniques. As the review of existing dementia cost studies indicates, most analyses have not attended to all cost elements, making selective use of direct costs and often omitting indirect costs altogether. Moreover, even when a broader array of costs and inputs are captured there have been minimal efforts to relate them to resident and program outcomes.

Improved costing methodologies are central to the optimization of residential programs for persons with dementia. As special care expands within nursing homes and throughout assisted living and other residential settings, there is increased interest by providers as to the cost effectiveness of specific program features. Among policy makers the cost implications to society are important as plans for future aging cohorts are increasing in the 21st century, leading to increased demands for institutional care. The impact of costs on quality of care will remain paramount to consumers and providers alike; while issues of regulation and reimbursement will continue to be high priorities of policy makers. The high costs of special care for persons with dementia reinforces the need for improved understanding of processes and measurement of costs in order to focus on areas where efficiencies can be achieved. With federal and state governments likely to continue to cover a great proportion of the costs for institutional care, and new private sector models for paying for long-term care emerging, there will be a growing demand for careful cost analyses for the allocation of increasingly scarce resources.

REFERENCES

Brodaty, H., & Peters, K. (1991). Cost effectiveness of a training program for dementia carers. *International Psychogeriatrics, 3*(1), 11-22.

Burner, S. T., Waldo, D. R., & McKusick, D. R. (1992). National health expenditures projections through 2030. *Health Care Financing Review, 14*(1), 1-29.

Chappell, H., & Dickey, C. (1993). Decreased rehospitalization costs through intermittent nursing visits to nursing home patients: *Journal of Nursing Administration, 23*(3), 49-52.

Collins, C., & Stommel, M. (1991). Out of pocket expenditures by family caregivers of dementia patients residing in the community. *Home Health Care Services Quarterly, 12*(4), 29-43.

Dranove, D., Shanley, M., & White, W. (1991). How fast are hospital prices really rising? *Medical Care, 29* (August), 690-696.

Drazen, E., Feeley, R., Metzger, J., & Wolfe, H. (1980). *Methods for evaluating costs of automated hospital information systems*. Department of Health and Human Services, National Center for Health Services Research, PHS No. 233-79-3000.

DuNah, R., Harrington, C., Bedney, B. & Carrillo, H. (1995). Variations and trends in state nursing facility capacity: 1978-93. *Health Care Financing Review, 17*(1), 183-199.

Ernst, J., & Hay, J. (1994). The U.S. economic and social costs of Alzheimer's disease revisited. *American Journal of Public Health, 84*(8), 1261-1264.

Foote, A., & Erfurt, J. (1991). The benefit to cost ratio of work-site blood pressure control programs. *Journal of the American Medical Association, 265*(10), 1283-1286.

Gertler, P., & Waldman, D. (1992). Quality-adjusted cost functions and policy evaluation in the nursing home industry. *Journal of Political Economy, 100*(6), 1232-1256

Glandon, G., & Shapiro, R. (1988). Benefit-cost analysis of hospital information systems: The state of the (non) art. *Journal of Health and Human Resource Administration, 11* (Summer), 30-92.

Harrow, B., Tennstedt, S., & McKinlay, J. B. (1995). How costly is it to care for disabled elders in a community setting? *The Gerontologist, 35*, 803-813.

Hay, J., & Ernst, R. (1987). The economic costs of Alzheimer's disease. *American Journal of Public Health, 77*, 1169-1175.

Holmes, D., Lindeman, D., Ory, M., & Teresi, J. (1994). Measurement of service units and costs of care for persons with dementia in special care units. *Alzheimer Disease and Associated Disorders, 8*(1), 328-340.

Hu, J., & Sandifer, F. (1981). Synthesis of cost-of-illness methodology. National Center for Health Services Research, PHS Contract No. 233-79-3010.

Leon, J. (1994). The 1990/1991 National survey of special care units in nursing homes. *Alzheimer Disease and Associated Disorders*, 8(1), 72-86.

Maslow, K. (1994). Current knowledge about special care units: Findings of a study by the U.S. Office of Technology Assessment. *Alzheimer Disease and Associated Disorders*, 8(1), 14-40.

Mauskopf, J., Bradley, C., & French, M. (1991). Benefit-cost analysis of Hepatitis B vaccine programs for occupationally exposed workers. *Journal of Occupational Medicine*, 33(6), 691-698.

McCloskey, J., Bulechek, G., Moorhead, S., & Daly, J. (1996). Nurses' use and delegation of indirect care interventions. *Nursing Economics*, 14(1), 22-23.

Mehr, D., & Fries, B. (1995). Resource use on Alzheimer's special care units. *The Gerontologist*, 35, 179-184.

Miller, R. H. (1994). Measuring special care unit inputs, costs and value. *Alzheimer Disease and Associated Disorders*, 8(1), 341-344.

Montgomery, R., & Kosloski, K. (1994). A longitudinal analysis of nursing home placement for dependent elders cared for by spouses vs. adult children. *Journal of Gerontology*, 49(2), 62-74.

Office of Technology Assessment. (1992) Special care units for people with Alzheimer's and other dementias: consumer education, research, regulatory, and reimbursement issues. Washington, D.C.: *U.S. Government Printing Office*.

Ory, M., & Leon, J. (1996). Dementia special care units: Recent findings and future directions. Presentation at the Annual Meeting of the Gerontological Society of America, Washington, D.C.

Phelps, C., & Mushlin, A. (1991). On the (near) equivalence of cost-effectiveness and cost-benefit analyses. *International Journal of Technology Assessment in Health Care*, 7(1), 12-21.

Rice, D. P., Fox, P. J., Max, W., Webber, P. A., Lindeman, D. A., Hauck, W. W., & Segura, E. (1993). The economic burden of Alzheimer's disease care. *Health Affairs*, 12(2), 164-176.

Rubin R., Gold, W., Kelley, D., & Sher, J. (1992). *The cost of disorders of the brain*. Washington, DC: The National Foundation for Brain Research.

Stommel, M., Collins, C., & Given, B., (1994). The costs of family contributions to the care of persons with Dementia. *The Gerontologist*, 34(2), 199-205.

Townsend, A. (1990). Nursing home care and family caregivers' stress. In M. Stephens, J., Crowther, S., Hobfoll, and D., Tennenbaum, (Eds.), *Stress and coping in later-life families*. New York: Hemisphere Publishing.

Trahey, P. (1991). A comparison of the cost-effectiveness of two types of occupational therapy services. *American Journal of Occupational Therapy*, 45(5), 397-400.

Tsevat, J., Wong, J., Pauker, S., & Steinberg, M. (1991). Neonatal screening for sickle cell disease: A cost-effectiveness analysis. *Journal of Pediatrics*, 118(4), 546-54.

Veluchamy, S., & Saver, C. (1990). Clinical technology assessment, cost-effective adoption and quality management by hospitals in the 1990s. *Quality Review Bulletin*, 16(6), 223-8.

Warner, K., & Luce, B. (1982). *Cost-benefit and cost-effectiveness analysis in health care: Principles, practice and potential.* Ann Arbor, MI: Health Administration Press.

Weeks, J., Tierney, M., & Weinstein, M. (1991). Cost effectiveness of prophylactic intravenous immune globulin in chronic lymphocytic leukemia. *New England Journal of Medicine, 325*(2), 81-6.

Weinberger, M., Gold, D. T., Divine, G., Cowper, P., Hodgson, L., Schreiner, P., & George, L. (1993). Expenditures in caring for patients with dementia who live at home. *American Journal of Public Health, 83*(3), 338-341.

Welch, H., Walsh, H., & Larson, E. (1992). Cost of institutional care in Alzheimer's disease: Nursing home and hospital use in a prospective cohort. *Journal of the American Geriatrics Society, 40*(3), 221-224.

Index

("i" indicates an illustration, 't' indicates a table, 'n' indicates a note)

Springer Publishing Company

New...

Assessing the Health Status of Older Adults

Elena Andresen, PhD, **Barbara Rothenberg,** MPA, MA, and **James G. Zimmer,** MD, Editors

This volume reviews widely used methods for measuring the health status of older adults and addresses the assets and limitations of the most useful instruments and procedures. Topics covered include physical and functional assessment, measurement of disease severity and comorbidity, cognitive or mental status screening, and depression screening.

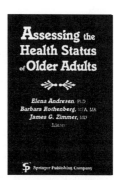

The text summarizes and critiques the seminal literature on health assessment for older adults and provides suggestions for choosing among competing instruments for a variety of settings and uses. Each chapter concludes with an annotated bibliography of the most important scientific publications for selected health status measures. This book is intended for gerontological and clinical practitioners, educators, and students.

Contents:

- Introduction
- Functional Assessment
- General Health Status Measures
- Measures of Severity of Illness and Comorbidity
- Cognitive Screening
- Depression Screening

1997   304pp   0-8261-9780-9   hardcover

536 Broadway, New York, NY 10012-3955 • (212) 431-4370 • Fax (212) 941-7842